Calcified Tissues 1965

Calcified Tissues 1965

Proceedings
of the Third European Symposium
on Calcified Tissues

held at

Davos (Switzerland), April 11th—16th, 1965

Sponsored by the

Laboratorium für experimentelle Chirurgie, Schweizerisches Forschungsinstitut, Davos

Edited by

H. Fleisch, H. J. J. Blackwood and M. Owen

with the assistance of

M. P. Fleisch-Ronchetti

SPRINGER-VERLAG · NEW YORK · INC.

1966

ISBN 978-3-642-85843-7 ISBN 978-3-642-85841-3 (eBook)
DOI 10.1007/978-3-642-85841-3

Softcover reprint of the hardcover 1st edition 1966

Library of Congress Catalog Card Number 65-27 964

Titelnummer 1323

Preface

The papers collected in this volume represent the formal proceedings of the Third European Symposium on Calcified Tissues which was held in Davos, Switzerland from 11th to 16th April 1965 under the sponsorship of the Laboratorium für experimentelle Chirurgie, Schweizerisches Forschungsinstitut Davos. This Symposium followed the now established tradition of the previous Symposia held in Oxford in 1963 and in Liège in 1964. Participation was again strictly on a residential basis. This year the Schatzalp Hotel provided a scenic and secluded meeting place high on a mountain side overlooking Davos yet close to the Forschungsinstitut in which the opening session of the Symposium was held.

The papers and communications published in the volume are arranged in order of presentation and are grouped under the five main themes selected for discussion by the Symposium, namely, "Cell function in the formation, maintenance and destruction of osseous tissue", "Response of calcified tissues to mechanical factors", "Mechanisms of mineralization and diseases related to mineral deposition", "Hormones and bone" and "Fundamental structure of dental hard tissues". The programme consisted of a number of review lectures given by invited speakers and of short communications in relation to each of the above themes. No attempt was made to record the discussions to the papers as, being a residential meeting, the more valuable and interesting interchanges took place informally in small discussion groups and not within the time schedule of the prearranged programme.

The Committees wish to express their thanks to the staff of the Laboratory for Experimental Surgery, Davos for their most valuable help and to all of the following who made this meeting possible through their financial support: Zentralverband schweizerischer Milchproduzenten; Nestlé Alimentana S.A., Cham et Vevey; Sandoz AG., Basel; Robapharm AG., Basel; Ciba AG., Basel; J. R. Geigy AG., Basel; F. Hoffmann-La Roche & Co. AG., Basel; Dr. A. Wander AG., Bern; Emser Werke AG., Domat/Ems; Laboratorien Hausmann AG., St. Gallen; Davos-Parsenn-Bahnen AG., Davos; Kleiner Rat des Kantons Graubünden; Landschaft Davos; Migros-Genossenschafts-Bund, Zürich; Schweizerische Unfallversicherungs-Gesellschaft, Winterthur; Treupha AG., Baden; Siegfried AG., Zofingen; Verkehrsverein Davos.

The European Symposium on Calcified Tissues is held annually and Professor P. Gaillard's invitation on behalf of the University of Leiden to meet in Holland in 1966 has been warmly accepted.

The editorial committee:
H. J. J. Blackwood
H. Fleisch
M. Owen

The organizing committee:
C. A. Baud — H. G. Haas
M. J. Dallemagne — L. Richelle
H. Fleisch — R. Schenk

Contents

Session I

Cell Function in the Formation, Maintenance and Destruction of Osseous Tissue

Chairmen: P. Gaillard, I. MacIntyre, H. J. Dulce, A. B. Borle

L. F. Bélanger, T. Semba, S. Tolnai, D. H. Copp, L. Krook and C. Gries
The Two Faces of Resorption 1

W. A. de Voogd van der Straaten
Some Remarks and Questions on Metabolic Patterns in the Family of Bone Cells . . . 10

Ch. M. Lapière
Remodelling of the Bone Matrix 20

M. E. Holtrop
The Origin of Bone Cells in Endochondral Ossification 32

M. Owen
RNA Synthesis in Growing Bone 36

J. S. Greenspan and H. J. J. Blackwood
Histochemical Studies of Chondrocyte Function in the Cartilage of the Mandibular Condyle of the Rat 40

A. B. Borle
Correlation between Morphological, Biochemical, and Biophysical Effects of Parathyroid Hormone on Cell Membranes 45

P. A. Thornton
Vitamin D-ascorbic Acid Association in Bone Metabolism 48

C. B. Sledge
Lysosomes and Cartilage Resorption in Organ Culture 52

G. Vaes
Acid Hydrolases, Lysosomes and Bone Resorption Induced by Parathyroid Hormone . 56

A. Dhem
Le forage des canaux de Havers 60

E. Rutishauser, W. Taillard and B. Friedli
Experimental Studies of the Non-inflammatory Vascular Pannus 63

L. V. Avioli and Ph. H. Henneman
Urinary Pyrophosphate in Disorders of Bone Metabolism 67

J. Jowsey
Bone Formation and Resorption in Bone Disorders 69

J. C. Birkenhager, J. van der Sluys Veer, R. O. van der Heul and D. Smeenk
Studies of Iliac Crest Bone from Controls and Patients with Bone Disease by Means of Chemical Analysis, Tetracycline Labelling and Histology 73

Session II

Response of Calcified Tissues to Mechanical Factors

Chairman: R. Amprino

C. A. L. Bassett
Electro-mechanical Factors Regulating Bone Architecture 78

G. Marotti and F. Marotti
Topographic-quantitative Study of Bone Tissue Formation and Reconstruction in Inert Bones 89

H. Wagner
Structure and Healing of Bone as a Response to Continuous and Discontinuous Strain and Stress 93

E. D. Sedlin and L. Sonnerup
Rheological Considerations in the Physical Properties of Bone 98

M. Brookes
Haemodynamic Data on the Osseous Circulation 101

N. E. Shaw
The Influence of Muscle Blood-flow on the Circulation in Bones 104

Session III

Mechanisms of Mineralization and Diseases Related to Mineral Deposition

Chairmen: S. M. Partridge, B. Engfeldt, W. D. Armstrong, J. P. Aubert and H. C. G. Bauer

F. G. E. Pautard
A Biomolecular Survey of Calcification 108

L. J. Richelle, C. Onkelinx and J.-P. Aubert
Bone Mineral Metabolism in the Rat 123

P. Lerch and C. Vuilleumier
Physico-chemical Methods for the Identification of Microcrystalline Basic Calcium Phosphates Prepared in Vitro 132

H. Newesely
Umwandlungsvorgänge bei Calciumphosphaten 136

J. MacGregor
Some Observations on the Nature of Bone Mineral 138

A. Ascenzi and E. Bonucci
The Osteon Calcification as Revealed by the Electron Microscope 142

H. J. Höhling, H. Themann and J. Vahl
Collagen and Apatite in Hard Tissues and Pathological Formations from a Crystal Chemical Point of View 146

H. J. Arnott
Studies of Calcification in Plants 152

R. Lagier, C. A. Baud and M. Buchs
Crystallographic Identification of Calcium Deposits as Regards to their Pathological Nature, with Special Reference to Chondrocalcinosis 158

A. Policard, C. A. Baud, A. Collet, H. Daniel-Moussard and J. C. Martin
Infrastructural and Crystallographic Study of Experimental Calcifications 162

S. M. Krane and M. J. Glimcher
Protein Phosphorus and Phosphokinases in Connective Tissue 168

W. M. McKernan and S. D. Dailly
The Relationship between Swelling of Hard Tissue Collagen in Acid and Alkali and the Presence of Phosphate Cross-links 171

R. Steendijk, J. Jowsey, A. van den Hooff and H. K. L. Nielsen
Microradiographic and Histological Observations in Primary Vitamin D-resistant Rickets 175

D. B. Morgan, C. R. Paterson, C. G. Woods, C. N. Pulvertaft and P. Fourman
Therapeutic Response and Effect on the Kidney of 100 Units Vitamin D Daily in Osteomalacia after Gastrectomy 178

T. G. Taylor, A. Williams and J. Kirkley
Changes in the Activities of Plasma Acid and Alkaline Phosphatases during Egg Shell Calcification in the Domestic Fowl 182

J. C. Stoclet and Y. Cohen
Calcium Exchanges in the Aorta of the Rat 186

G. D. McPherson
Estimation of the 24 Hour Exchangeable Calcium Pool in Children Using ^{48}Ca . . . 189

L. Miravet et D. Hioco
Transfert du calcium intestinal chez l'homme dans les maladies déminéralisantes de l'os 193

L. Lutwak
Absorption of Calcium in Man: Effect of Disease, Hormones and Vitamin D 198

J.-F. Dymling
Therapeutic Results in Renal Tubular Osteomalacia with Special Reference to Calcium Kinetics 202

G. Milhaud et J. Bourichon
Etude du métabolisme du calcium chez l'homme à l'aide de calcium 45: l'ostéopétrose et l'ostéopsathyrose 207

D. A. Smith and C. J. Mackenzie
Calcium Clearance and Re-absorption in Patients with Osteoporosis, Renal Stone and Primary Hyperparathyroidism 211

Session IV

Hormones and Bone

Chairmen: P. Fourman and P. H. Henneman

G. Nichols, jr.
Bony Targets of Non-"skeletal" Hormones 215

B. E. C. Nordin
Hormones and Calcium Metabolism 226

H. A. Soliman, C. J. Robinson, G. V. Foster and I. MacIntyre
Mode of Action of Calcitonin 242

E. Uehlinger
Of the Influence of Thyroxine, Thiouracil, Cortisone, Estrogen and Testosterone on Endochondral Ossification Utilizing Autoradiography 243

J. A. Fernandez de Valderrama and L. M. Munuera
The Effect of Cortisone and Anabolic Agents on Bone 245

W. M. Rigal and W. M. Hunter
Sites and Mode of Action of Growth Hormone 250

G. F. Mazzuoli and L. Terrenato
Intestinal Absorption and Skeletal Dynamic of Calcium in Acromegaly 254

Session V

Fundamental Structure of Hard Dental Tissues

Chairman: H. J. J. Blackwood

R. M. Frank
Ultrastructure of Human Dentin 259

E. P. Katz, G. Mechanic and M. J. Glimcher
Preliminary Studies of the Ultracentrifugal and Free Zone Electrophoresis Characteristics of Neutral Soluble Proteins of Bovine Embryo Enamel 272

A. Boyde
The Development of Enamel Structure in Mammals 276

List of participants

Allgöwer, M., Kantonsspital, Chur, Schweiz.

Amprino, R., Istituto di Anatomia Umana, Università, Bari, Italia.

Armstrong, W. D., Department of Physiological Chemistry, University of Minnesota, Minneapolis, Minn., USA.

Arnott, H. J., Cell Biology Institute, University of Texas, Austin, Texas, USA.

Ascenzi, A., Istituto di Anatomia Patologica, Università, Pisa, Italia.

Aubert, J.-P., Institut Pasteur, Paris, France.

Avioli, L. V., Seton Hall College, Division of Endrocrinology, Jersey City, N. J., USA.

Bachra, B. N., Laboratory of Physiological Chemistry, Leiden, Holland.

Bassett, C. A. L., Department of Research Orthopaedics, Columbia University, College of Physicians and Surgeons, New York, N. Y., USA.

Baud, C. A., Institut de Morphologie, Ecole de Médecine, Genève, Suisse.

Bauer, G. C. H., Hospital for Special Surgery, New York, N. Y., USA.

Bélanger, L. F., Department of Histology, University of Ottawa, Ottawa, Canada.

Bengtsson, A., Department of Pathology, University, Uppsala, Sweden.

Bersin, T., Laboratorium Hausmann AG., St. Gallen, Schweiz.

Birkenhäger, J. C., Department for Diseases of Metabolism, University Hospital, Leiden, Nederland.

Birkenhäger-Frenkel, D. H., Antoni van Leeuwenhoekhuis, Amsterdam, Nederland.

Bisaz, S., Laboratorium für experimentelle Chirurgie, Schweizerisches Forschungsinstitut, Davos, Schweiz.

Blackwood, H. J. J., Royal Dental Hospital, School of Dental Surgery, London, England.

Bohr, H., Orthopaedic Hospital, Copenhagen, Denmark.

Bolognani, L., Istituto di Chimica Biologica, Università, Pavia, Italia.

Bonucci, E., Istituto di Anatomia Patologica, Università, Pisa, Italia.

Bordier, P., Centre du Métabolisme Phosphocalcique, Hôpital Lariboisière, Paris, France.

Borle, A. B., Department of Physiology, University of Pittsburgh, Pittsburgh, Pa., USA.

Boyde, A., Department of Anatomy, London Hospital Medical College, London, England.

Brookes, M., Department of Anatomy, Guy's Hospital Medical School, London, England.

Chalmers, J., Orthopaedic Department, Royal Infirmary, Edinburgh, Scotland.

Cimasoni, G., Institut Dentaire, Genève, Suisse.

Collet, A., Cerchar B. P. 27, Creil (Oise), France.

Coutelier, L., Laboratoire de Chirurgie Orthopédique et Traumatologie, Louvain, Belgique.

Czitober, H., I. Medizinische Universitätsklinik, Wien, Österreich.

Dallemagne, M. J., Institut de Thérapeutique Expérimentale, Liège, Belgique.

Dhem, A., Laboratoire de Chirurgie Orthopédique et Traumatologie, Louvain, Belgique.

Dingle, J. T., Strangeways Research Laboratory, Cambridge, England.

Dulce, H. J., Institut für angewandte physiologische Chemie und klinische Chemie, Berlin, Deutschland.

Dupont, D., Institut de Morphologie, Ecole de Médecine, Genève, Suisse.
Dymling, J. F., Malmö General Hospital, Malmö, Sweden.
Engfeldt, B., Department of Pathology II, University, Uppsala, Sweden.
Ezra-Cohn, H., Nuffield Orthopaedic Centre, Oxford, England.
Fitton Jackson, S., Strangeways Research Laboratory, Cambridge, England.
Fleisch, H., Laboratorium für experimentelle Chirurgie, Schweizerisches Forschungsinstitut, Davos, Schweiz.
Foster, G. V., Postgraduate Medical School, London, England.
Fourman, P., The School of Medicine, Leeds, England.
François, P., Institut de Thérapeutique Expérimentale, Liège, Belgique.
Frank, R. M., Institut Dentaire, Faculté de Médecine, Strasbourg, France.
Gaillard, P., Laboratorium voor Cytologie en Experimentele Histologie, Universiteit, Leiden, Nederland.
Greenspan, J. S., Royal Dental Hospital, School of Dental Surgery, London, England.
Haas, H. G., Medizinische Universitätsklinik, Bürgerspital, Basel, Schweiz.
Hartles, R. L., School of Dental Surgery, University, Liverpool, England.
Hattyasy, D., Leninkörut 66, Szeged, Hungary.
Hekkelman, J. W., Laboratorium voor Cytologie en Experimentele Histologie, Universiteit, Leiden, Nederland.
Henneman, Ph. H., Seton Hall College, Division of Endocrinology, Jersey City, N. J., USA.
Hess, R., Ciba AG., Basel, Schweiz.
Heuck, F., Katharinenhospital, Stuttgart, Deutschland.
Hioco, D., Centre du Métabolisme Phosphocalcique, Hôpital Lariboisière, Paris, France.
Höhling, H. J., Institut für medizinische Physik, Münster, Deutschland.
Holtrop, M. E., Laboratorium voor Cytologie en Experimentele Histologie, Universiteit, Leiden, Nederland.
Horn, H. D., Urologisch-Balneologische Forschungsstelle, Bad Wildungen, Deutschland.
Hooff, A. van den, Jan Swammerdan Instituut, Amsterdam, Nederland.
Huggler, A., Kantonsspital, Chur, Schweiz.
Jasinski, B., Robapharm AG., Basel, Schweiz.
Jasinski, W. K., Institute of Oncology, Warsaw, Poland.
Jeffree, G. M., Pathology Research Laboratory, University, Bristol, England.
Johnson, N. W., Dental Research Unit, Bristol, England.
Jowsey, J., Mayo Clinic, Rochester, Minn., USA.
Knese, K. H., Institut für Biologie, Landw. Hochschule Hohenheim, Stuttgart-Hohenheim, Deutschland.
Koskinen, E. V. S., Clinic for Orthopaedics and Traumatology, University, Helsinki, Finland.
Krane, S. M., Massachusetts General Hospital, Boston, Mass., USA.
Kshirsagar, S. G., M.R.C. Bone-seeking Isotopes Research Unit, Churchill Hospital, Oxford, England.
Kuhlencordt, F., Stoffwechsellaboratorium, I. Medizinische Universitätsklinik, Hamburg-Eppendorf, Deutschland.
Lagier, R., Institut Universitaire de Pathologie, Hôpital Cantonal, Genève, Suisse.
Lapière, Ch. M., Institut de Médecine, Département de Clinique et de Pathologie Médicales, Université, Liège, Belgique.
Lemaire, R., Clinique Chirurgicale, Université, Liège, Belgique.
Lentner, C., J. R. Geigy AG., Basel, Schweiz.
Lerch, P., Institut de Radiophysique Appliquée, Lausanne, Suisse.

Lindholm, B., Sahlgren's Hospital, Metabolic Laboratory, Medical Clinic II, Göteborg, Sweden.

Little, K., Nuffield Orthopaedic Centre, Oxford, England.

Lutwak, L., Cornell University, Sage Hospital, Ithaca, N. Y., USA.

MacGregor, J., Bioengineering Unit, University of Strathclyde, Glasgow, Scotland.

MacIntyre, I., Postgraduate Medical School, London, England.

Marotti, G., Istituto di Anatomia Umana, Università, Bari, Italia.

Matrajt, H., Centre du Métabolisme Phosphocalcique, Hôpital Lariboisière, Paris, France.

Matturri, L., Istituto di Anatomia e Istologia Patologica, Università, Milano, Italia.

Mazzuoli, G., Istituto di Patologia Medica, Università, Policlinico Umberto I, Roma, Italia.

McKernan, W. M., British Glues and Chemicals Ltd., Gelatine Division, London, England.

McPherson, D., Hospital for Special Surgery, New York, N. Y., USA.

Mechanic, G., Orthopaedic Research Laboratories, Massachusetts General Hospital, Boston, Mass., USA.

Milhaud, G., Institut Pasteur, Paris, France.

Miravet, L., Centre du Métabolsime Phosphocalcique, Hôpital Lariboisière, Paris, France.

Morgan, D. B., Department of Chemical Pathology, The Medical School, Leeds, England.

Morscher, E., Orthopädische Klinik, Universität, Basel, Schweiz.

Moukhtar, M. S., Institut Pasteur, Paris, France.

Müller, M., Kantonsspital, St. Gallen, Schweiz.

Newesely, H., Forschungsgruppe für Mikromorphologie, Fritz-Haber-Institut, Berlin, Deutschland.

Nichols, G., Department of Medicine, Harvard Medical School, Boston, Mass., USA.

Nordin, B. E. C., The General Infirmary, Leeds, England.

O'Dell, D., Strangeways Research Laboratory, Cambridge, England.

Onkelinx, C., Institut de Thérapeutique Expérimentale, Liège, Belgique.

Owen, M., M.R.C. Bone-seeking Isotopes Research Unit, Churchill Hospital, Oxford, England.

Partridge, S. M., Low Temperature Station, Cambridge, England.

Pautard, F. G. E., The Astbury Department of Biophysics, University, Leeds, England.

Perren, S., Laboratorium für experimentelle Chirurgie, Schweizerisches Forschungsinstitut, Davos, Schweiz.

Price, C., Pathology Research Laboratory, University, Bristol, England.

Probst, J.-Y., Sandoz AG., Basel, Schweiz.

Richelle, L., Institut de Thérapeutique Expérimentale, Liège, Belgique.

Rose, G. A., Department of Medicine, General Infirmary, Leeds, England.

Rowles, S. L., Birmingham Dental Hospital, Birmingham, England.

Rutishauser, E., Institut de Pathologie Générale et Anatomie Pathologique, Université, Genève, Suisse.

Schenk, R., Anatomisches Institut, Basel, Schweiz.

Schibler, D., Laboratorium für experimentelle Chirurgie, Schweizerisches Forschungsinstitut, Davos, Schweiz.

Sedlin, E. D., Department of Orthopaedic Surgery, University, Göteborg, Sweden.

Shaw, N. E., Royal National Orthopaedic Hospital, Institute of Orthopaedics, Stanmore, Mddx., England.

Sledge, C. B., Strangeways Research Laboratory, Cambridge, England.

Sluys Veer, J. van der, Department of Endocrinology and Metabolism, University Hospital, Leiden, Holland.

Smeenk, D., Department of Endocrinology and Metabolism, University Hospital, Leiden, Holland.

Smith, D. A., Department of Medicine, Gardiner Institute, Western Infirmary, Glasgow, Scotland.

Soliman, H., Postgraduate Medical School, London, England.

Steendijk, R., Kinderkliniek, Binnengasthuis, Amsterdam, Nederland.

Stoclet, J. C., Faculté de Pharmacie, Laboratoire de Pharmacodynamie, Paris, France.

Strandh, J., Department of Pathology II, University, Uppsala, Sweden.

Straumann, F., Institut Straumann, Waldenburg, Schweiz.

Taylor, T. G., Department of Physiological Chemistry, University, Reading, England.

Terrenato, L., Istituto di Patologia Medica, Università, Policlinico Umberto I, Roma, Italia.

Thornton, P. A., VA Hospital, University of Kentucky, Lexington, Ky., USA.

Trautz, O. R., New York University, College of Dentistry, New York, USA.

Uehlinger, E., Pathologisches Institut der Universität, Zürich, Schweiz.

Vaes, G., Laboratoire de Chimie Physiologique, Université, Louvain, Belgique.

Valderrama, J. F. de, Zurbano 39, Madrid, España.

Vaughan, J., M.R.C. Bone-seeking Isotopes Research Unit, Churchill Hospital, Oxford, England.

Vittali, P., Chirurgische Universitätsklinik, Köln-Merheim, Deutschland.

Voogd van der Straaten, W. A. de, Laboratorium voor Cytologie en Experimentele Histologie, Universiteit, Leiden, Nederland.

Vuilleumier, C., Institut für anorganische und physikalische Chemie, Universität, Bern, Schweiz.

Wagner, H., Orthopädische Universitätsklinik, Münster, Deutschland.

Wasserman, R. H., Institute of Biological Chemistry, University, Copenhagen, Denmark.

Weigel, W., Robapharm AG., Basel, Schweiz.

Wernly, M., 1 Sonnenbergstraße, Bern, Schweiz.

Zinn, M., Bad Ragaz, Schweiz.

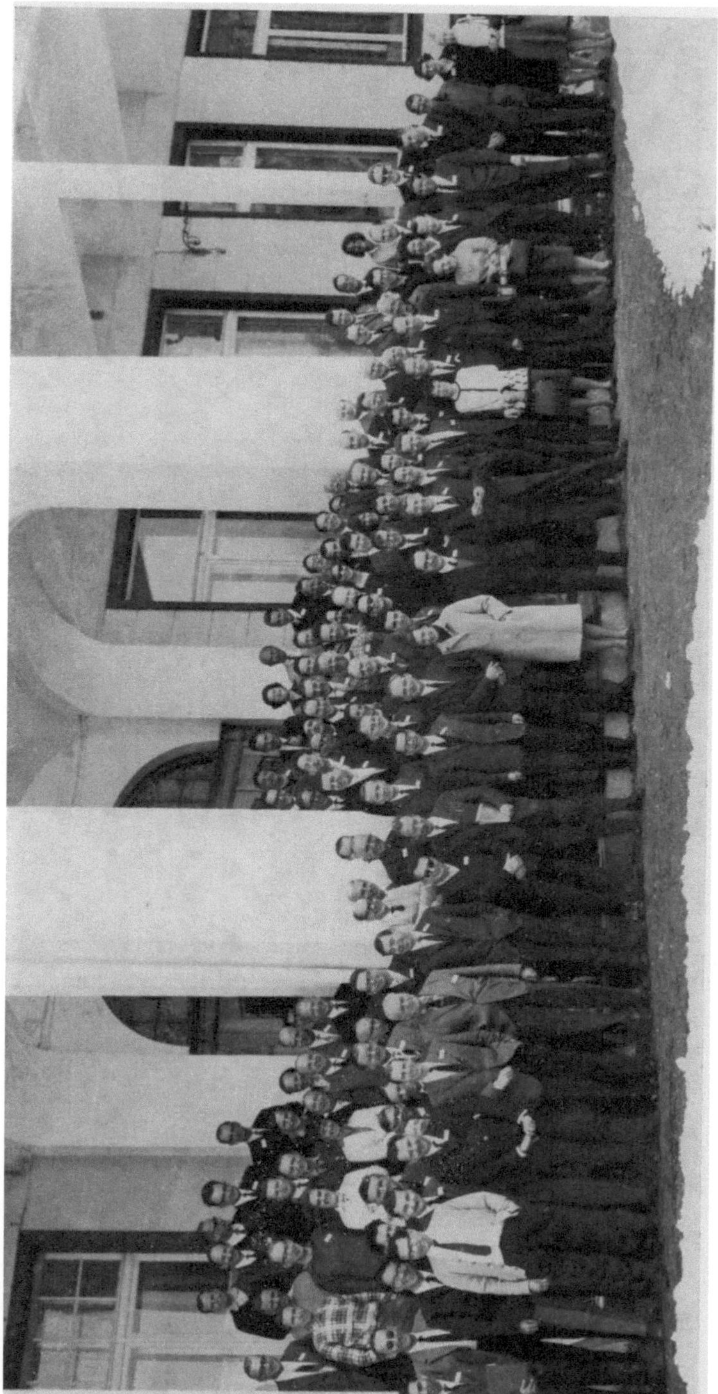

The Two Faces of Resorption

L. F. BÉLANGER, T. SEMBA *, S. TOLNAI

Department of Histology and Embryology, Faculty of Medicine, University of Ottawa, Ottawa, Canada

D. H. COPP

Department of Physiology, Faculty of Medicine, University of British Columbia, Vancouver, B. C., Canada

L. KROOK, C. GRIES

Department of Pathology and Bacteriology, New York State Veterinary College, Ithaca, N. Y., U. S. A.

1. Development of the concept of osteolysis

Recent reviews and textbooks state that "the osteoclast is the agent of bone destruction" (LACROIX, 1961), that this cell is "actively involved in some way in the resorption of bone" (HANCOX and BOOTHROYD, 1963) or else that there is "much interesting controversy about the origin, the nature and the function of these cells" (HAM and LEESON, 1961) and that "indeed, the process of bone resorption is not understood as thoroughly as we might wish" (HAM and LEESON, 1961). "On the other hand, resorption may take place in the absence of osteoclasts for instance in the so-called creeping replacement in bone transplants" (COPENHAVER, 1964).

The concept of non-osteoclastic resorption has been itself, "creeping" through the years, towards the home of the bone investigator; perhaps this meeting will be the occasion when it will find its way inside . . .

The idea of "remodeling absorption" from within, proposed by JOHN HUNTER towards the end of the 18th century (HOME, 1800) might have been an early step in this direction. After cauterization of portions of bone, HUNTER reported that "the earthy part of the living bone in contact with the dead portion, was first absorbed". Living cells within the bone were apparently needed for this process.

Much later several investigators were attracted by changes in the staining properties of the organic matrix in relation with interstitial loss of substance. These were manifested by basophilia (ZAWISCH-OSSENITZ, 1927; KIND, 1951; RUTH, 1954, 1961) or by intensified staining for mucopolysaccharides (HELLER-STEINBERG, 1951; ENGEL, 1952; GAILLARD, 1955 a, b).

Changes in the appearance of the osteocytes and also in the size and shape of lacunae and canaliculi were observed by von RECKLINGHAUSEN (1910) (oncosis),

* Post-Doctorate Fellow of the Medical Research Council of Canada.

JAFFE (1933), KIND (1951) and LIPP (1954, 1956), with the light microscope and more recently by BAUD (1962) with the electron microscope.

RUTISHAUSER and MAJNO (1951) made the interesting observation that during its hypertrophic or oncotic phase, the osteocyte produced alkaline phosphatase. The subsequent death of the osteocyte, leaving empty lacunae which oftentimes fill with calcium salt (SHERMAN and SELAKOVITCH, 1957; SISSONS, 1964) has been related by DUFOUR (1952) and by URIST *et al.* (1963) to osteoporosis and other rarefying diseases of the skeleton. Empty lacunae have also been recognized as a conspicuous feature of old age (FROST, 1960; SISSONS, 1964).

Recently, LIPP (1959) has detected the presence of aminopeptidase in some of the osteocytes. On the other hand, BÉLANGER and MIGICOVSKY (1963 a) have shown that these cells contained an enzyme capable of digesting gelatin. Furthermore, BÉLANGER *et al.* (1963 b) have been able to associate the same areas with toluidine blue metachromasia and also with organic matrix and salt depletion as revealed by alpharadiography (BÉLANGER and BÉLANGER, 1959) and X ray microradiography (BÉLANGER

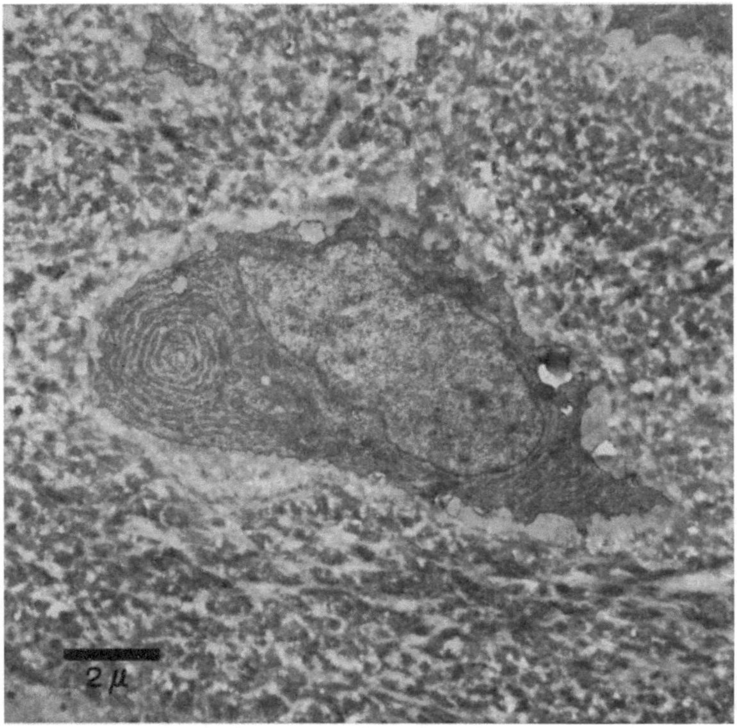

Fig 1. Peripheral osteocyte from the mid-diaphysis of an 2 days-old chick embryo. The cell is apparently closely encased by the surrounding matrix. Endoplasmic reticulum, ribosomes and mitochondria are prominent features of the cytoplasma

et al., 1963 a). To designate specifically this intimate form of resorption related to osteocytic activity, the abused term *osteolysis* has been proposed (BÉLANGER *et al.*, 1963 b; BÉLANGER, in press).

Jowsey (1963) and Jowsey *et al.* (1964) have reported on the basis of microradiographic studies of a variety of bone depleting conditions, "that the osteocytes may be capable of controlling the amount of mineral and also perhaps, the amount of matrix, deposited in the tissue adjacent to them". At the Second Parathyroid conference held at Noordwijk in August 1964, Talmage (in press) who had already demonstrated that the removal of hydroxyproline from bone followed a pattern quite similar to that of the mineral components (Talmage, 1962), reported that numerous enlarged osteocytes were observed early in bone fragments cultured with parathormone.

2. Electron microscopy of bone cells of the chick

Further aspects of this osteocytic activity have been uncovered by electron microscopy during the past year.

Very intense osteolysis has already been observed in the bones of young chicks (Bélanger *et al.*, 1963 b). This type of material being not too hard, can be processed for electron microscopy with a minimum of pretreatment.

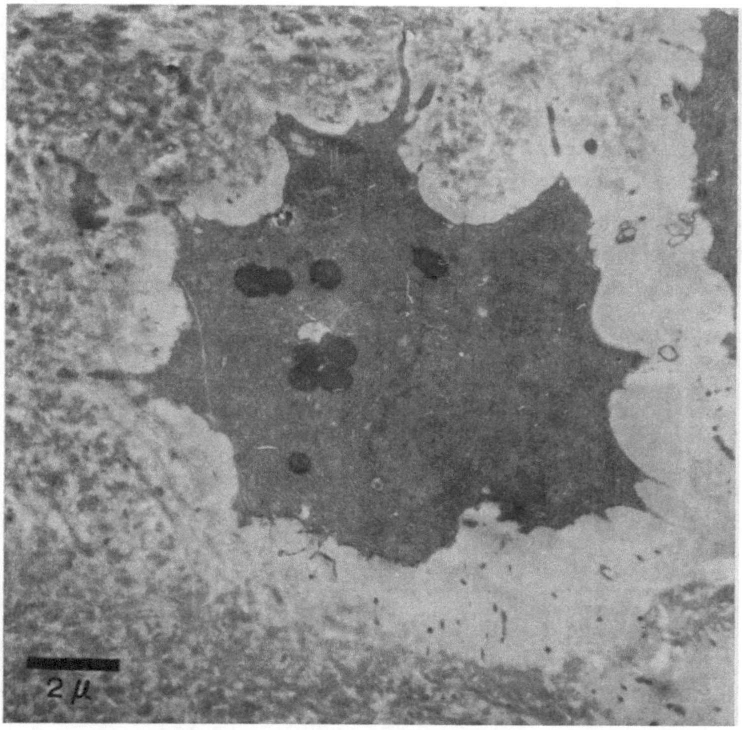

Fig. 2. A centrally located osteocyte in the same specimen as above. The lacuna is wide and apparently confluent with an adjacent one. Vesicles containing osmiophilic material (lysosomes?) are prominent features of the cytoplasma

In collaboration with Teruhiko Semba and Susan Tolnai, small fragments of the mid-diaphysis of the tibia from II days chick embryos were fixed in Palade's isotonic osmic mixture at 5 °C and then partly demineralized in an aqueous isotonic solution of the disodium salt of ethylene-diamine tetra-acetic acid (EDTA) at pH 7.4. Sections of ca. 800 Å were cut in epoxy resin and submitted to electron microscopy.

The low power pictures obtained so far have revealed that the ovoid cells (osteoblasts) located at the immediate outer border of the peripheral trabeculae contained mitochondriae and an extensive endoplasmic reticulum network, as already described elsewhere in mammalian tissue (DUDLEY and SPIRO, 1961; CAMERON *et al.*, 1963).

Young osteocytes located immediately inside the bone matrix (Fig. 1) revealed similar features of the cytoplasma. These cells generally filled the lacunae in which they were contained. Osteocytes located further away from the border, inside larger lacunae (Fig. 2) showed apart from the above features, some osmiophilic vesicles of different sizes, which might well be lysosomes. This observation is of interest in view of the previous histochemical demonstration of protease activity over the more mature osteocytes (BÉLANGER and MIGICOVSKY, 1963 a).

3. The effects of acute parathyroid stimulation

Parathyroid stimulation by perfusion of dogs and sheep with EDTA, over periods of a few hours only, such as performed by D. H. COPP at the University of British Columbia (COPP, 1963) has produced effects in cancellous bone particularly visible in alpharadiographs (BÉLANGER, in press). The number of enlarged osteocytes was increased in the parietal bone after 4 hrs. Moreover, the surrounding matrix displayed already at this early stage, a remarkable loss of density.

4. The effects of prolonged parathyroid stimulation

We were highly privileged during the years 1964—65 to be associated with DRS. LENNART KROOK and CHRISTIAN GRIES from the Veterinary College of Cornell University in studies involving horses which were fed a diet containing an optimum

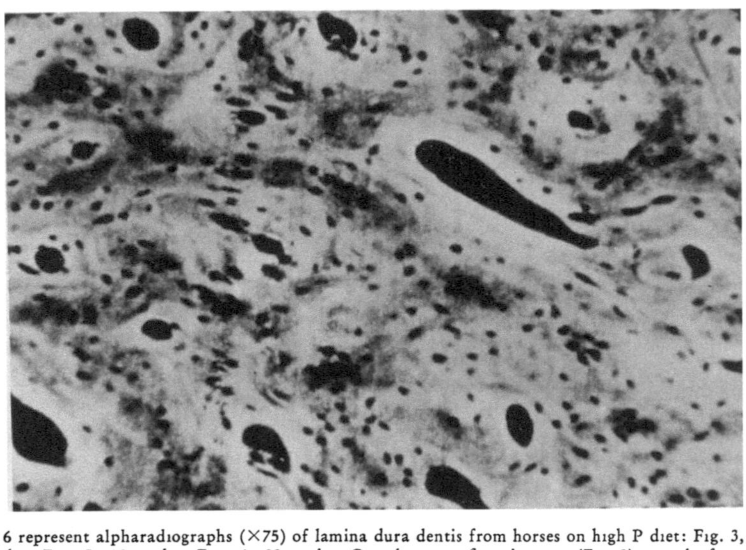

Fig. 3

Figs. 3, 4, 5, 6 represent alpharadiographs (×75) of lamina dura dentis from horses on high P diet: Fig. 3, 4 weeks, Fig. 4, 7 weeks; Fig. 5, 12 weeks; Fig. 6, 30 weeks. Osteolysis at first intense (Fig. 3); newly-formed tissue decreasing (Fig. 4, larger canals); compact bone replaced by spongy bone (Fig. 5); becoming more and more immature and abnormal (Fig. 6)

amount of calcium (about 15 gm/day/horse) and an excessive amount of phosphorus (about, $3^1/_2$ times as much).

The animals were killed after periods of 4, 7, 10, 12 and 30 weeks of abnormal feeding. The clinical observations have been similar to those already published by Krook and Lowe (1964). After 4 weeks, very minor signs of osteitis fibrosa were present but the parathyroids were enlarged about 3 times. After 8 weeks, extremely severe osteitis fibrosa was recognized and in the colourful language of the senior veterinary pathologist (K), "the parathyroids were almost as big as the testicles of a dachshund".

The bone response was uneven throughout the body. On the other hand, the horses which were the youngest at the onset of the experiment were the most severely affected. Changes in the mandibles and maxillae were observed sooner and progressed at a more rapid rate than those in the metacarpi (Krook and Lowe, 1964) and long bones. Increased radiolucency was particularly evident in the bones of the skull and face. Complete resorption of the *lamina dura dentis* was evident after 30 weeks.

Comparative alpharadiographs of the periodontal portion of the mandible and maxilla examined in the light of histochemical staining and with the knowledge of the mechanism of bone growth provided by radioautography (Bélanger and Migicovsky, 1963 b) have been very instructive.

Short term studies have demonstrated that only mesenchymal cells, preosteoblasts or "osteoprogenitors" (Tonna, 1965; Bélanger and Migicovsky, 1963 b; Young 1963) are originally labeled. The presence of radioactive osteoblasts and osteocytes occurring later is an indication of growth movements and also of tissue replacement in areas where the adult condition has already been achieved.

In 3 weeks-old chicks, the replacement rate of metaphyseal trabeculae of the tibia has been established at 4 days (Bélanger and Migicovsky, 1963 b). In the lamina dura of the horse jaw, this time is unknown. However, a constant cell movement must be similarly taking plase from the border of the osteonic canal, towards the areas of lower tissue density where osteolysis occurs and where the cells die. If osteolysis and peripheral accretion are balanced, a static histological, histochemical and radiological picture is maintained. On the other hand, if osteolytic stimuli such as hyperparathyroidism are present, resorption is presumably greater than accretion.

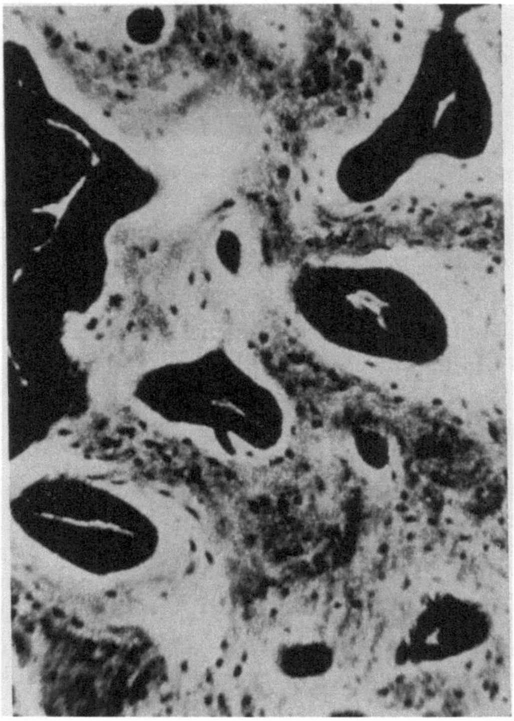

Fig. 4

The result should be a progressive loss of bone manifested by an enlargement of the osteonic canal and a gradual loss of bone substance.

Alpharadiographs of demineralized sections of normal bone have revealed that the areas where osteolysis is occurring are characterized by the presence of enlarged

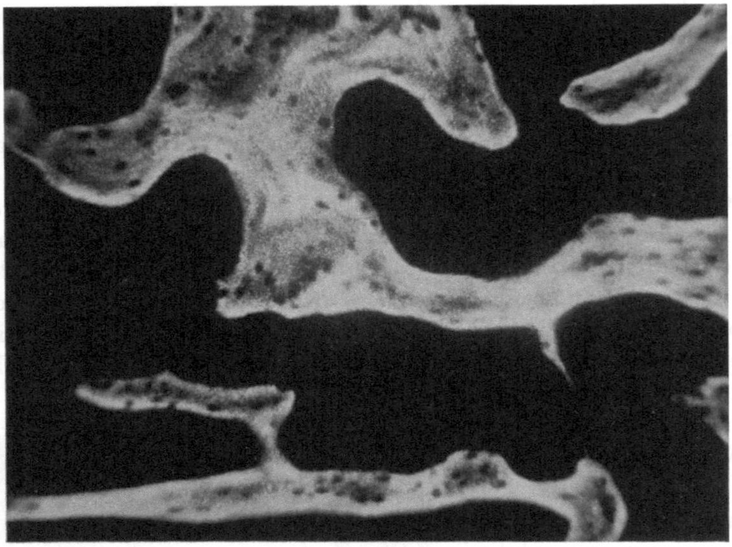

Fig. 5

and oftentimes confluent lacunae surrounded by low-density matrix (Belanger *et al.*, 1963 b). Newly-formed portions of the tissue, at the border of osteonic canals consist of denser matrix containing small lacunae (Bélanger *et al.*, 1963 b). The lower-density matrix of the osteolytic sites stains more intensely with the periodic acid-Schiff and exhibits toluidine blue and azur metachromasia, indicative of a concentration of mucopolysaccharides in these areas (Bélanger *et al.*, 1963 b).

In the present series, the periodontal bone (lamina dura) was still fairly compact after 4 weeks (Fig. 3). The canals were small but there was already a considerable intensification of osteolysis.

After 7 weeks (Fig. 4), the areas of osteolysis were more extensive and characterized by lower density of matrix corresponding to more widespread p.a.-Schiff staining.

After 12 weeks (Fig. 5), the canalicular arrangement of the lamina dura had in great part disappeared and the newly-formed bone was of the trabecular type. The central portion of the trabeculae showed the characteristic manifestations of osteolysis. At this stage consequently, bone formationhad regressed to a more primitive form, but this younger type of bone could still be considered as normal bone. At this stage also, some less dedifferentiated areas, showed the disappearance of the p.a.-Schiff positive areas characteristic of osteolytic resorption. Numerous, irregular cementing lines separated the areas of new growth. The newly-formed bone contained only osteocytes of small size and many lacunae were empty.

After 30 weeks, the trabeculae were thin and either uniformly dense of fibrillar (Fig. 6). The tissue surrounding this abnormal bone was also de differentiated and inhabited mostly by mesenchymal cells.

Osteoclasts which had been sparsely observed at 4 and 7 weeks, were more numerous at 12 weeks. They attained almost tumoral frequency at 30 weeks and appeared most active along the abnormal new trabeculae.

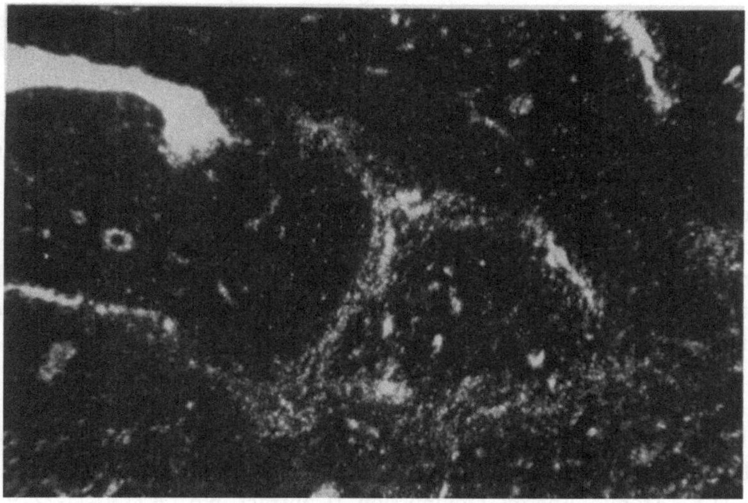

Fig. 6

5. The role of osteoclasts

These observations bring us to consider the role of osteoclasts and the factors which are responsible for the occurrence of these cells.

In an excellent review, Hancox (1956) lists a series of generalized and localized factors as responsible for the appearance of osteoclasts. In the first group, hyperparathyroidism, hypervitaminosis A, the administration of glucose or lead and a diet low in calcium have been reported. "Remodeling", bone fractures, ectopic bones or teeth, degenerated deciduous roots, circulatory disorders, infections, introduction of inert material in the root canals of teeth, have been recognized as so many local factors.

The introduction of Plutonium (Arnold and Jee, 1957) or Yttrium (Neuman *et al.*, 1960; Jowsey, 1963) into the organism, has produced beautiful demonstrations of surface resorption in the presence of osteoclasts.

Grafts such as performed by Barnicot (1948) and also in vitro transplantation and culture of bone specimens (Gaillard, 1955 a, b; Goldhaber, 1962) have been followed by stimulation of osteoclastic activity.

Irving and Handelman (1963) have recently published interesting results with devitalized autologous bone grafts. A multinucleated giant cell reaction was initiated from mesenchymal cells whether the grafted bones were mineralized or demineralized. The host response did not seem to be affected by parathormone.

All these events and also the results of our current observations on horses seem to have something in common: *The presence of abnormal skeletal tissues* either bone, cartilage or the components of the teeth.

6. Conclusions

At this point we would like to propose the following conclusions:

(1) Normal adult bone is a constantly renewed tissue in which resorption is equally matched by accretion.

(2) Intimate resorption (osteolysis), taking place away from the bone surfaces seems to occur. The mature osteocytes are probably responsible for this phenomenon. One of the factors involved is the production by these cells, of a protease possibly linked to lysosome activity.

(3) The mature osteocytes seem to respond readily (within a few hours) to endogenous parathyroid stimulation. The role of these cells in the maintenance of calcium homeostasis, is perhaps more important than previously realized.

(4) Osteoclasia appears as a specialized response to the presence of abnormal skeletal material, either of general or local origin. The osteoclasts which probably originate from primitive cells, may be akin to the giant multinucleated cells of connective tissue. Like those, their major role may be to take part in the maintenance of the integrity of the body.

Acknowledgements

The authors are indebted to MRS. L. F. BÉLANGER for skilled technique; also to the Medical Research Council of Canada, to the Canada Department of Agriculture and to the U.S. Atomic Energy Commission (Contract No. AT(30-1)-2779) for financial assistance. Para-Thormone was graciously supplied by Eli Lilly and Co. (Canada) Ltd., Toronto.

References

ARNOLD, J. S., and W. S. S. JEE: Bone growth and osteoclastic activity as indicated by radioautographic distribution of Pu^{239}. Amer. J. Anat. **101**, 367 (1957).

BARNICOT, N. A.: The local action of the parathyroid and other tissues on bone in intracerebral grafts. J. Anat. **82**, 233 (1948).

BAUD, C. A.: Morphologie et structure inframicroscopique des ostéocytes. Acta anat. **51**, 209 (1962).

BÉLANGER, L. F.: Osteolysis: An outlook on its mechanism and etiology. In Parathyroid Hormone, Ultrastructure, Secretions and Functions. GAILLARD, P. G., and R. V. TALMAGE (eds.). Chicago: University of Chicago Press (in press).

—, and C. BELANGER: Alpharadiography: A simple method for determination of mass concentration in cells and tissues. J. biophys. biochem. Cytol. **6**, 197 (1959).

—, and B. B. MIGICOVSKY: Histochemical evidence of proteolysis in bone: The influence of Parathormone. J. Histochem. Cytochem. **11**, 734 (1963 a).

— — Bone cell formation and survival in H^3-thymidine-labeled chicks under various conditions. Anat. Rec. **145**, 385 (1963 b).

—, J. ROBICHON, and C. BÉLANGER: Mounting hard tissues for microradiography. Experientia **19**, 163 (1963 a).

— —, B. B. MIGICOVSKY, D. H. COPP, and J. VINCENT: Resorption without osteoclasts (Osteolysis). In Mechanisms of Hard Tissue Destruction. SOGNNAES, R. F. (ed.). Washington: Amer. Ass. Advanc. Sci. 1963 b, p. 531.

CAMERON, D. A., H. A. PASCHALL, and R. A. ROBINSON: The ultrastructure of bone cells. In Bone Biodynamics. FROST, H. M. (ed.). Boston: Little, Brown 1963, p. 91.

COPENHAVER, W. M.: Bailey's Textbook of Histology (15th ed.). Baltimore: Williams and Wilkins 1964.

COPP, D. H.: The hormones of the parathyroid glands and calcium homeostasis. In Bone Biodynamics. FROST, H. M. (ed.). Boston: Little, Brown 1963, p. 441.

Dudley, H. R., and D. Spiro: The fine structure of bone cells. J. biophys. biochem. Cytol. **11**, 627 (1961).

Dufour, J. J.: Etat pré-fractural du col fémoral. Helv. chir. Acta **19**, 15 (1952).

Engel, M. B.: Mobilization of mucoprotein by parathyroid extract. A. M. A. Arch. Path. **53**, 339 (1952).

Frost, H. M.: In vivo osteocyte death. J. Bone Jt Surg. **42 A**, 138 (1960).

Gaillard, P. J.: Parathyroid gland tissue and bone in vitro. I. J. exp. Cell Res. Suppl. **3**, 154 (1955 a).

— Parathyroid gland tissue and bone in vitro. III. Proc. kon. ned. Akad. Wet. **C 58**, 286 (1955 b).

Goldhhaber, P.: Some current concepts of bone physiology. New Engl. J. Med. **266**, 870 (1962).

Ham, A. W., and T. S. Leeson: Histology (4th ed.). Philadelphia: J. B. Lippincott 1961.

Hancox, N.: The osteoclast. In The Biochemistry and Physiology of Bone. Bourne, G. H. (ed.). New York: Academic Press 1956, p. 213.

—, and B. Boothroyd: Structure-function relationships in the osteoclast. In Mechanisms of Hard Tissue Destruction. Sognnaes, R. F. (ed.). Washington: Amer. Ass. Advanc. Sci. 1963, p. 497.

Heller-Steinberg, M.: Ground substance, bone salts and cellular activity in bone formation and destruction. Amer. J. Anat. **89**, 347 (1951).

Home, E.: Experiments and observations on the growth of bones; from the papers of the late Mr. Hunter. Trans. med. chir. Knowledge **2**, 277 (1800).

Irving, J. T., and C. S. Handelman: Bone destruction by multinucleated giant cells. In Mechanisms of Hard Tissue Destruction. Sognnaes, R. F. (ed.). Washington: Amer. Ass. Advanc. Sci. 1963, p. 515.

Jaffe, H. L.: Hyperparathyroidism (Recklinghausen's disease of bone). Arch. Path. **16**, 63 (1933).

Jowsey, J.: Microradiography of bone resorption. In Mechanisms of Hard Tissue Destruction. Sognnaes, R. F. (ed.). Washington: Amer. Ass. Advanc. Sci. 1963, p. 447.

—, B. L. Riggs, and P. J. Kelly: Mineral metabolism in osteocytes. Proc. Mayo Clinic **39**, 480 (1964).

Kind, H.: Studien zur Frage der Osteolyse. Beitr. path. Anat. **111**, 283 (1951).

Krook, L., and J. E. Lowe: Nutritional secondary hyperparathyroidism in the horse, with a description of the normal equine parathyroid gland. Path. vet. suppl. **1** (1964).

Lacroix, P.: Bone and cartilage. In The Cell, Vol. V. Brachet, J., and A. E. Mirsky (eds.). New York: Academic Press 1961, p. 219.

Lipp, W.: Neuuntersuchungen des Knochengewebes. II. Histologisch erfaßbare Lebensäußerungen der Knochenzellen. Acta anat. **22**, 151 (1954).

— Neuuntersuchungen des Knochengewebes. III. Histologisch erfaßbare Lebensäußerungen der Osteozyten in embryonalen Knochen des Menschen. Anat. Anz. **102**, 361 (1956).

— Aminopeptidase in bone cells. J. Histochem. Cytochem. **7**, 205 (1959).

Neuman, W. F., B. J. Mulryan, and G. R. Martin: A chemical view of osteoclasis based on studies with yttrium. Clin. Orthop. **17**, 124 (1960).

Recklinghausen, F. von: Über Rachitis und Osteomalacie. Jena 1910.

Ruth, E. B.: Further observations on histological evidence of osseous tissue resorption. Anat. Rec. **118**, 347 (1954).

— Basophilic islands in osseous tissue and their relation to resorption. Anat. Rec. **140**, 307 (1961).

Rutishauser, E., and G. Majno: Physiopathology of bone tissue: The osteocytes and fundamental substance. Bull. Hosp. Jt Dis. **12**, 468 (1951).

Sherman, M. S., and W. G. Selakovitch: Bone changes in chronic circulatory insufficiency. J. Bone Jt Surg. **39 A**, 892 (1957).

Sissons, H. A.: Histological studies of normal and osteoporotic bone. In L'ostéoporose. Hioco, D. J. (ed.). Paris: Masson 1964.

Talmage, R. V.: Parathyroid function: A calcium replacement mechanism. Amer. Zoologist **2**, 353 (1962).

Talmage, R. V.: Cytological and biochemical changes resulting from fluctuations in endogenous parathyroid hormone levels. In Parathyroid Hormone, Ultrastructure, Secretions and Functions. Gaillard, P. G., and R. V. Talmage (eds.). Chicago: University of Chicago Press (in press).
Tonna, E. A.: Osteoclasts and the aging skeleton: A cytological, cytochemical and autoradiographic study. Anat. Rec. **137**, 251 (1960).
Urist, M. R., N. S. MacDonald, M. J. Moss, and W. A. Skoog: Rarefying disease of the skeleton: Observations dealing with aged and dead bone in patients with osteoporosis. In Mechanisms of Hard Tissue Destruction. Sognnaes, R. F. (ed.). Washington: Amer. Ass. Advanc. Sci. 1963, p. 385.
Young, R. W.: Nucleic acids, protein synthesis and bone. Clin. Orthop. **26**, 147 (1963).
Zawisch-Ossenitz, C.: Über Inseln von basophiler Substanz in den Diaphysen langer Röhrenknochen. Z. mikr.-anat. Forsch. **10**, 472 (1927).

Some Remarks and Questions on Metabolic Patterns in the Family of Bone Cells

W. A. de Voogd van der Straaten

Laboratorium voor Celbiologie en Histologie, Rijksuniversiteit Leiden, Leiden, Nederland

In order to speak sensibly about metabolic patterns in the family of bone cells at least three general points have to be clarified. The first point concerns the way in which the word family is used; the second point concerns the concept of metabolic pattern *in general;* and the last point concerns the interconnection between some pure scientific and methodological questions in our special field.

1. By definition the members of a family are relatives, and they remain so even if they are miles apart. Now the *different types* of cells found in bone tissue, the bone cells, are relatives but they are not miles apart; on the contrary the members of the family of bone cells live closely together and form a functional and structural unit. In what I am going to say about bone cells, however, I will not look upon them *as relatives* but as *different types of labourers* in a "family factory".

2. It is common knowledge that the *morphologically comparable* cellular elements of a tissue e. g. osteocytes, are not by necessity all in the same functional state at the same time. Without discussing the background of this phenomenon, I think that none of us would attribute these variations to differences in metabolic pattern. What then is covered by this term and what is the special meaning of the word pattern? Or to restate this problem in a positive way, why do we in all probability suppose different metabolic patterns to be existent in osteoblasts and osteoclasts even if we have no pertinent biochemical data at hand? To my mind a list of biochemical differences would not *necessarily* imply different metabolic patterns. Such a list would deserve our full attention and would be a challenge, stimulating our ingenuity in making connections between these biochemical differences and the *essential* differences in function, the cells are known to have in the tissue. It is only from the moment that we have succeeded in making reasonable *connections* that we are allowed to speak of different metabolic patterns. To press this point a little further, it is clearly a matter of convention how to define the term metabolic pattern. In fact I prefer an opera-

tional definition linking up the specific biochemical organization and the specific function of the cell. However we will soon find out that our definition is a little pedantic as our present day knowledge hardly allows for even one single good example.

3. The final preliminary point will carry us forward to the heart of our subject. The number of publications concerning the metabolism of bone cells is increasing, and it is already apparent that there is a wide difference in scope and method among the various approaches. Concerning differences in scope there are two extremes. At one end we find investigations disclosing the activity of the cellular enzymatic apparatus. At the other end investigations dealing with the fate of certain substrates. Figuratively speaking one could say that the first group deals with the metabolic highway system of the cells, the other group with the real traffic on that highway system. *This picture will make clear to us that the conditions of the highways and the intensity of the traffic do not necessarily run parallel.*

Concerning differences in method, we can more or less arbitrarily differentiate into methods that carry no considerable risk of changing the metabolic parameters under investigation and methods that do. To my mind histochemical and enzymological investigations performed on previously intact bone tissue fall within the group of low risk. However metabolic investigations using slices or otherwise wounded pieces of bone tissue ask for a more critical attitude. And in fact without any data at hand one can foresee that e. g. by damaging the delicate network of osteocytes serious harm is probably done.

In this connection unpublished data from HEKKELMAN (personal communication) have illustrative value: He observed that pieces of diaphyseal rabbit bone (roughly $15 \times 5 \times 2 = 150$ mm^3) put in Hanks balanced salt solution lose a considerable amount

Table 1. *The total amount of nucleic acid obtained after 2 hours of incubation and expressed as µg/ml incubation fluid from $^1/_3$ g of bone*

	2 °C	37 °C	P_D
Hanks (ph 7.4)	2.7 ± 0.77 (6 exp.)	6.6 ± 1.96 (6 exp.)	< 0.002
Hanks without glucose (ph 7.4)	3.2 ± 0.4 (6 exp.)	4.3 ± 1.2 (12 exp.)	< 0.01
P_D.	insignificant	< 0.01	

Table 2. *The activity of isocitric dehydrogenase obtained in the medium after 2 hours of incubation: mµ moles/min/g of bone*

	2 °C	37 °C	P_D
Hanks (ph 7.4)	6.28 ± 2.2 (6 exp.)	13.2 ± 5.6 (6 exp.)	$0.02 > p > 0.01$
Hanks without glucose (ph 7.4)	4.82 ± 1.3 (9 exp.)	6.42 ± 4.41 (16 exp.)	insignificant
P_D.	insignificant	$0{,}02 > p > 0.01$	

of nucleic acid and enzymes as e. g. isocitric and lactic dehydrogenase. The output was found to depend on the temperature of incubation and the presence or absence of glucose; see Tables 1 and 2.

Moreover the yield was not far below that obtained after homogenization followed by extraction, and to take HEKKELMAN's own words, "the phenomenon suggests a pumping out of cellular material".

In a recent interesting publication (PECK *et al.*, 1964) we find another aspect of the same problem. The authors describe the isolation of bone cells from rat calvaria in buffered collagenase. The cells obtained passed successfully viability tests and proved fit for cultivation. From cytochemical alkaline phosphatase reactions they argue that their harvest probably contained osteoblasts and osteocytes. Moreover radioassay of CO_2 and lactate after confrontation with labelled glucose under aerobic conditions revealed metabolic traits reminiscent of "intact" bone tissue. However they observed no bone formation in tissue culture and were not able to prevent dedifferentation and/or overgrowth by "fibroblasts". The latter point is not surprising at all. Is the absence of bone formation surprising? Taking the acceptable view that bone formation is a complex process dependent on the interplay of very subtle intra and extra cellular conditions, the experiments clearly show that somewhere these conditions were not fulfilled. However taking the biochemical data really to mean that the collagenase isolated cells have preserved their original metabolic organization, we come to the conclusion that perhaps even full knowledge concerning the metabolism of the individual cells will always be *fundamentally insufficient* to explain the formation of bone as a tissue.

There is still another example to be considered in the clarification of my third preliminary point. Starting with the assumption that destruction is in general easier to understand than construction, one may be tempted to look upon the process of osteoclastic bone resorption as a nut easy to crack. In fact it is not uncommon for the specialist in tissue culture to be consulted about a method for cultivating osteoclasts in pure strain for investigational purposes. The bare facts are that such a culture is non existent and probably even impossible. GAILLARD (1961) has repeatedly observed in PTE treated cultivated radius rudiments that the numerous typical osteoclasts disappear from the moment the bony shaft is totally resorbed. A good explanation seems to be that the development or the preservation of typical osteoclasts depends among other things on the presence of bone and/or breakdown products of bone. In the light of work of BÉLANGER we arrive at the same conclusion; however he adheres to the restricting view that the *development* of the osteoclasts demands the presence of bone. Returning to the observation of GAILLARD and leaving undiscussed what, in this situation, the fate of the osteoclasts might be, we conclude that the student of osteoclastic function, working with isolated cells, would in all probability waste his effort on *cells in transition.*

Now coming to my main point and starting from the metabolic schemes known from general biochemistry, what lines can be drawn in black and what lines have to be dotted or even omitted? This specially concerns carbohydrate metabolism, which is responsible for at least 3 different tasks in bone tissue: 1. Generation of energy; 2. Provision of the cells with precursors to be used in the synthesis of proteins, mucopolysaccharides and pentose containing compounds of biological importance such as the pyridine nucleotides and RNA and DNA; and 3. Production of organic acids supposed to be important in the solubilization of matrix mineral.

It is from histochemical investigations that we have at least some data concerning the different types of cells (BALOGH *et al.*, 1961; HERRMANN-ERLEE, 1962). BALOGH worked with long bones of 4-week-old mice; HERRMANN-ERLEE with 15 day-old mouse radius rudiments. In reproducing their semi-quantitative data I restrict myself to some data concerning the carbohydrate metabolism of the cells of the inner periosteum and the osteoblasts, the osteocytes and the osteoclasts. Taking together data from both authors and omitting a number of minor discrepancies they demonstrate from *each* of the main pathways a number of enzymes to be active. However it is quite remarkable that they observed no 6-p-G Dehydrogenase activity as this is the second enzyme in the pentose phosphate cycle of which the initial enzyme, the G-6-p Dehydrogenase, was found to be active. The data of BALOGH show in fact disappointingly little difference between the different types of cells. However HERRMANN-ERLEE finds Succinic dehydrogenase to be active only in the osteoclasts and osteoblasts at the ossification ring. In BALOGH's data the osteoclasts do not hold a monopoly, but here this enzyme is more active than in the other types of cells. Moreover and in sharp contradistinction to BALOGH, she finds no Lactic dehydrogenase in osteoclasts. Finally she was unable to demonstrate α-glycerophosphate dehydrogenase activity in the cell types mentioned, with the only exception again of the osteoblasts at the ossification ring.

Summarizing, no convincing argument is found to doubt the completeness of the carbohydrate metabolizing machinery. Moreover the osteoclasts and the osteoblasts at the diaphyseal-metaphyseal junction seem to keep a special position. *However the data are absolutely insufficient to construe different metabolic patterns in the sense I have defined.* Concerning the special position of the osteoclasts I would like to add another point: Both authors found the osteoclasts deprived of Glutamic Dehydrogenase activity, and as you know this enzyme belongs to the domain of protein catabolism.

Before passing on to some investigations concerning metabolic pathways in bone cells it will repay to discuss, whether essential cellular potencies must find *by necessity* some reflection in the conditions of the metabolic pathways. I will try to formulate an answer on the basis of a special example: In the Liège symposium we have heard VAES's paper on acid Hydrolases and Lysosomes in bone cells (VAES, 1965). Moreover in Leyden we have seen his successfull work on the PTE intensified release of Lysosomal enzymes from cultivated mouse calvaria. I will take the position that in all probability his finding will prove to be of essential importance in the understanding of the process of bone resorption. Now one cannot foresee that the intracellular presence of even a high number of Lysosomes can be read in some way or another from certain peculiarities in the metabolic pathways. However it is possible that the production of the acid hydrolases and of the organic acids, necessary to bring the released enzymes in their pH optimum, or even the mechanism of extrusion, do ask for certain provisions that indeed can be read from the pathways. My answer then is, that perhaps many peculiarities in the metabolic pathways of bone cells will become explainable, provided data from other origins become available.

With only a few exceptions data concerning the main metabolic routes in bone tissue are not specific to the different types of cells; on the contrary they mostly reflect the combined contribution of different types.

In his thesis "Bone metabolism and the action of Parathyroid extract" HEKKELMAN gave us an excellent survey, describing the 1963 situation. Leaving out some important controversial points in the literature, we meet a picture in which 1. the glycolytic pathway, the pentose phosphate cycle and the Krebs cycle are operative. 2. However concerning the oxidative phosphorylation nearly nothing is known. 3. The activities of the pentose shunt dehydrogenases are suprisingly high in diaphyseal rabbit bone tissue as compared with e. g. kidney, liver and brain tissue. Moreover the strikingly high relative activity of pyridine nucleotide transhydrogenase — being as it is, involved in the reoxydation of NADPH — seems to underline the importance of the NADP dependent dehydrogenases in bone. 4. On the other hand the relatively low activity of Succinic Cytochrome C reductase suggests a less important role of the tricarboxylic acid cycle. 5. Concerning the citrate metabolism, especially under the influence of PTH, the problem about the balance between citrate synthesis and oxidation is still open to some controversy. 6. Finally, in this picture we meet already some connections between carbohydrate metabolism and protein synthesis, especially collagen synthesis. These connections concern carbohydrate inermediates being precursors of some amino acids and furthermore the ribose synthesis being prerequisite to RNA synthesis and so indirectly to protein synthesis; see Fig. 1.

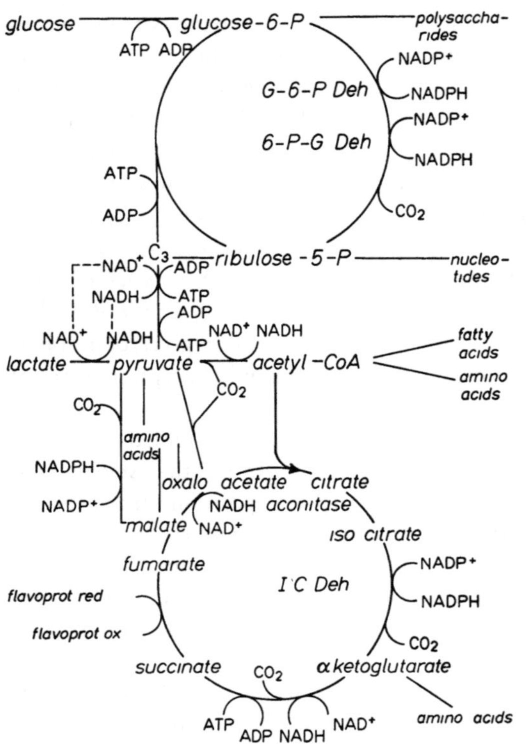

Simplified scheme of the main metabolic pathways

Fig. 1. A simplified scheme of the main metabolic pathways, according to J. W. HEKKELMAN: Bone metabolism and the action of parathyroid extract, 1963. Note: NAD(H) = DPN(H); NADP(H) = TPN(H)

Now although the data concerning the action of PTH on bone tissue belong to a subgroup of our universe of discourse, they are of direct relevance, because they reveal in all probability the *key points* of bone metabolism. Moreover, though not being essential, work on the main pathways is mainly done by students in the PTE field.

And so an essential contribution to our picture is HEKKELMAN's hypothesis stating that PTE induces a decrease of the amount of NADP and/or NADPH *available* for catabolic processes in the bone cells (HEKKELMAN, 1963, 1965). His argument hinges on phenomena concerning the *extractability* of Isocitric dehydrogenase from diaphyseal bone homogenates and more specially on the influence of NADP or NADPH — additional or naturally present — on this extractability. In fact he did no direct determinations of the cofactors mentioned.

It will be interesting now to compare this picture with a number of observations communicated at the 2nd Parathyroid symposium held in 1964 in the Netherlands:

A most interesting paper on the influence of PTE on bone metabolism and the levels of Nicotinamide nucleotides was given by VAN REEN (1965). He determined the pyridine nucleotides in the epiphyseal — metaphyseal area of rabbit femora fluorometrically and found quite to his own surprise the NADP content in the tissue of PTE pretreated animals to be increased by a factor 2.25. The NAD content was not changed significantly, NADH and NADPH were decreased by a factor 0.7.

His surprise does not primarily concern a possible controversy with HEKKELMAN's data but far more a seeming incompatibility of a PTE induced increase of NADP and the well established PTE induced increase of citrate concentration in bone. (At least this holds as long as one supposes the activity of the NADP dependent Isocitric dehydrogenase to be of importance in the balance of citrate production and oxidation.) In fact in VAN REEN's opinion the "old" concept of a metabolic block at the Isocitric dehydrogenase level cannot be considered as the final answer in explaining the accumulation of citrate in bone.

In trying to reflect a little upon this new situation it is good to keep in mind, that in most organs NADP is present mainly in the reduced state, the reverse being true for NAD. In bone tissue, according to VAN REEN, the ratio NADP/NADPH comes near to unity; under the influence of PTE there is a dramatic shift towards the oxidized state.

Returning then to HEKKELMAN's hypothesis concerning the action of PTE, it has been my contribution to show that in Gaillard's system of cultivated mouse radius rudiments, *additional* NAD or NADP are capable of inhibiting the development of the morphological effect of the hormone. Moreover the same was found to apply for a number of NADP-ase inhibitors, suggesting that by artificially keeping up the NADP level the hormone effect is hampered in its development (DE VOOGD VAN DER STRAATEN, 1965). Finally I have been able to demonstrate that PTE induces in radius rudiments a decreased binding of ^{14}C-Nicotinic Acid, a compound being preeminently the precursor of NAD and NADP; see Fig. 2. Summarizing, my observations seem to be in favour of HEKKELMAN's hypothesis and rather difficult to reconcile with VAN REEN's data.

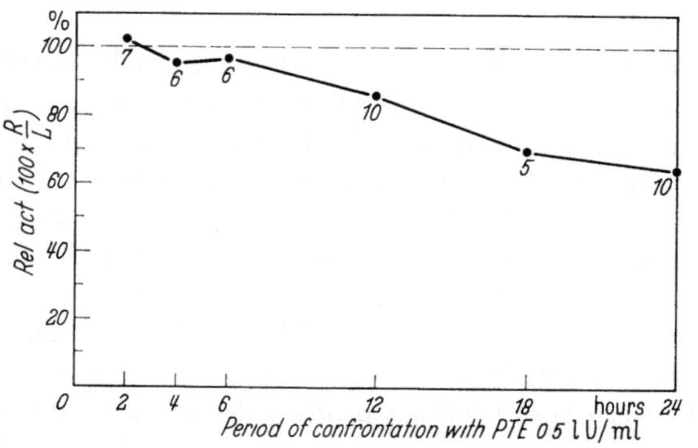

Fig. 2. The effect of PTE 0.5 IU/ml on the Nicotinic acid-7-^{14}C binding capacity of mouse radius rudiments in vitro. The radii were taken from 15-day-old embryo's; the left hand radii were cultivated in standard medium, the corresponding right hand radii being confronted with PTE. In all experiments this period of cultivation was followed by a 1 hour period of confrontation with labelled Nicotinic acid. The graph presents the relative activities of the washed bone shafts of the experimental radii, the activities of the corresponding control shafts being taken as 100

Against this controversial background there seems to be some need for a "unifying concept". Looking again upon VAN REEN's data we meet so to say an "internal discrepancy", possibly even pointing to a way out; see Fig. 3.

This "discrepancy" is found in the tremendous rise in NADP without any accompanying rise in the amount of the reduced form. And from the very fact that on the contrary NADPH decreases under the influence of PTE one gets the feeling that the oxidized and the reduced state do not keep the simple relation to one another one should perhaps suppose to exist in an uncomplicated chain of oxido-reductions. In

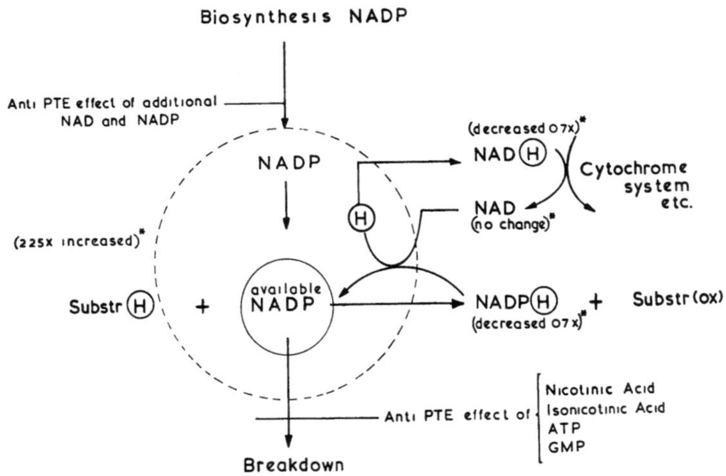

Fig. 3. The concept of 2 NADP fractions; the scheme presents some findings of VAN REEN (*) communicated at the 2nd Parathyroid symposium, 1964. Moreover the function of NADP and NAD in dehydrogenation reactions is given. Finally the supposed mechanism of action of a number of PTE antagonizers is indicated

fact the decrease of NADPH alone, could possibly point to a hormone induced increase of pyridine nucleotide transhydrogenase activity as this enzyme takes away the hydrogen from the NADPH and transports this hydrogen to NAD. However in trying to solve the problem from *this* side one finds there is no explanation for the *increase* of NADP. The "unifying concept" then could be, that we have to discriminate between the NADP "present" and the NADP *really available* for the catabolic enzymes in the metabolic machinery. In align with this idea we suppose that the observed rise of the NADP level concerns the fraction of NADP "*present but not available*". To go one step further, one could suppose that the "screen" between both fractions protects the *non available* fraction against enzymatic breakdown thus accounting for an increase. Behind this idea we find the concept of cellular compartmentalization. Clearly at the moment this concept is, in our situation only a formalism, although HEKKELMAN and I are speculating that the non available fraction, if existing at all, could be hidden in the nucleus of the cells.

In relation to what I have said I would like to report furthermore an important observation made by (COHN and GRIFFITH, 1965) working with slices of the distal ends of rabbit femora. They found NAD and NADP specifically capable of stimulating the $C^{14}O_2$ evolution from Fumarate-1,4-C^{14}. Using Citrate-1,5-C^{14} this effect failed to appear. In slices from PTE pretreated animals the CO_2 evolution is less than in control slices and this hormone effect is *not* overcome by NADP. Further analysis revealed that the rate of conversion from Fumarate to Malate is independent of NADP, however in the presence of NADP less Malate *accumulates*. This already makes clear that the NADP probably acts in the Malate-Pyruvate region. Detailed analysis of the reaction-rates involved in the conversion of Fumarate to Lactate and CO_2 indeed revealed, that the NADP effect concerns the activity of the NADP-Malate oxidase (Malic enzyme). COHN and GRIFFITH conclude that their bone preparation contains a pyridine nucleotide stimulated pathway for decarboxylation of *Dicarboxylic* acids.

I hope to have impressed upon you the central position the pyridine nucleotides take in recent concepts concerning bone metabolism. However I would do scant justice to todays knowledge, by concealing important information concerning a possible influence the nucleus of the bone cell can have upon the processes we have discussed. It is very well possible that this information will throw, among others, a new light upon the pyridine nucleotide problem.

In this connection I will deal now with recent investigations of GAILLARD, concerning the combined effect of PTE and Actinomycin D or Puromycin on cultivated radius rudiments (GAILLARD, 1965). Full details being published I give only the essentials. From his former work we know that PTE induces dramatic morphological and functional changes in radii of 15 day-old mouse embryos (GAILLARD, 1960, 1961). The morphological changes concern the bony shaft, the cartilage and the connective tissue proper. Among other changes, seven fully reproducible morphological phenomena were found to be characteristic for the action of PTE on radius explants; they are listed in fig. 4. Now on the basis of the generally accepted opinion that acute and chronic conditions of hyperparathyroidism are among others characterized by a defective synthesis of specific proteins by osteogenic cells, it was decided to study the combined effect of PTE and some inhibitors of protein synthesis. To put it in more detail, it was thought that by eliminating the central or peripheral parts of the cellular protein synthetic apparatus, information could be obtained concerning the role of this apparatus in the development of the hormone effect. This approach was *not* based on any preconceived idea concerning possible specific interaction between hormone and inhibitor whatsoever. On the contrary I even foresee that *because of this unspecificity* this type of approach will prove applicable to other fields as well.

The antibiotic Actinomycin D was chosen because it is known to interfere with the continuous flooding of the cytoplasm with nuclear m-RNA. Puromycin interferes with the last steps of protein formation at the ribosomal level. Concerning the way of application of these antibiotics a few remarks have to be made: Actinomycin was given in a concentration of 0.005 γ per ml of the medium for 6 hours prior to the confrontation of the explants with PTE 0.1 IU/ml. Puromycin however was given simultaneously with the PTE in concentrations of 0.1 or 0.01 γ/ml. In both set-ups the whole experiment lasted for 48 hours. Finally it is important to known that the concentrations were below the level of noticeable toxicity. The concentration of PTE was put at 0.1 IU/ml because this is a "borderline" concentration below which the intensity of the phenomena falls down steeply.

In this situation Actinomycin D proved to inhibit the development of all the morphological phenomena of hormone action listed in Fig. 4. However Puromycin proved able to interfere with the development of the phenomena 1 ± 4 only. In particular the hormone-induced proliferation of connective tissue inside the shaft was found to escape the inhibitory action of Puromycin entirely.

From these important observations GAILLARD draws a number of direct and indirect conclusions: 1. First of all that for the expression of the complete effect of PTE on the explants the unhampered production of certain proteins is necessary. 2. Moreover that the action of PTE is more closely associated with the production of m-RNA than with the Puromycin sensitive synthetic activities at the ribosomal level.

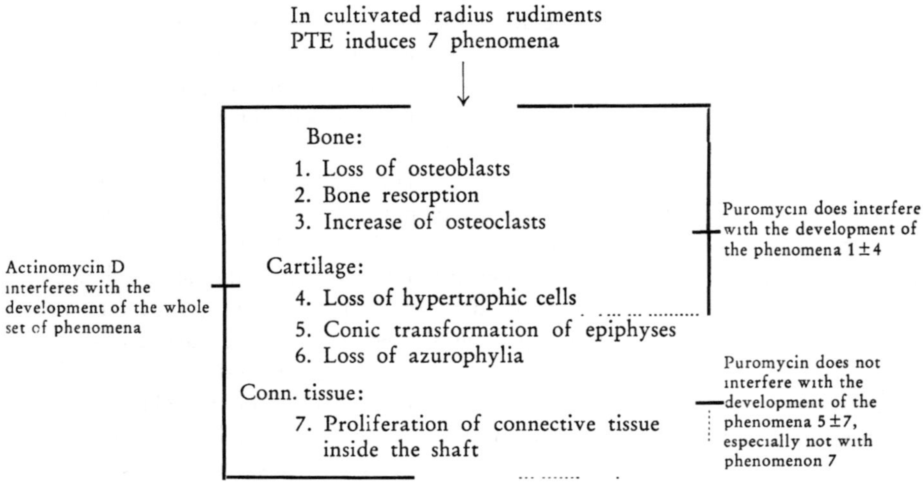

Fig. 4. The 7 morphological changes, characteristic for the action of PTE on cultivated mouse radius rudiments according to GAILLARD and the antagonistic effect of Actinomycin D and Puromycin

At this point I would like to bring again to your attention the idea that PTE could act by inducing quantitative changes in the NAD and/or NADP biosynthetic apparatus. 3. The observation that the hormone-induced proliferation of connective tissue is, so to say, "Puromycin resistant" brings GAILLARD to a most interesting consideration. This finding seems to suggest that different receptors might exist for the biosynthetic mechanism of cell reproduction and for the production of specific secretions of a proteinaceous character. And although in this special case the postulated receptors have to be localized in different types of cells, the question rises whether we have to generalize and to postulate two different systems in *each* individual cell. Perhaps we find a morphological substrate of this concept in the well known dichotomy in free and membrane attached ribosomes.

In the light of GAILLARD's observations RASMUSSEN's (1964) idea that Actinomycin D interferes with the PTE stimulated differentiation of osteoclasts, thus interfering with osteoclastic bone resorption, seems to be oversimplified. In fact the lesson to be drawn from GAILLARD's experiments is, that the hormone effect is polymorphic and that it does not fit into a concept dealing primarily or even exclusively with osteoclastic function.

Although not directly connected with this subject I would like to make a final digression. In thinking about protein synthesis and the production of proteins for specified different purposes outside the cell, we are confronted with a serious lack of knowledge concerning the mechanism of extrusion. It is certainly dubious whether every protein leaves the cell by the mechanism of reversed pinocytosis. However, taking the rather generalized position that the cell has many "exits" allowing for a transport even from the nuclear envelope through the endoplasmatic reticulum into the extracellular space, again we meet a difficulty as the sites of protein synthetic action are at "the other side", the ribosomal side, of the membranous screen. Although this all belongs to elementary cytology it does not detain me from making the "moralizing" statement that concepts concerning the specific protein synthetic activity of bone cells need to take into account these problems of transport. This holds specially if we are dealing with exogenous influences, such as the action of PTE, on these cellular activities.

In what I have said, I have tried to fulfil the promise of the title of my paper, nothing more. However I do hope that you recognized that it was said in the voice and with the special interest of a cellular biologist.

References

Balogh, K., Jr., H. R. Dudley, and R. B. Cohen: Oxidative enzyme activity in skeletal cartilage and bone. Lab. Invest. **10**, 839 (1961).

Cohn, D. V., and F. D. Griffith: The influence of parathyroid extract on oxidative and decarboxylative pathways in bone. The parathyroid glands, ultra structure, secretion and function. Chicago: The University of Chicago Press 1965.

Gaillard, P. J.: The influence of parathormone on the explanted radius of albino mouse embryo's. Proc. kon. ned. Akad. Wet. **C 63**, 25 (1960).

— The influence of parathyroid extract on the explanted radius of albino mouse embryo's. II. Proc. kon. ned. Akad. Wet. **C 64**, 119 (1961).

— Protein metabolism and the effect of parathyroid on bone. Texas reports on Biology and Medicine Suppl. I, **23**, 259 (1965).

Hekkelman, J. W.: Bone metabolism and the action of parathyroid extract. Thesis. Leiden 1963.

— An enzymological study of bone metabolism and its regulation by parathyroid hormone. In Calcified Tissues. Richelle, L. J., and M. J. Dallmagne (eds.). Liège: Université de Liège 1965, p. 393.

Herrmann-Erlee, M. P. M.: A histochemical investigation of embryonic long bones: the effect of parathyroid hormone on the activity of a number of enzymes. Proc. kon. ned. Akad. Wet. **C 65**, 22 (1962).

Peck, W. A., S. J. Birge, and S. A. Fedak: Bone cells: Biochemical and biological studies after enzymatic isolation. Science **146**, 1476 (1964).

Rasmussen, H., C. Arnaud, and C. Hawker: Actinomycin D and the response to parathyroid hormone. Science **144**, 1019 (1964).

Reen, R. van: The influence of parathyroid extract on bone metabolism and the levels of Nicotinamide nucleotides. The parathyroid glands, ultra structure, secretion and function. Chicago: The University of Chicago Press 1965.

Vaes, G.: Hydrolytic enzymes and Lysosomes in bone cell. In Calcified Tissues. Richelle, L. J., and M. J. Dallemagne (eds.). Liège: Université de Liège 1965, p. 51.

Voogd van der Straaten, W. A. de: The possible role of NADP in the action of parathyroid hormone on bone. The parathyroid glands, ultra structure, secretion and function. Chicago: The University of Chicago Press 1965.

Remodelling of the Bone Matrix

CH. M. LAPIÈRE

Institut de Médecine, Département de Clinique et de Pathologie Médicales
et
Laboratoire de Dermatologie Expérimentale, Université de Liège, Hôpital de Bavière,
Liège, Belgique

Introduction

Bone, the supporting frame of vertebrate animals is made of a two-phase material, the collagen matrix and the hydroxyapatite crystals. The organization of the collagen fibers and of the crystals is such that these two materials with different elastic moduli and strength carry out their mutual function organized as trabeculae and account for the mechanical properties of bone (CURREY, 1964). Strongly regulated mechanisms involving synthesis and degradation of the matrix and of the crystal lattice, are probably responsible for such a high degree of organization.

Until recently, little has been known about the way collagen is synthesized and degraded in bone while some progress has been made in the last few years concerning these processes in soft connective tissues. This difference in the amount of information is mainly due to the difficulty in applying to calcified tissues the techniques of investigation used for the study of collagen metabolism in soft connective tissues. There is, however, no reason to think that the main steps of formation and removal of the collagen fibers are completely different in bone compared to soft collagenous structures. Indeed the osteoblast is only a particular form of fibroblast and the osteoclast a specialized histiocyte. The main difference between soft and calcified connective tissue lies in the composition of the ground substance. Semi-liquid and highly permeable in soft connective tissues, it is mostly rigid in bone, immobilizing fibers and cells in a crystalline jail. This difference must change the relationship of the collagen framework with its surrounding medium. It surely has some side effect on the metabolism of the fibers. It is, however, too early to take this into consideration. In the present discussion we shall only consider the problem related to the synthesis and the breakdown of the matrix in calcified tissues.

Composition and organization of the bone matrix

The dry weight of bone is composed of 65—70% of inorganic crystals of calcium and phosphate and 30—35% of an organic matrix in which the collagen accounts for as much as 90—95% (EASTOE, 1956). It represents so much of the organic phase of the bone that any changes in it must represent modifications of the matrix. The collagen of bone is not different in amino acid composition, except for its hydroxylysine content, from this protein found in skin or other organs according to data of PIEZ and LIKINS (cited in GROSS, 1963 b). According to GLIMCHER (1965), bone collagen would however be composed of only α chains. It does not seem to form as much β or γ sub-units as skin collagen.

Without considering in detail any concepts of calcification we want to call attention to the fact that the crystals are very closely related to the collagen fibers (S. F. JACKSON, 1957; GLIMCHER *et al.*, 1957). The nucleation could arise around a phosphate group bound to definite regions of the collagen (GLIMCHER and KRANE,

1962; KRANE and GLIMCHER, 1962). This is not a particular property of bone collagen but a function displayed by any collagen in its native type fibrous form (GLIMCHER, 1959). It indicates that besides the collagen system, there must exist in soft and calcified connective tissues some other component controling calcification. We will not deal with this problem although we recognize that its role in the organization of the collagen in calcified tissues might be of the greatest importance.

In contrast to the loose and commonly random arrangement of the collagen fibers in most soft connective tissue, in bone the collagen framework is organized in tubules (osteons) or in lamellae. These are the units of bone which adapt to external mechanical stresses by a process of remodelling as emphasized by WOLFF in 1892 (cited by GLIMCHER, 1959). An understanding of how organization and remodelling of bone is feasible from a biochemical point of view will only be possible when its basic phenomena are known, that is how synthesis of calcified structures occurs and how breakdown is realized.

Synthesis and organization of collagenous structure in soft and calcified connective tissues

The collagen in soft connective tissues can be fractionated by varying the salt concentration or the pH of the extracting medium (HARKNESS *et al.*, 1954; JACKSON, 1957; GROSS, 1958 a, 1959; HARKNESS, 1961). These fractions of the tissue collagen belong to different pools of molecules. Their size depends on the metabolic activity of the fibroblasts of the tissue (GROSS, 1958 b) and can be related to the age of the molecules (GROSS, 1958 c). The experiments of HARKNESS *et al.* (1954) of JACKSON (1957) and JACKSON and BENTLEY (1960) show that radioactive collagen appears at different rates in the various fractions after injecting a labelled amino acid. These results correlate with the hypothesis of GROSS (1959) proposing that the extractability of the collagen depends on its stage of aggregation, which would be partially a function of its age. Immediately after its synthesis the newly formed collagen liberated in the extracellular space is extractable in isotonic saline at neutral pH and low temperature (5 °C). After these molecules are organized in the connective tissue, an increased ionic strength is required to separate another fraction of the loosely arranged fibers. More collagen molecules can be further separated from the bulk of the remaining insoluble fibers by lowering the pH to 3.5. With increasing time the proportion of extractable collagen decreases indicating an increase of organization.

By a combination of the methods of isotopic labeling of the collagen and fractionation of these molecules by different salt solutions we can follow the process of synthesis and organization of the fibers in connective tissues. We have used this technique to investigate the metabolism of the collagen in remodelling tissues (LAPIÈRE and GROSS, 1963; LAPIÈRE *et al.*, 1965; LAPIÈRE *et al.*, in press). These experiments in the tadpole and more recent results provide us with information which can be schematically summarized in Fig. 1.

The proposed interpretation is the following. The precursor amino-acids are taken from the local pool inside the fibroblast where they are incorporated into the peptide chains of the collagen. In the cell this collagen is bound to the microsomes (GREEN and LOWTHER, 1959). At this stage it is not extractable (I_1). Shortly after, it is liberated into the extracellular space where we find it in the pool of fibers. At the temperature of the body all the collagen seems to be organized in fibers. The extraction procedure removes some collagen from this pool.

Whether the extractable collagen arises from fibers of different age or from outside layers around different fibers is not yet known. Some autoradiographic studies of

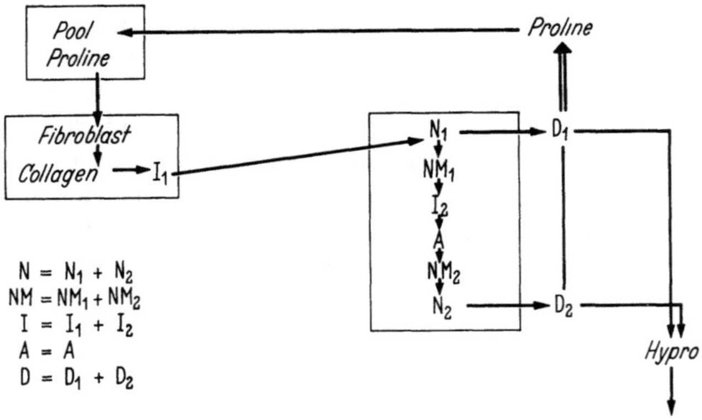

Fig. 1. N represents the neutral isotonic saline extracted collagen; NM the neutral hypertonic extracted fraction; A the acid one and I the insoluble. D refers to degradation products

HAY and REVEL (1963) show that the newly formed collagen is concentrated in regions of different metabolic activity. According to TANZER and HUNT (1964), in the lathyritic chick embryo the newly formed bone collagen is organized in fibrillar aggregates which can be solubilized. Following JACKSON and BENTLEY (1960) it seems reasonable to admit a dual origin of the salt extracted collagen. It could arise from newly formed fibrils and from the outside layer of previously deposited collagenous elements which are increasing in size by accretion of newly synthesized molecules. In tadpole tissues, the extracellular collagen can be fractionated in different pools. The proposed composition of these fractions is summarized at the bottom of Fig. 1. For each of them, in terms of incorporation of the labelled precursor, the "1" form is labelled much faster and more heavily than the "2" form.

The isotonic saline extract (N) contains the newly formed collagen (N_1) but also, mainly in remodelling tissues, larger amounts of a pre-existent unlabelled collagen (N_2). The hypertonic saline (NM) is also composed of two pools, one of which (NM_1) becomes labelled later than its proposed precursor (N_1). It has to be distinguished from another pool (NM_2) larger in size but labelled much later. The more organized collagen which is not extractable under our experimental conditions, (I_2), comes next in the metabolic chain. It has to be differentiated from the very small but highly radioactive collagen bound to the microsomes in cells (I_1) which is not extractable. The acid extractable collagen (A) always has the lowest specific activity among all the fractions. It might derive from the I_2 pool. Although the proposed scheme is based on the analysis of isotope dilution experiments, it remains partly hypothetical because it has not yet been possible to separate the different pools of molecules forming each fraction. However it gives an indication that the structured collagen fibers in the connective tissues are organized according to some factors related to aging and to the metabolic activity of the tissue. This metabolic behaviour of the extracellular collagen is different in soft connective tissues which are in a steady state and those which are remodelling. In steady state tissues, a short metabolic pathway seems to be predominant. The newly formed collagen molecules are degraded to a large extent before their incorporation in organized fibers. This is represented schematically in Fig. 1 by a pathway passing from I_1 to N_1 and D_1. In remodelling tissues, the newly synthesized molecules are used for building new fibers while the pre-existing old fibers become solubilized and lysed. The net result is that the newly formed collagen remains for a much longer time in the pool of the fibers. It is represented in Fig. 1 by a metabolic pathway starting at I_1 and passing from N_1 to N_2 to finish at D_2.

These metabolic pathways are based on the extractability of the collagen. This property depends on the stability of the structured fibers which seems to be a function of intermolecular bonds. Maturation processes occuring also at the molecular level have been demonstrated by ORHECKOWITCH *et al.* (1960) and PIEZ *et al.* (1961).

Since the work of NEUBERGER and SLACK (1953) it is known that bone has a collagen metabolism as active as any other connective tissue. Further studies (FLANAGAN and NICHOLS, 1964) have shown that bone is potentially capable of synthesizing significant amounts of protein. This overall metabolic activity of bone has not been analysed in the same way as that in soft connective tissue. Indeed the collagen of normal bone cannot be usefully fractionated by salt solutions of different ionic strength or pH.

Some metabolic studies using salt fractionation of the collagen have however been made in animals treated with lathyritic drugs. In this experimental condition more collagen is extractable in cold hypertonic saline (LEVENE and GROSS, 1959). This seems to be related to some abnormality of the process of maturation of the collagen molecule, which lacks intramolecular bonds (MARTIN *et al.*, 1961) and forms unstable aggregates (GROSS, 1963 a). Isotope incorporation studies (TANZER and GROSS, 1964) demonstrate that the collagen in lathyritic bone is heterogenous, suggesting that lathyritic collagen originates from 2 or more collagen pools.

The problem in studying the metabolism of bone arises from the complexity of this biological material. It is composed of elements of different age. Each of them consists of different layers of calcified collagen which have been formed by the progressive deposition of the matrix and the crystals. Obvious differences in the metabolic activity of the mineral part of these units can be demonstrated either by microradiographic or autohistoradiographic techniques (MARSHALL *et al.*, 1959; MCLEAN and ROWLAND, 1963). Simultaneously with different degree of mineralization, the density of the organic matrix is also variable from one osteon to the other and within the same element from the center to the periphery (SMITH, 1963). In these elementary units of bone the collagen layers vary in direction from the central cavity to the compact peripheral tissue (GLIMCHER, 1959). These elementary units of bone can be divided into different regions according to their density of calcification (ROBINSON, 1960). This author calculated for different regions of an osteon the probable concentration of its components. He proposed a model in which a unit volume of bone of different degrees of calcification would have an amount of matrix almost constant while the relative proportion of calcium and water would vary in opposite direction one to the other. On this hypothesis, HERMAN and RICHELLE (1961) have calculated that the density of bone from different regions would range from 1.7 to 2.3. They designed a technique to separate these constituents of bone according to their stage of calcification. Samples of bone are finely ground in a high speed specially designed grinder. The fine particles (about 5 μ large) are separated into fractions of different density by flotation in liquids of different composition. Using this technique they have been able to demonstrate that calcium metabolism is partly related to the exchange properties of these different fractions with the body fluid (RICHELLE and BRONNER, 1963). Hormones which are known to modify the composition of bone affect these components at different rates (RICHELLE, 1964). These results emphasize a difference in reactivity of the fractions of bone demonstrating the efficacy of the technique to investigate the metabolism and the organization

Table 1. *Calcium and Collagen in Bone Fractionated by Gradient Density*

	Fractions							Total bone 100 mg.
	1.7	1.8	1.9	2.0	2.1	2.2	2.3	
Calcium	0.48 (0.11)[1]	0.66 (0.15)	0.72 (0.17)	2.18 (0.51)	10.79 (2.52)	77.10 (18.03)	8.08 (1.89)	100% (23.39)
Collagen	2.5 (0.44)	3.7 (0.65)	6.4 (1.12)	7.3 (1.27)	26.9 (4.69)	45.1 (7.87)	8.2 (1.43)	100% (17.45)
Calcium / Collagen	0.25	0.23	0.15	0.40	0.54	2.29	1.32	1.34

[1] Between brackets, amount in mg. per fraction.

Table 1. Distribution of calcium and collagen in total bone of sixty day old rats and in fractions obtained by gradient density of ground bone (Upper values of each section in percent of the total and lower figures in mg from 100 mg. of bone)

Table 2. *Specific Activity (S. A.) of the Collagen Hydroxyproline in Bone Fractionated by Gradient Density*

Time in hours	Total Bone[1]	Hydroxyproline Relative specific activity[2] Fractions						
		1.7	1.8	1.9	2.0	2.1	2.2	2.3
0.5	328	13.4	10.4	3.8	2.0	0.79	0.31	0.12
1	451	10.2	4.9	1.7	3.5	0.66	0.23	0.21
3	649	10.7	6.0	2.1	0.9	0.50	0.15	0.15
6	660	10.2	11.5	2.5	2.0	0.42	0.13	0.08
12	516	11.3	14.9	4.5	3.2	0.87	0.16	0.06
24	791	9.4	12.9	5.4	4.0	1.30	0.15	0.05
36	719	5.2	10.2	3.9	2.1	0.79	0.15	0.07
48	919	4.3	7.4	2.0	3.3	1.25	0.25	0.07

[1] S.A. of hydroxyproline in dpm/μM.
[2] Represent the factor by which the S.A. of the hydroxyproline of the total bone must be multiplied to obtain the real S.A. of the hydroxyproline in the fraction.

Table 2. Explanation in the text. The maximum relative specific activity of the collagen in the fractions is framed inside of the heavy lines

of the calcified tissues. Together with RICHELLE and ONCKELINX we are applying this technique of investigation to the study of bone collagen metabolism in rats.

The particles of different density from diaphysal bone of 60 day old rats contain different proportions of the total collagen and calcium (Table 1) in increasing amount from the lightest fraction (1.7) to the one of density 2.2 An almost identical proportion of collagen and calcium is located in the heaviest particles. The ratio of calcium to collagen is low in the first three fractions. It increases to a maximum in the fraction with the greatest volume, (2.2), but it becomes lower again in the densest fraction.

To consider if these fractions are related to the metabolism of the collagen in bone we have labelled the collagen with a radioactive tracer and measured the radioactivity in the bone fractionated by gradient density.

Sixty day old rats were injected with ^{3}H proline and killed at increasing times after injection of the tracer. The long bones were collected and immediately cooled on ice. Diaphyses cleaned of marrow were ground and separated into fractions of different densities. After hydrolysis in 6 N HCl, the amount of hydroxyproline was measured and this amino acid purified by thin layer chromatography in the presence of cold carrier. The radioactivity of the samples was measured in a liquid scintillation counter. The results are illustrated in Table 2 for different time points up to 48 hours. The S.A. of the hydroxyproline of the unfractionated bone is tabulated in dpm/μM. The values for the hydroxyproline of each fraction are multiples of the S.A. of the hydroxyproline of the unfractionated bone. This method of computing the data allows us to locate the migration of the label. The only variable is the time elapsed since the synthesis of the collagen.

The S.A. of the hydroxyproline in the unfractionated bone is increasing with time, faster during the first hours than later. It is the expression of the overall turnover of the collagen in the bone. The location of the maximum S.A. of the collagen in the fractions gives more information. We see immediately that the S.A. of the collagen varies widely according to the density of the fractions and also to the time elapsed since the injection of the tracer. Half an hour after the injection of the labelled precursor, the lightest fraction (1.7) has the highest specific activity. There is however some label in all the fractions. With increasing time, up to 3 hours, the collagen of the lightest fraction (1.7) keeps the highest S.A. In the meantime the S.A. of the other fractions decreases. These data would indicate that the newly synthesized collagen is contained in the 1.7 fraction. The radioactivity in the other fraction could represent some contamination of the samples by labelled non protein bound hydroxyproline disappearing progressively by dilution. Six hours after the injection of the label, the S.A. of the collagen in the fraction 1.8 increases, indicating the appearance of the labelled molecules coming from the 1.7 fraction. Twelve hours are required to see the same change in the 1.9 and 2.0 fractions and 24 hours in the 2.1. At that time the relative S.A. of the 1.7 fraction drops because more labelled molecules are then located in the other fractions. The same appears after 36 hours for the 1.8 and 1.9 fractions. The labelled collagen seems to move to the 2.2 fraction only after 48 hours. More than two days are required for the label to reach the last fraction. The progressive reduction of the relative S.A. of the collagen when it passes from one fraction to the other is due to the dilution of the newly formed bone collagen in fractions of increasing size.

The general meaning of this metabolic study is illustrated in Table 2 by the conformation of the area between the dark lines. It represents the location of the maximum relative specific activity of the collagen for each fraction in relation to time. Mainly located in the lightest fraction it moves progressively toward the heaviest one. These results are in agreement with the hypothesis that the collagen framework of bone is synthesized as a non or slightly calcified matrix which undergoes progressive changes related to aging and mineralization.

On the basis of our knowledge of the organization of the collagen fibers in soft connective tissues, these data allow us to propose a schematic representation of what could be the relationship collagen — mineral — water in bone (Fig. 2). When

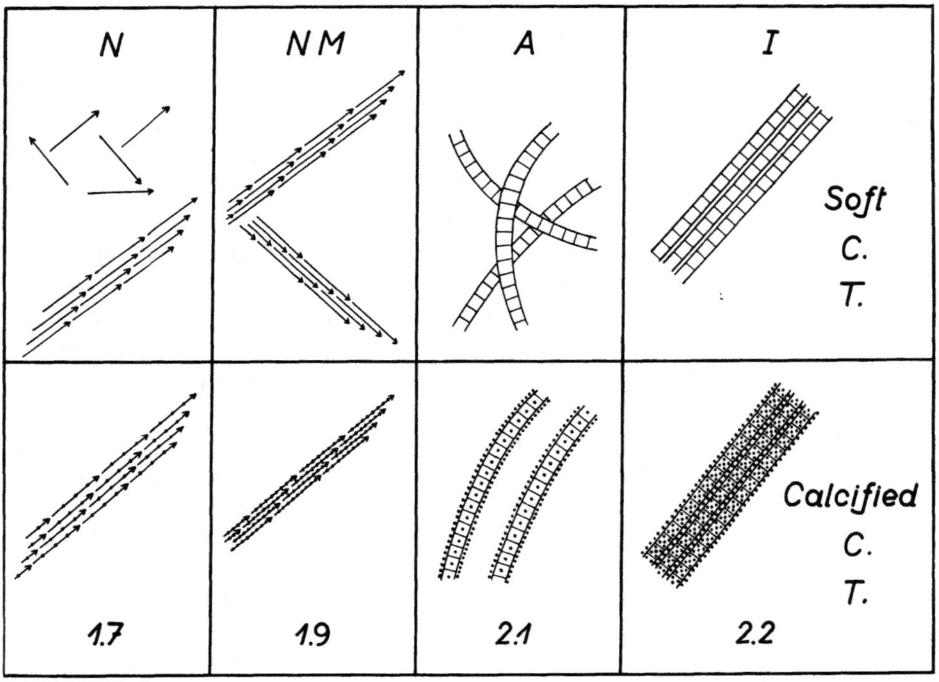

Fig. 2. Schematic illustration of the organization of collagen fractionated from soft and calcified connective tissues. From left to right are represented the neutral isotonic salt extractable collagen (N) compared to the least calcified 1.7 bone collagen, the neutral hypertonic salt extracted collagen (NM) from more compact fibers and the 1.9 denser more calcified bone structures, the fibers extracted in acid medium (A) and the calcified fibrous 2.1 element, finally, the bulk of the insoluble fibers (I) and of the 2.2 most calcified bony structures

collagen is synthesized in bone, it appears in the extracellular space as a very loose arrangements of molecules comparable to the N fraction of soft connective tissue. These loose fibers undergo immediate calcification as seen with the electron microscope (S. F. JACKSON, 1957). They may already have been present inside the osteoblast according to SCOTT and GLIMCHER (1963). As they are loose fibers and slightly calcified they contain a large amount of bound water and therefore have a light density. As time passes after the formation of this new bone, the amount of water decreases in the fibers while the deposition of calcium salt increases. This process can be compared to the maturation of the fibers in soft connective tissue. Their increased organization requires a hypertonic medium for extraction (NM). This condensation process has been demonstrated *in vitro* by GROSS (1958 c). A further evolution of the process of maturation and calcification of the newly formed element would lead to closer association of calcium salts and collagen fibers (2.1) in a way rather similar to the increase in density and the progressive insolubilization of fibers in non calcified connective tissues (A). The bulk of the osteons would be composed of fully mineralized structures (2.2) which can be compared to the mass of insoluble fibers in soft connective tissues (I).

The percent distribution of the collagen in these different fractions of soft and calcified tissues is somewhat analogous. There is little collagen in the isotonic saline (N) extract and in the lightest bone fraction (1.7), some more in the hypertonic extract (NM) and in the 1.9 fraction, even more in the acid and the 2.1. One main fraction contains the bulk of the collagen, the insoluble one in soft connective tissues and the 2.2 fraction of bone.

It is obvious that only metabolic studies using fractionation techniques will allow us to go further in our understanding of the organization of calcified tissues. The above partial results of a larger experiment designed to study the formation and removal of the bone matrix brings to our attention the similarity in the mechanism of synthesis, organization and distribution of the collagen framework in bone and soft connective tissues. This identity might be based on general properties of the collagen molecules. Bone seems to be in this respect, only a special problem of the molecular biology of the connective tissues.

Collagen breakdown in soft and calcified connective tissues

During growth, bone is under constant, rapid remodelling. This function is accomplished by the three types of bone cells, osteoblasts, osteocytes and osteoclasts. This remodelling seems to be required for some part of the homeostatic control of the calcium ion concentration in body fluid (McLean and Rowland, 1963) according to the dual mechanism of the control of calcium balance proposed by McLean and Urist (1961). As a part of this mechanism, bone cells are capable of tunelling compact bone to induce the formation of new haversian canals. This function, which continues even in the absence of the parathyroids (Jowsey *et al.*, 1958) seems to be related to the activity of osteoclasts. More recently Bélanger *et al.*, (1963) demonstrated that bone can also be degraded by the activity of osteocytes in a process called osteolysis. It is enhanced by parathormone as well as the osteoclastic activity *in vivo*.

The best example of fast removal of calcified connective tissue is found in tissue culture (Goldhaber, 1958; Gaillard, 1959). The breakdown of the collagen matrix of bone cultivated *in vitro* has been shown by Stern *et al.* (1963) by measuring an increasing amount of solubilized hydroxyproline. That bone cells were capable of secreting an enzymatic system having collagenolytic activity was demonstrated in tissue culture by Gross and Lapière (1962) and further studied in detail by Walker *et al.* (1964). Dissecting the results of these experiments, we find that all the conditions for claiming the presence of a collagenase system were fulfilled. The collagen used is in fibrous form in a native state and little of it is degraded by large amounts of trypsin. The pH of the reaction mixture remains at neutrality and a considerable proportion of the breakdown product is dialysable. The reaction goes to completion, breaking down all the collagen present. Finally, the production of this lytic enzyme is enhanced by parathormone proportionally to the duration of the treatment.

With G. VAES, we have been able to demonstrate some collagenolytic activity in homogenates of bone from calvaria of new born rats. This enzymatic activity is also increased by treatment with parathormone. We are, however, not yet able to correlate these results with the activity of a collagenase-like enzyme. WOODS and NICHOLS (1963, 1964) have demonstrated a similar enzymatic system in homogenates of bone cells.

The only isolated animal collagenase is the enzyme collected from tissue culture of tadpole skin (LAPIÈRE and GROSS, 1963). This enzyme is now purified (NAGAI *et al.*, 1963) and characterized (NAGAI *et al.*, 1964). It possesses all the characteristics required for being a true collagenase. It lyses the native collagen at a constant rate under physiological conditions. Its activity on the collagen molecule is very specific and limited.

Although this enzyme is present in tissue culture we have never been able to demonstrate its presence in living tissues. On the other hand we found a slight amount of protease-like activity on native collagen (LAPIÈRE and GROSS, 1963). Because of these findings we became very careful about the conditions under which the enzyme assay has to be carried out in order to detect a collagenase-like enzyme in the presence of proteolytic enzymes.

The enzyme has to be active on native collagen. Denaturation to gelatin occurs in certain circumstances. There are certain limits of pH and temperature outside of which the collagen does not remain native. This is demonstrated by an experiment in which different samples of radioactive highly purified skin collagen (either in fibrous form or in solution) are placed for several hours at 37 °C in buffered solution of pH ranging between 2.8 and 9.4. After bringing the pH back to 7.5 the activity of trypsin is used to check the native or denatured state of the collagen. A small and rather constant amount of dialysable labelled collagen fragments are liberated from the samples preincubated between limits of pH ranging from 4.8 to 9.1. Below and above these limits, collagen is degraded to gelatin and therefore becomes susceptible to the proteolytic activity of trypsin.

Assaying fractionated bone extract on native collagen we found collagenolytic activity at pH 5.5 and 7.0 both in the non particulate part of the homogenate and in the light and heavy particles. However we do not feel that this activity is collagenase-like because it does not fulfill all the conditions of enzyme kinetics in the same way as the bacterial or the tadpole collagenase.

We know that bacterial collagenase lyses collagen at a fast rate while trypsin at pH 7.0 and pepsin at pH 5.5 have only very limited activity (Fig. 3). When we study the regression lines of concentration or time dependence activity of these three enzymes we can see that none of them would pass through the origin. This may mean that the substrate, the native collagen in its fibrous form, is not homogeneous. A small part of it (5—12%) is more susceptible to enzyme attack. It could represent a portion of the collagen which is not organized in dense fibers. The activity of trypsin on native collagen is indeed much more significant (80%) when the collagen is in solution. With respect to these considerations we have to accept that we can only call by the name "collagenase" an enzyme displaying sufficient activity on native collagen whatever its stage of aggregation might be. As far as I know, none of the works published until now has given evidence of such an enzyme in homogenates of bone or of any other tissues.

It is interesting to consider such a difference in activity of enzymes depending on the degree of polymerisation of the collagen. It can be related to the observation that in soft connective tissues the degradation seems to occur from the pools of collagen

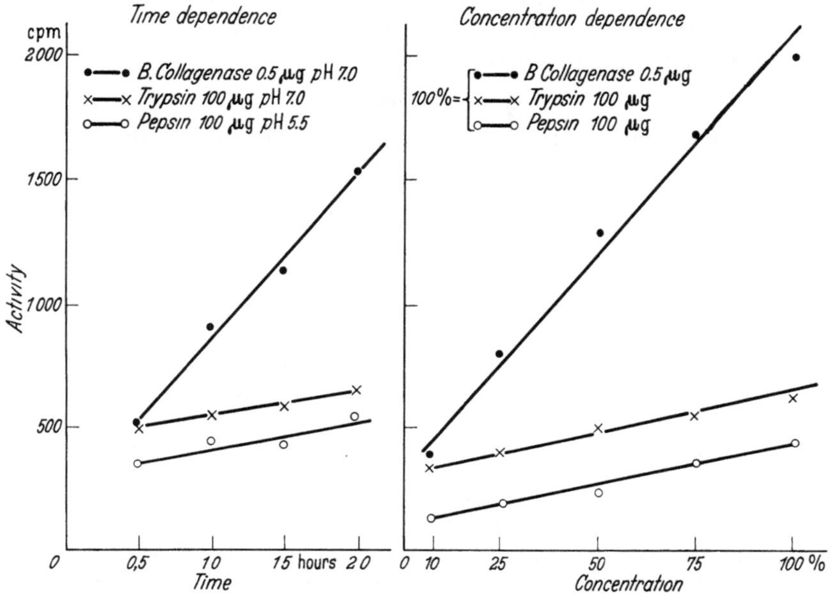

Fig. 3. Concentration and time dependence activity of bacterial collagenase (purified), trypsin (Calbiochem) and pepsin (Calbiochem) on ^{14}C collagen fibers (S.A. 20.500 cpm/mg.). Results expressed in cpm liberated above blank

which are the most easily extractable, the less organized. This form of collagen increases in tissues having rapid degradation processes. This has been inferred from studies in the metamorphosing tail of the tadpole (Lapière and Gross, 1963) in the uterus (Woessner and Brewer, 1963) and in the carrageenan granuloma (Jackson, 1957). In these resorbing tissues (Weber, 1957; Woessner and Brewer, 1963) and in resorbing bone (Vaes, 1964) there is also an increased amount of acid cathepsins. These enzymes could be involved in completing the breakdown of collagen after it is phagocytised by specialised cells. Electromicrograph pictures of histiocytes containing considerable amounts of fragmented fibrils have been shown to occur in the resorbing tail of the tadpole (Usuku and Gross, 1965). Pictures having comparable meaning have been published by Hancox and Boothroyd (1963) for the osteoclasts of resorbing bone.

On the basis of these different findings one might suggest that collagen degradation in soft and calcified tissues is a two step mechanism. In the first the collagen matrix would be disorganized by an extracellular enzyme having collagenase activity. Further activity of intracellular enzymes would complete the breakdown to liberate free and peptide bound collagen aminoacids.

Conclusion and summary

Although much work is still needed before the metabolism of the bone matrix can be understood, preliminary experiments indicate a close similarity with the metabolism of the collagen in soft connective tissues. Synthesis, organization or enzymatic breakdown are to a considerable extent analogous.

Fractionation studies of soft and calcified tissues separate the collagen in fractions of different organization according to their age. These fractions seem to be related one to the other in a process of maturation quite similar in both tissues.

Enzymatic breakdown of the collagen in skin and bone is demonstratable in tissue culture. There exists identical difficulty in isolating a collagenolytic enzyme from living soft and calcified connective tissues.

Acknowledgements

This work has been supported in part by Grant AM 07250 of the National Institute of Arthritis and Metabolism of the U.S. Public Health Service.

The author wishes to acknowledge the many valuable discussions with DRS. JEROME GROSS and MARVIN TANZER and the criticism of the manuscript by the latter.

References

BÉLANGER, L. F., J. ROBICHON, B. B. MIGICOVSKY, D. H. COPP, and J. VINCENT: Resorption without osteoclasts (osteolysis). In Mechanisms of Hard Tissue Destruction. SOGNNAES, R. J. (ed.) Washington: Amer. Ass. Advanc. Sci. 1963, p. 531.

CURREY, J. D.: Three analogies to explain the mechanical properties of bone. Biorheol. **2**, 1 (1964).

EASTOE, J. E.: The organic matrix of bone. In The Biochemistry and Physiology of Bone. BOURNE, G. H. (ed.). New York: Academic Press 1956, p. 81.

FLANAGAN, B., and G. NICHOLS: Direct measurements of human bone metabolism in normal and hyperparathyroid subjects. Clin. Res. **12**, 266 (1964).

GAILLARD, P. J.: Parathyroid gland and bone *in vitro*. Develop. Biol. **1**, 152 (1959).

GLIMCHER, M. J.: Molecular biology of mineralized tissues with particular reference to bone. Rev. mod. Phys. **31**, 359 (1959).

— The organization of collagen in bone. In Symposium international sur la biochimie et la physiologie du tissu conjonctif. DELAUNAY, A. (ed.). (In press.)

—, A. J. HODGE, and F. O. SCHMITT: Macromolecular aggregation states in relation to mineralization: the collagen hydroxyapatite system as studied *in vitro*. Proc. nat. Acad. Sci. **43**, 860 (1957).

—, and S. M. KRANE: Studies of the interaction of collagen and phosphate. I. The nature of inorganic orthophosphate binding. In Radioisotopes and Bone. LACROIX, P., and A. M. BUDY (eds.). Oxford: Blackwell Scientific Publications 196x2, p. 393.

GOLDHABER, P.: The effect of hyperoxia on Bone Resorption in Tissue Culture. A. M. A. Arch. Path. **66**, 635 (1958).

GREEN, N. M., and D. A. LOWTHER: Formation of collagen hydroxyproline *in vitro*. Biochem. J. **71**, 55 (1959).

GROSS, J.: Studies on the formation of collagen. I. Properties and fractionation of neutral salt extracts of normal guinea pigs connective tissue. J. exp. Med. **107**, 247 (1958 a).

— Studies on the formation of collagen. II. The influence of growth rate on neutral salt extracts of guinea pigs dermis. J. exp. Med. **107**, 265 (1958 b).

— Studies on the formation of collagen. III. Time-dependent solubility changes of collagen *in vitro*. J. exp. Med. **108**, 215 (1958 c).

— On the significance of the soluble collagens. In Connective Tissue, Thrombosis and Atherosclerosis. PAGE, I. H. (ed.). New York: Academic Press 1959, p. 77.

— An intermolecular defect of collagen in experimental lathyrism. Biochim. biophys. Acta **71**, 250 (1963 a).

— Comparative biochemistry of collagen. In Comparative Biochemistry, A Comprehensive Treatise. FLORKIN, M., and H. S. MASON (eds.). New York: Academic Press 1963 b, p. 307.

—, and CH. M. LAPIERE: Collagenolytic activity in amphibian tissues: A tissue culture assay. Proc. nat. Acad. Sci. **48**, 1014 (1962).

HANCOX, N. M., and B. BOOTHROYD: Structure-function relationships in the osteoclast. In Mechanisms of Hard Tissue Destruction. SOGNNAES, R. J. (ed.). Washington: Amer. Ass. Advanc. Sci. 1963, p. 497.

HARKNESS, R. D.: Biological functions of collagen. Biol. Rev. **36**, 399 (1961).
—, A. M. MARKO, H. M. MUIR, and A. NEUBERGER: The metabolism of collagen and other proteins of the skin of rabbits. Biochem. J. **56**, 558 (1954).
HAY, E. D., and J. P. REVEL: Autoradiographic studies of the origin of the basement lamella in *Amblyostoma*. Develop. Biol. **7**, 152 (1963).
HERMAN, H., et L. RICHELLE: Le calcium échangeable de la substance minérale de l'os étudiée à l'aide du Ca-45. VII. Activité comparée de fractions d'os total de densité différente. Bull. Soc. Chim. Biol. **43**, 273 (1961).
JACKSON, D. S.: Connective tissue growth stimulated by carrageenin. I. The formation and removal of collagen. Biochem. J. **65**, 277 (1957).
—, and J. P. BENTLEY: On the nature of the extractable collagens. J. biophys. biochem. Cytol. **7**, 37 (1960).
JACKSON, S. F.: The structure of developing bone in the embryonic fowl. Proc. roy. Soc. B **146**, 270 (1957).
JOWSEY, J., R. E. ROWLAND, J. H. MARSHALL, and F. C. MCLEAN: The effect of parathyroidectomy on haversian remodeling of bone. Endocrinology **63**, 903 (1958).
KRANE, S. M., and M. J. GLIMCHER: Studies of the interaction of collagen and phosphate. II. Nucleotidase activity and binding of nucleotide phosphorus. In Radioisotopes and Bone. LACROIX, P., and A. M. BUDY (eds.). Oxford: Blackwell Scientific Publications 1962, p. 419.
LAPIÈRE, CH. M., A. BRUSCHI, M. L. TANZER, and J. GROSS: Metabolic behaviour of the collagen in steady state and remodelling tissues. In Calcified Tissues. RICHELLE, L. J., et M. J. DALLEMAGNE (eds.). Liège: Collection des colloques de l'Université de Liège 1965, p. 275.
—, and J. GROSS: Animal collagenase and collagen metabolism. In Mechanisms of Hard Tissue Destruction. SOGNNAES, R. J. (ed.). Washington: Amer. Ass. Advanc. Sci. 1963, p. 663.
—, C. ONKELINX, and L. J. RICHELLE: Collagen metabolism in skin and bone. In Symposium international sur la biochimie et la physiologie du tissu conjonctif. DELAUNAY, A. (ed.). (In press.)
LEVENE, CH. I., and J. GROSS: Alteration in state of molecular aggregation of collagen induced in chick embryos by β-aminopropionitrile (Lathyrus factor). J. exp. Med. **110**, 771 (1959).
MARSHALL, J. H., R. E. ROWLAND, and J. JOWSEY: Microscopic metabolism of calcium in bone. II. Quantitative autoradiography. Radiat. Res. **10**, 213 (1959).
MARTIN, R. G., J. GROSS, K. A. PIEZ, and M. S. LEWIS: On the intramolecular cross linking of collagen in lathyritics rats. Biochim. biophys. Acta **53**, 599 (1961).
MCLEAN, F., and R. E. ROWLAND: Internal remodeling of compact bone. In Mechanisms of Hard Tissue Destruction. SOGNNAES, R. J. (ed.). Washington: Amer. Ass. Advanc. Sci. 1963, p. 371.
—, and M. R. URIST: An introduction to the physiology of skeletal tissue. In Bone. Chicago: The University of Chicago Press 1961.
NAGAI, Y., CH. M. LAPIERE, and J. GROSS: Isolation and partial characterization of an animal collagenolytic enzyme. Fed. Proc. **22**, 648 (1963).
— — — Purification and characterization of amphibian collagenolytic enzyme. Abstract 6th. International Congress of Biochemistry, N. Y. 1964.
NEUBERGER, A., and H. G. B. SLACK: The metabolism of collagen from liver, bone, skin and tendon in the normal rat. Biochem. J. **53**, 47 (1953).
OREKHOVITCH, V. N., V. O. CHPIKITER, V. I. MAZOUROV, et O. V. KOUNINA: Procollagènes. Classification, métabolisme, action des protéinases. Bull. Soc. Chim. biol. **42**, 505 (1960).
PIEZ, K. A., M. S. LEWIS, G. R. MARTIN, and J. GROSS: Subunits of the collagen molecule. Biochim. biophys. Acta **53**, 596 (1961).
RICHELLE, L. J.: One possible solution to the problem of the biochemistry of bone mineral. Clin. Orthop. **33**, 211 (1964).
—, and F. BRONNER: The calcium exchange reaction of bone *in vitro*. Effect of parathyroid extract. Biochem. Pharmacol. **12**, 647 (1963).
—, C. ONKELINX, and J. P. AUBERT: Mineral metabolism in the rat. This Book 1965, p. 123.

ROBINSON, R. A.: Chemical analysis and electronmicroscopy of bone. In Bone as a Tissue. RODAHL, K., J. T. NICHOLSON, and E. M. BROWN (eds.). New York: Mac Graw Hill 1960, p. 186.
SCOTT, B. L., and M. J. GLIMCHER: Intracellular pathway and extrusion of collagen in the osteoblasts of developing bone. J. appl. Phys. **34**, 2524 (1963).
SMITH, J. W.: Age changes in the organic fraction of bone. J. Bone Jt Surg. **45 B**, 761 (1963).
STERN, B. D., G. L. MECHANIC, M. J. GLIMCHER, and P. GOLDHABER: The resorption of bone collagen in tissue culture. Biochem. biophys. Res. Commun. **13**, 137 (1963).
TANZER, M. L., and J. GROSS: Collagen metabolism in the normal and lathyritic chick. J. exp. Med. **119**, 275 (1964).
—, and R. D. HUNT: Experimental lathyrism. An autoradiographic study. J. Cell Biol. **22**, 623 (1964).
USUKU, G., and J. GROSS: Morphologic studies of connective tissue resorption in the tailfin of metamorphosing bullfrog tadpole. Develop. Biol. **11**, 352 (1965).
VAES, G.: Acid hydrolases and lysosomes in bone cells. Abstract 1st Meeting Federation European Biochemical Societies. London 1964, p. 83.
WALKER, D. G., CH. M. LAPIERE, and J. GROSS: A collagenolytic factor in rat bone promoted by parathyroid extract. Biochem. biophys. Res. Commun. **15**, 397 (1964).
WEBER, R.: On the biological function of cathepsins in tail tissue of Xenopus larvae. Experientia **13**, 153 (1957).
WOESSNER, J. F., and T. H. BREWER: Formation and breakdown of collagen and elastin in the human uterus during pregnancy and postpartum involution. Biochem. J. **89**, 75 (1963).
WOODS, J. F., and G. NICHOLS: Collagenolytic activity in mammalian bone. Science **142**. 386 (1963).
— — The intracellular location of bone "collagenase". Fed. Proc. **23**, 550 (1964).

The Origin of Bone Cells in Endochondral Ossification

MARIJKE E. HOLTROP

Laboratorium voor Celbiologie en Histologie, Rijksuniversiteit, Leiden, Nederland

In developing long bone the area of endochondral ossification consists of a variety of tissues in which various developmental processes take place: cartilage cells arrange themselves into cell columns; hypertrophic cartilage cells are formed; all kinds of bone cells appear, osteoblasts, osteocytes and osteoclasts; the adjacent connective tissue and bloodvessels also take an active part in the process by penetrating and invading the developing cartilage tissue.

In this rather complex system it is very difficult to determine which cells actually differentiate into bone cells. The possibility to make an experimental approach to this problem came within reach following some transplantation experiments with fragments of ribs from young mice. It was found that an intramuscular transplant of a well defined part of the developing area of a rib (*viz.* a piece of cartilage including the zone of the cell columns), progressed to complete endochondral ossification within two weeks of transplantation (Fig. 1). First a zone of hypertrophic cartilage cells was formed and a layer of bone was deposited around this zone. Connective tissue and bloodvessels then penetrated the bony border from the outside, invaded the hypertrophic cartilage cells and finally bone was deposited alongside the remnants of the cartilage matrix. So, following the intramuscular grafting of pure cartilage together with its adhering perichondrium, osteoblasts, osteocytes and osteoclasts appeared after some time.

So with this knowledge the question can be asked again — what is the origin of the bone cells?

For the special circumstances outlined above we can put the question somewhat differently. Did the newly formed bone cells originate from the host (connective tissue and/or muscle), or could they be derived from the donor tissue (cartilage and/or perichondrium)?

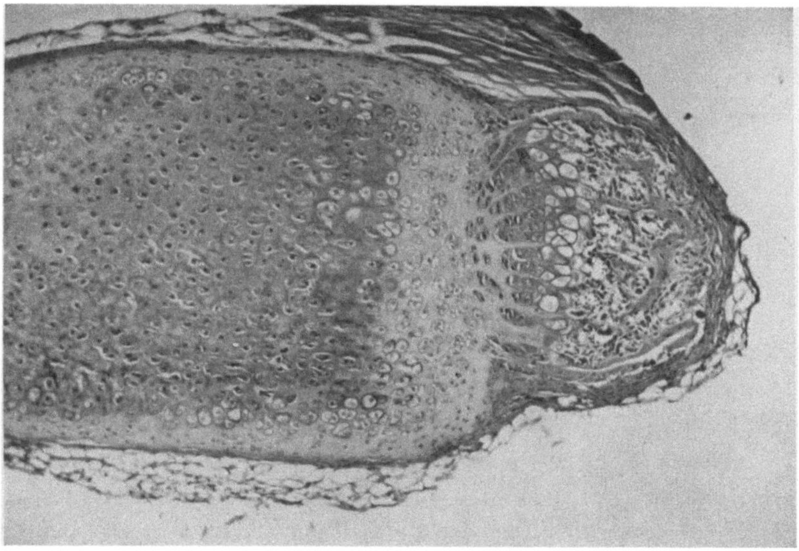

Fig. 1. Endochondral ossification observed within two weeks after intramuscular homotransplantation of a fragment of mouse ribcartilage including the zone of cell columns

To solve this problem it is necessary to distinguish donor cells and host cells. This can be achieved most completely by applying the *in vitro* cultivation technique. In this way the host is eliminated totally and every development occurring in the cultivated donor tissue must certainly be brought about by the donor cells.

Thus, fragments of ribcartilage similar to those used in the grafts, derived from 18-day-old mouse embryos, were cultivated on a coagulum according to a modified watchglass technique. After 17 days of cultivation hypertrophic cartilage cells were formed and alongside this zone a border of bone was deposited (Fig. 2). From these experiments it is obvious that the donor tissue has indeed the potency to form bone. However, this result does not prove that in *grafts* the donor tissue also produces bone. In order to get some information on this point donor cells were made distinguishable from host cells by labelling the donor tissue with ^{3}H-thymidine prior to transplantation; in this way the fate of the donor cells during their presence in the host could be determined.

Under these circumstances, we have to take into account the possibility that a donor cell could release its label when dying, and a host cell could then pick up the label. In such event a considerable dilution of the label would, however, take place. For this reason only heavily labelled cells were considered to be derived from the graft.

Donor mice were injected with ^{3}H-thymidine and fragments of ribcartilage including the zone of cell columns were excised and transplanted according to the usual technique. Autoradiographs of the donor tissue before transplantation showed that tritiated thymidine was readily taken up, predominantly by cells in the zone of cell columns. Twelve days after transplantation the grafts showed endochondral

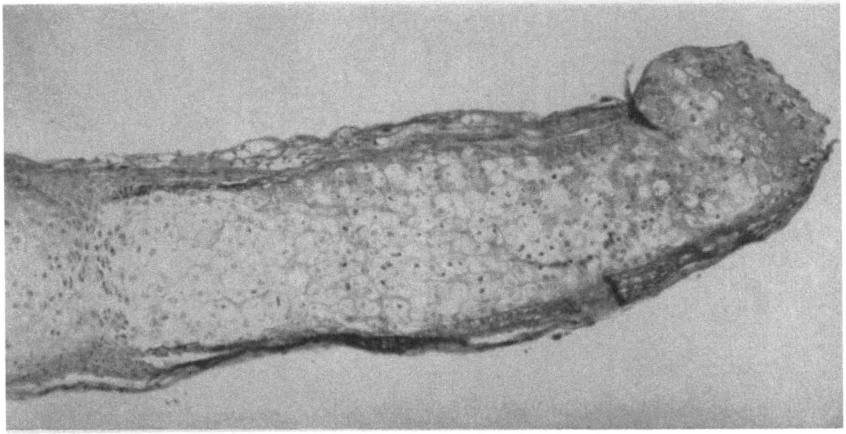

Fig. 2. Ribcartilage including the zone of cell columns derived from a 18-day-old mouse embryo as observed after 17 days of cultivation on a coagulum. Hypertrophic cartilage is formed and bone is deposited alongside

ossification in the manner already described. Autoradiographs showed that hardly any label was left in the zone of the cell columns. But some heavily labelled osteoblasts, and also some heavily labelled osteocytes were found.

This experiment shows, therefore, that not only in tissue culture, but also in grafts, the donor tissue is capable of forming bone.

The question now arises as to whether the bone cells originate from the perichondrium or from the cartilage, or from both.

It would seem reasonable that they had originated from the perichondrium as in fact some perichondrium cells were labelled before transplantation. However, some further observations led us to assume that *cartilage cells* might also be precursors of bone cells.

Information concerning this supposition was obtained by repeating the transplantation experiments, but this time using grafts of ribfragments of cartilage without any perichondrium at all. Cutting off the perichondrium of mouse ribs proved difficult as they were too small to handle easily. It was found that the ribs of rats could be completely parted from the perichondrium while enough cartilage remained for transplantation. It was still doubtful how these 'maltreated' fragments would behave after transplantation but surprisingly enough, two weeks after transplantation of such fragments endochondral ossification developed in exactly the same way as the grafts with adhering perichondrium had done.

In order to determine what happened to the cartilage cells during their presence in the host, in the next experiment, the donor tissue was labelled with ^{3}H-thymidine. Ribfragments including the zone of cell columns but deprived of perichondrium, were transplanted according to the usual technique. Autoradiographs of the fragments before transplantation showed that the label was taken up by some cells of the zone

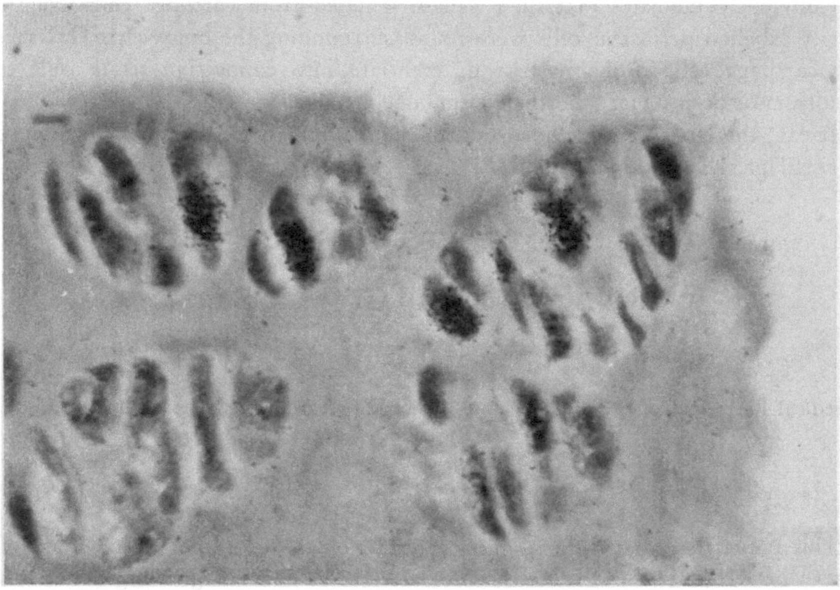

Fig. 3. Cell columns in rat ribcartilage deprived of the perichondrium and labelled with ^{3}H-thymidine

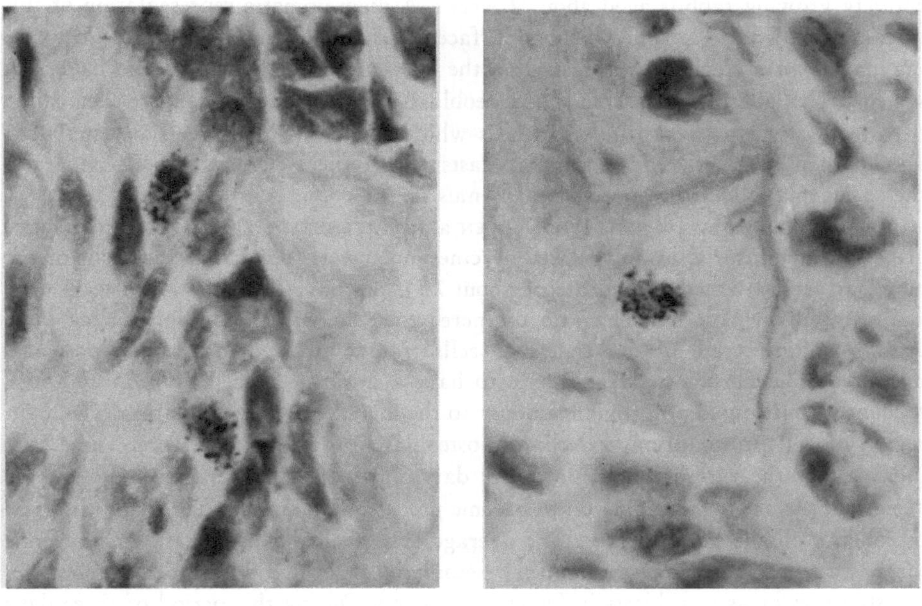

Fig. 4. A labelled transplant deprived of perichondrium, observed two weeks after grafting. The original transplant was fully comparable with the situation given in Fig. 3. In the graft labelled osteoblasts and osteocytes can be seen

of cell columns and most important no perichondrium appeared to have been left on the fragments at all (Fig. 3).

Two weeks after transplantation of such cartilaginous fragments, the grafts were taken out of the host and autoradiographs were prepared. Examination of the ossified part of the grafts revealed heavily labelled osteoblasts and osteocytes (Fig. 4). This obviously indicates that these cells originated from cartilage cells. Moreover, heavily labelled periosteal cells were found surrounding the bony cap. This suggests that cartilage cells probably first differentiate into connective tissue cells (perichondrium or periosteum) and then form bone afterwards.

It can, therefore, be concluded that to the list of possible precursors of bone cells, the cartilage cell should be added.

RNA Synthesis in Growing Bone

M. Owen

Medical Research Council, Bone-Seeking Isotopes Research Unit, The Churchill Hospital, Oxford, England

Introduction

This paper describes the preliminary results of an autoradiographic study of the pattern of RNA synthesis in cells which are associated with growing bone surfaces. The system studied is the periosteal surface of the shaft of the femur of young actively growing rabbits aged about 2 weeks. A diagrammatic representation of this surface is shown in Fig. 1 a. The bone surface has characteristic loops typical of forming haversian systems. Osteoblasts line the surface of the bone and the haversian systems. The layer of cells behind the osteoblasts on the bone surface have been called preosteoblasts, a term also given to cells which are within the haversian canals but not on their surfaces. A layer of fibroblasts with typical elongated nuclei separates the osteogenic cellular layer from nearby muscle.

In previous work, (Owen, 1963; Owen and Macpherson, 1963) the rate of bone growth was measured using tritiated glycine and it was found that the front of the bone surface advanced at the rate of about 70 μ per day. The situation after 4 days is illustrated in Fig. 1 b. The rate of increase of the cell population during bone growth and the rate of movement of cells from one stage to another was also measured. The fibroblasts were shown to have a low rate of cell division and consequently contributed a negligible amount to the increase in cell population. The main region of cell proliferation was the pre-osteoblasts on the bone surface. These cells increased at the rate of about 33% per day, and spent on average 3 days on the periosteal surface before going on to become preosteoblasts within haversian canals or osteoblasts on the bone surface. The average time spent by osteoblasts on the bone surface was also three days before they became incorporated within the bone matrix as osteocytes or as osteoblasts in haversian systems. During this period of three days it was also shown that the osteoblasts produced on average between two and three times their own volume of bone matrix.

We were interested to learn something about the pattern of RNA synthesis in this system consisting as it does of a fairly uniform population of highly differentiated cells, the osteoblasts, engaged in active protein synthesis, predominantly collagen, (each cell producing on average just less than its own volume of matrix per day) and their precursors, the preosteoblasts, which are presumably a mixed population of cells in different stages of differentiation and cell division.

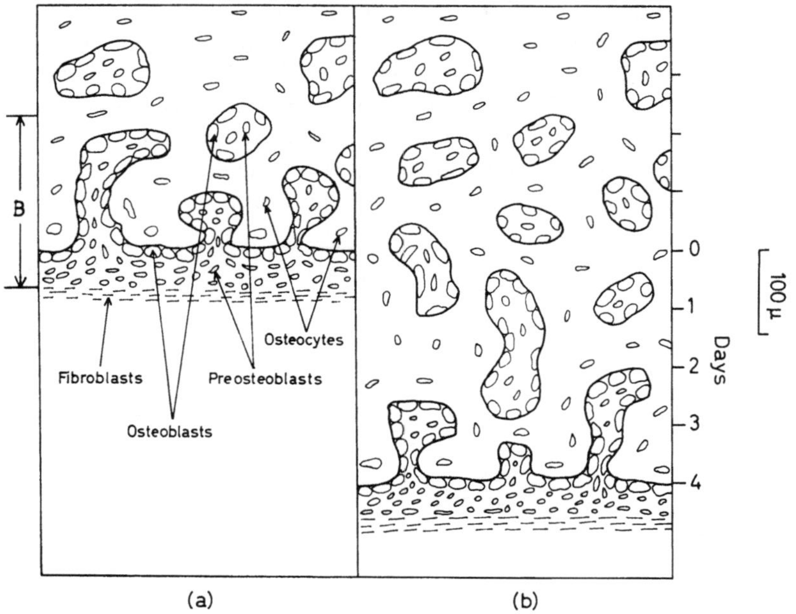

Fig. 1. Diagrammatic representation of the periosteal surface of the shaft of the femur of a two-week old rabbit illustrating (a) the various layers of cells on the bone surface and (b) bone growth over a period of 4 days

Materials and methods

Suckling rabbits between one and two weeks of age were chosen according to weight, 110 to 130 grams. Tritiated uridine, (Uridine-5-T, specific activity 24.4 c/mM) obtained from The Radiochemical Centre, Amersham was used as an RNA precursor. An intraperitoneal injection of uridine, 5 μc/gram, was given and the rabbits killed at intervals varying from 15 mins. to 4 days after injection. Autoradiographs were prepared as previously described (Owen, 1963). Exposure times were 10 days. In some cases a second injection of about one hundred fold non-radioactive uridine was given 1 hour after the initial injection of the radioactive material, in order to determine the effect of this on the pattern of uptake with time.

Counts were made of the number of grains per nucleus and per cytoplasm for preosteoblasts and osteoblasts on the bone surface and in haversian canals within a band of bone of width B on the periosteal surface, Fig. 1 a. The width of B varied according to the time interval at which the animal was killed. Up to 8 hours after injection B was 200 μ wide. At the later time intervals the width of B was increased to take account of bone growth, see Fig. 1 b. Cells *on* the bone surface, i. e. within the loops out to the first layer of fibroblasts, were counted separately to those within the haversian canals. Counts were corrected for background which was less than 1.0 grain per cell.

Results

There was radioactive labelling generally throughout all osteoblasts and preosteoblasts. Labelling of fibroblasts was not above background in the autoradiographs studied. The results for grains per nucleus and grains per cytoplasm are shown for osteoblasts in Fig. 2 and for preosteoblasts in Fig. 3. The results for the osteoblasts, Fig. 2, show that there is an initial rapid appearance of labelled RNA in the nucleus which reaches a maximum between one and two hours after injection and then remains approximately constant at this level up to 4 days. The appearance of labelled RNA in the cytoplasm with time occurs more slowly and reaches a maximum at about 24 hours and thereafter there appears to be a slight fall off by 3 and 4 days after injection. Over the time period studied there was no detectable difference in the results for osteoblasts on the surface or in haversian canals.

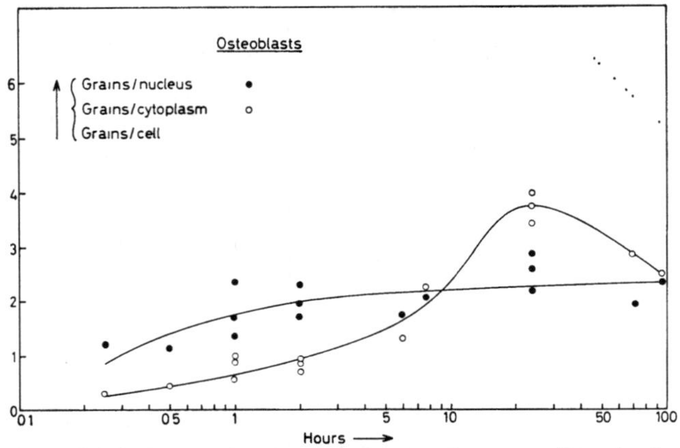

Fig. 2. Uptake of ^{3}H-Uridine with time after injection as measured on autoradiographs, in osteoblasts on the periosteal surface of the shaft of a two-week old rabbit femur

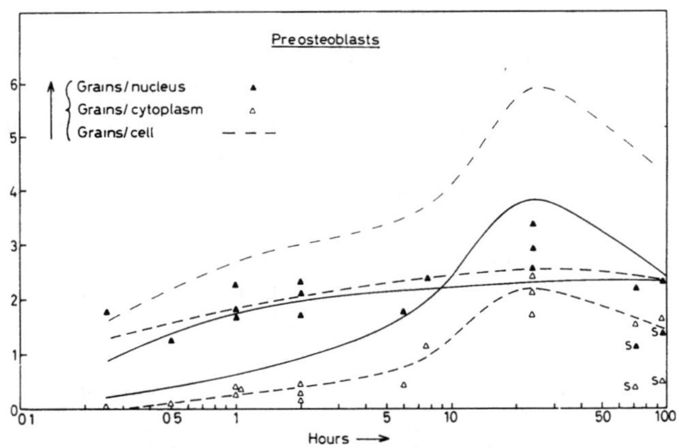

Fig. 3. Uptake of ^{3}H-Uridine with time after injection as measured on autoradiographs, in preosteoblasts on the periosteal surface of the shaft of a two-week old rabbit femur. The dashed curves are for the preosteoblasts. The curves for the osteoblasts from Fig. 2 are also shown for comparison

The results for the preosteoblasts, Fig. 3, show a very similar pattern. For comparison the curves for the osteoblasts from Fig. 2 have been included in Fig. 3. The curves for the grains per nucleus for both the osteoblasts and the preosteoblasts are not significantly different. The curves for the grains per cytoplasm have a similar shape but the results for the preosteoblasts are considerably below those of the osteoblasts. In the case of the preosteoblasts the results for the cells on the surface were lower than those in the haversian canals at the two longest time intervals, 3 and 4 days. In Fig. 3 the results for the cells on the surface are designated by S, the other points are for the cells in haversian canals. This probably reflects some cell division which takes place mainly in the cells on the periosteal surface.

An injection of non-radioactive uridine one hour after radioactive uridine had no detectable effect on the curves for RNA in the nucleus or cytoplasm of either cell types.

Discussion

A detailed discussion of these results is not possible in the space allotted and a few points only will be made. The present results are in agreement with previous reports concerning the study of RNA synthesis in the cells of bone in so far as a comparison can be made (BURCHARD *et al.*, 1959; YOUNG, 1963). Previous autoradiographic studies similar to the present one, however, have been made on other cell types mostly in vitro. The type of experiment performed has usually involved incubation of the cells for a short period in medium containing the radioactive precursor followed by a period in non-radioactive medium. Experiments have been carried out mostly on rapidly dividing populations (Hela cells and fibroblasts) though some experiments on a non-multiplying cell (macrophages) have also been made (WATTS and HARRIS, 1959; HARRIS, 1959; FEINENDEGEN *et al.*, 1960; PERRY, 1960). In spite of the difference in experimental design it is significant that the 'in vitro' results for different systems and our 'in vivo' results for osteoblasts and preosteoblasts show the same common features. The results from both types of experiments show that there is an initial rapid labelling of RNA in the nucleus and a time lag before radioactivity is detected in the cytoplasm. It is generally accepted that synthesis of most RNA takes place in the nucleus and that cytoplasmic RNA is derived from this, although there is still some controversy on this issue (PRESCOTT, 1964).

It is of interest to determine the amount of RNA turnover which occurs in cells in conjunction with protein synthesis, where turnover of RNA is defined as a balanced process of synthesis and degradation of RNA. It ought to be possible to make a direct measurement of turnover in RNA using a radioactively labelled precursor as in the present experiment, by determining the extent to which the radioactive label is retained in the RNA. Some of the conditions in the present experiment are favourable for such a measurement, for example we can be fairly certain in the case of the osteoblasts that we are looking at the same population of cells over the period of 4 days and that there has been a negligible amount of cell division in these cells. From the upper curve in Fig. 2 it can be seen that about 25% of the labelled RNA turns over in 3 days. However this figure is likely to be a lower limit since reutilization of degradation products, which is known to occur, will mask the effect of turnover.

In fact interpretation of experiments of the present kind are very difficult due mainly to 'pool effects' and reutilization phenomena, (WATTS and HARRIS, 1959; WATTS, 1964 a; WATTS, 1964 b). There is good evidence, mainly from tissue culture studies, to show that RNA precursors, such as labelled nucleosides, are first rapidly incorporated into intracellular pools of intermediate-sized molecules. RNA synthesis then proceeds using these labelled intermediates and, depending upon the size of a particular intracellular pool, the labelling of RNA may continue for some time after a pulse of labelled nucleoside has been given. This is referred to as the 'pool effect'. Dilution of these pools by non-radioactive precursors is not always easily obtained and as shown in the present experiment a second injection one hour later of non-radioactive Uridine one hundred fold, failed to produce any detectable effect in the pattern of RNA synthesis and presumably in the dilution of the pool of labelled intermediates. It is clear that the cells in the system being studied show a large pool effect since labelling of RNA does not reach a maximum until 24 hours after injection.

References

Burchard, J., R. Fontaine et P. Mandel: Métabolisme des acides ribonucléiques de l'os de lapin et de rat in vivo. C. R. Soc. Biol. **153**, 334 (1959).
Feinendegen, L. E., V. P. Bond, W. W. Shreeve, and R. B. Painter: RNA and DNA metabolism in human tissue culture cells studied with tritiated cytidine. Exp. Cell Res. **19**, 443 (1960).
Harris, H.: Turnover of nuclear and cytoplasmic ribonucleic acid in two types of animal cell, with some further observations on the nucleolus. Biochem. J. **73**, 362 (1959).
Owen, M.: Cell population kinetics of an osteogenic tissue I. J. Cell Biol. **19**, 19 (1963).
—, and S. MacPherson: Cell population kinetics of an osteogenic tissue II. J. Cell Biol. **19**, 33 (1963).
Perry, R. P.: On the nucleolar and nuclear dependence of cytoplasmic RNA synthesis in Hela cells. Exp. Cell Res. **20**, 216 (1960).
Prescott, D. M.: Cellular sites of RNA synthesis. In Progress in Nucleic Acid Research and Molecular Biology. Davidson and Cohn (eds.). New York: Academic Press 1964, p. 33.
Watts, J. W.: Turnover of nucleic acids in a multiplying animal cell. Biochem. J. **93**, 297 (1964 a).
— Turnover of nucleic acids in a multiplying animal cell. Biochem. J. **93**, 306 (1964 b).
—, and H. Harris: Turnover of nucleic acids in a non-multiplying animal cell. Biochem. J. **72**, 147 (1959).
Young, R. W.: Nucleic acids, protein synthesis and bone. Clin. Orthop. **26**, 147 (1963).

Histochemical Studies of Chondrocyte Function in the Cartilage of the Mandibular Condyle of the Rat

J. S. Greenspan, H. J. J. Blackwood

Royal Dental Hospital of London School of Dental Surgery, London, England

Introduction

The cartilage of the mandibular condyle has not been used extensively as a site at which to investigate the processes of cell differentiation, maturation and endochondral ossification. The investigation reported here is part of a more comprehensive study of the cellular dynamics, cytochemistry and ultrastructure of this tissue. The aim of this study is to extend our knowledge of the normal and pathological behaviour of the mandibular condyle and of the general biological processes with which its cells are concerned.

The cartilage can be divided into three distinct cell zones, namely the articular, proliferative and hypertrophic zones. The articular zone provides an articular covering for the cartilage. The proliferative zone is concerned with growth and chondrogenesis, and the hypertrophic zone shows the characteristics changes of cell hypertrophy and matrix production which precede ossification in cartilage. This latter zone can be further divided into the premineralised and mineralised zones.

Material and methods

The mandibular condylar cartilages were removed from 48 male and female Wistar rats of varying ages (19 days insemination age 1, 4, 8, 12, 14, 16 and 18 days post-partum). Undemineralised cryostat sections of the cartilages were subjected to a range of functional and analytical histochemical procedures including techniques for mitochondrial oxidative enzymes, lysosomal and non-lysosomal hydrolytic enzymes, proteins, carbohydrates and lipids. The position of the mineralising front was determined microradiographically and confirmed by the von Kossa method.

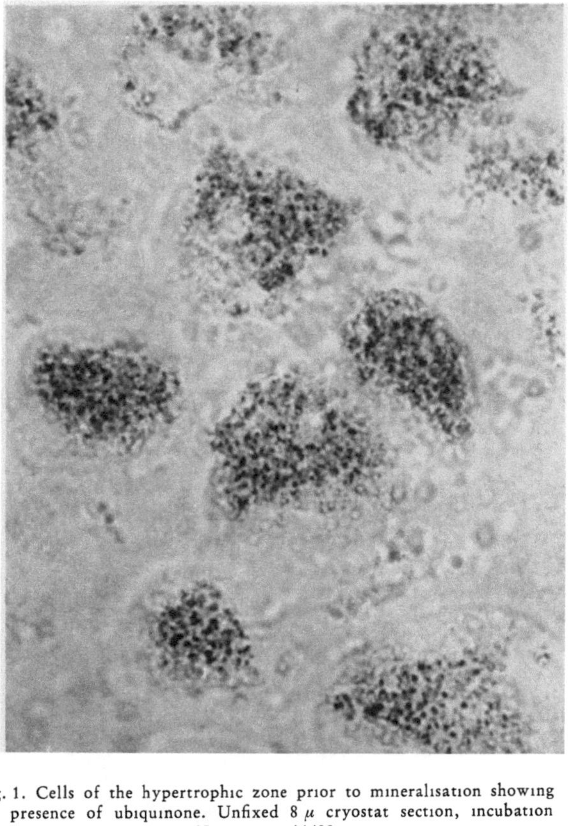

Fig. 1. Cells of the hypertrophic zone prior to mineralisation showing the presence of ubiquinone. Unfixed 8 μ cryostat section, incubation 15 minutes. ×400

Observations

Mitochondrial enzyme activity was low in the proliferative zone but increased slightly in the adjacent area of the hypertrophic zone and in the articular zone. Activity increased markedly with chondrocyte maturation and reached maximum levels in the hypertrophic zone several cells distant from the mineralising front (Fig. 1) Within the mineralising zone activity decreased. The correlation of the levels of these enzymes with matrix production as evidenced by their increasing activity in the cells of the hypertrophic zone and their decreased activity in the mineralising zone supports the view that the primary function of these cells is probably matrix production.

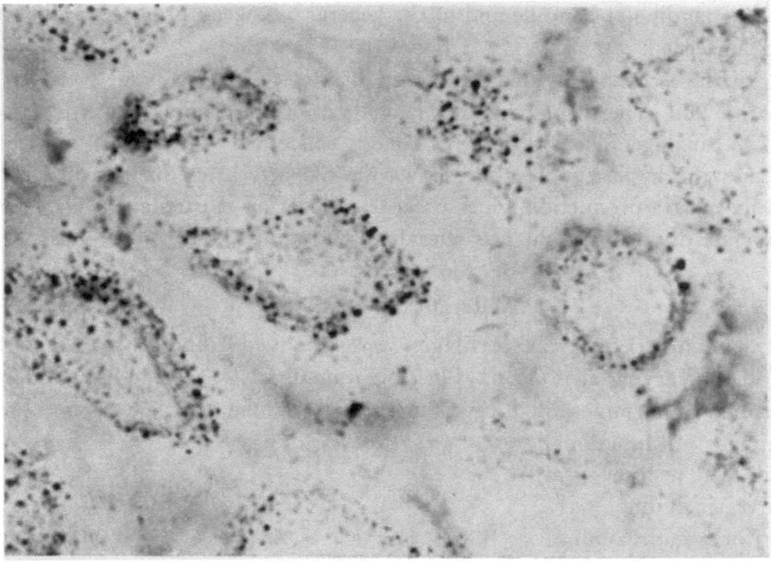

Fig. 2. Cells within the mineralising zone of the cartilage showing granular staining for acid phosphatase. Unfixed 8 μ cryostat section, AS.TR phosphate, fast dark blue R salt, pH 5.5, incubation time 15 minutes. ×400

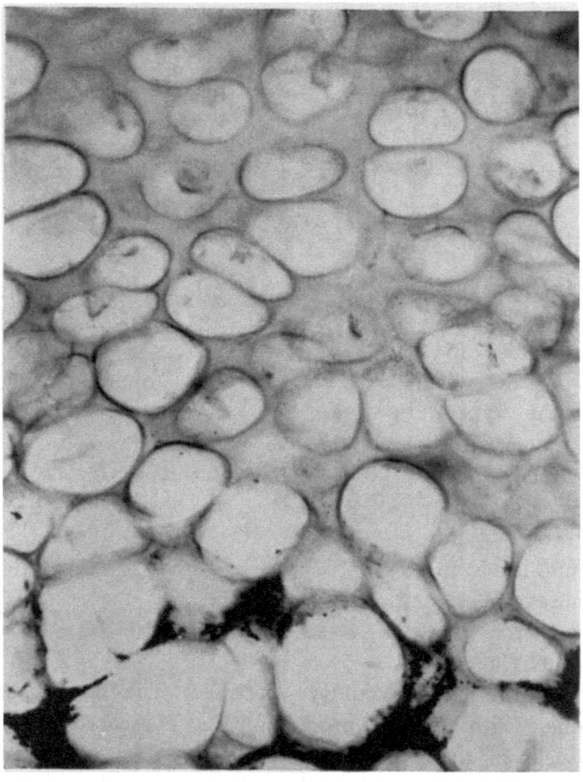

Fig. 3. von Kossa reaction showing the level of mineralisation in the hypertrophic zone of the cartilage. Unfixed 8 μ cryostat section. ×160

Acid phosphatase appeared in increasing amounts in the maturing chondrocytes of the hypertrophic zone up to the point of commencing mineralisation. Surviving chondrocytes in the mineralising cartilage showed a lower level of activity (Fig. 2).

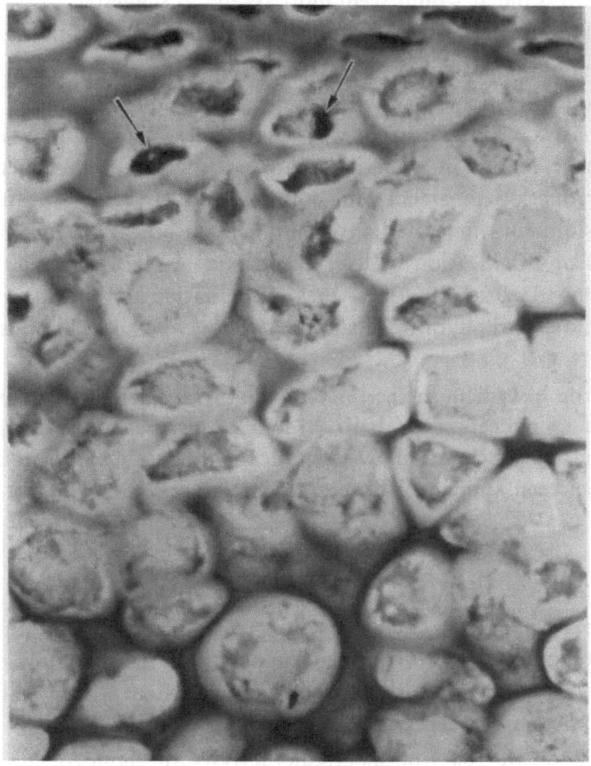

Fig. 4. Serial section to Fig. 3 showing a similar field stained by the PAS procedure. Glycogen (arrow) is present in the chondrocytes but has disappeared prior to mineralisation. 8 μ cryostat section post-fixed in 90% alcohol/formalin. ×160

Non-specific esterase activity was present in the same distribution as acid phosphatase and showed as small positive granules in the chondrocyte cytoplasm. Similar granules were seen in the acid phosphatase preparations. These observations indicate the presence of lysosomes in the chondrocytes which would be in accord with recent views on the mechanism of cartilage resorbtion (Fell, 1964; Sledge and Dingle, 1965). On the other hand the chondrocytes in the mineralising zone are probably dying cells so it is possible that the acid hydrolase positive bodies could represent autophagic vacuoles (de Duve, 1963).

Alkaline phosphatase appeared in mature chondrocytes just prior to mineralisation and was stronger in chondrocytes within the mineralising zone. The highest levels of alkaline phosphatase were seen in osteoblasts and in periosteal cells of the condylar process. These findings confirm for this tissue the well documented association of alkaline phosphatase with cells involved in calcification (see Cabrini, 1961 for review).

Glycogen appeared in increasing amounts in maturing chondrocytes and was at a maximum in cells of the hypertrophic zone at some distance from the mineralising front, but disappeared from these cells before mineralisation actually commenced (Fig. 3 and 4). This suggests that glycogen is probably not directly involved in the calcification process but it would seem more likely, as suggested by Weatherall *et al.* (1964), that it is concerned with mucopolysaccharide synthesis and matrix production.

Weak sudanophilia was present in the cartilage matrix of the hypertrophic zone prior to its mineralisation but somewhat stronger sudan staining occurred in the mineralising matrix. The reaction was completely abolished, however, by prior extraction of the sections in a methanol/alcohol mixture. The latter procedure also resulted in a reduction in alcian blue staining at these sites. The substance or substances responsible for these findings could well be the same as that described by Irving at sites of calcification in long bones and in teeth (Irving, 1959; Wuthier and Irving, 1964; Irving, 1965). A likely explanation for these staining reactions is that a lipid/acidic carbohydrate complex is involved and this possibility is being investigated further.

In general the histochemical activity of the surface articular zone of the cartilage was low which is in keeping with its structure and the purely mechanical function which this zone appears to fulfil. No significant differences in histochemical activity was observed between animals of different ages and sex.

Summary

Histochemical changes coincident with cell differentiation and endochondral ossification were studied in the condylar cartilages of the mandible of young Wistar rats. Undemineralised cryostat sections were subjected to a range of functional and analytical histochemical procedures.

The results indicate that the metabolic activity of chondrocytes is roughly proportional to matrix production. The presence of glycogen is correlated with this metabolic activity rather than with mineralisation, whereas the presence of alkaline phosphatase is strictly correlated with actual or impending mineralisation. Lysosomal enzymes are present in chondrocytes. A sudanophilic substance which may not be lipid in nature is also associated with sites of mineralisation.

References

Cabrini, R. L.: Histochemistry of ossification. In International Review of Cytology. No. XI. Bourne, G. H., and J. H. Danielli (eds.). 1961, p. 283.

Duve, C. de: The Lysosome Concept. In Lysosomes. de Reŭck, A. S. A., and M. P. Cameron (eds.). London: Churchill 1963, p. 1.

Fell, H. B.: Organ culture and the physiology of skeletal tissues. In Bone and Tooth. Blackwood, H. J. J. (ed.). Oxford: Pergamon Press 1964, p. 311.

Irving, J. T.: A histological staining method for sites of calcification in teeth and bone. Arch. oral Biol. **1**, 89 (1959).

— Bone matrix lipids and calcification. In Calcified Tissues. Richelle, L. J., and M. J. Dallemagne (eds.). Liège: Université de Liège 1965, p. 313.

Sledge, C. B., and J. T. Dingle: Oxygen induced resorption of cartilage in organ culture. Nature (Lond.) **205**, 140 (1965).

WEATHERALL, J. A., J. P. BAILY, and S. M. WEIDMANN: Sulphated mucopolysaccharides and calcification. In Bone and Tooth. BLACKWOOD, H. J. J. (ed.). Oxford: Pergamon Press 1964, p. 227.
WUTHIER, R. E., and J. T. IRVING: Lipids in developing calf bone. J. dent. Res. **43**, 814 (1964).

Correlation between Morphological, Biochemical, and Biophysical Effects of Parathyroid Hormone on Cell Membranes

A. B. BORLE

Department of Physiology, University of Pittsburgh School of Medicine, Pittsburgh, Pa., U. S. A.

We have previously reported that parathyroid hormone (PTH) added to HeLa cells decreased cellular adhesion to glass, produced cell clumping (increased mutual adhesion of the cells) as well as the appearance of blebs and microvilli of the cell membrane (BORLE and NEUMAN, 1965). Monkey kidney cells seem to respond to PTH as well. One unit of PTH/ml of medium produced a large number of vacuoles in the cytoplasm and an enlargement and swelling of the Golgi apparatus (Fig. 1 and 2). Sequential observations suggest that the vacuoles are formed by pinocytosis.

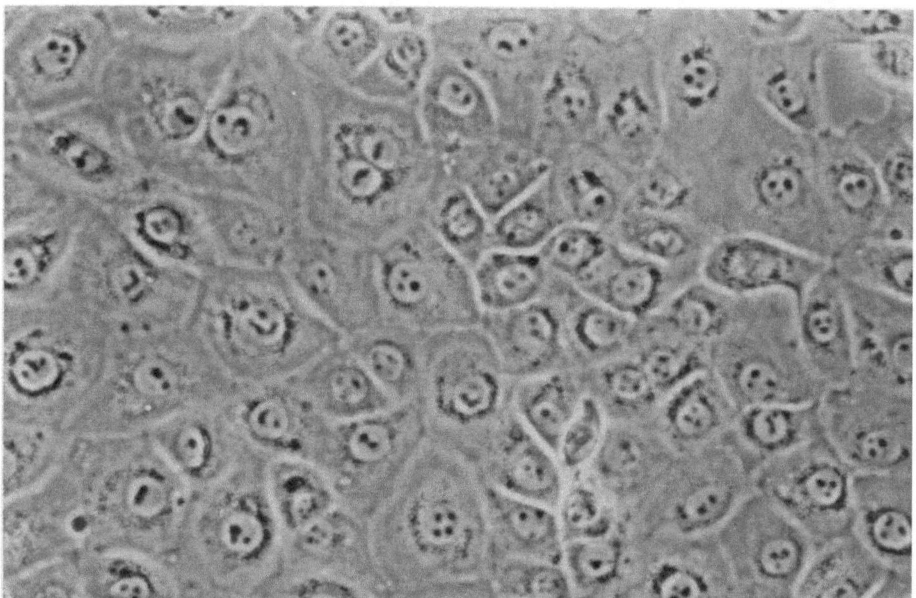

Fig. 1. Monkey kidney cells, control culture

Metabolic Studies: Both of these cell strains were incubated in Krebs-Ringer bicarbonate buffer to determine whether the morphological modifications produced by PTH would be associated with metabolic changes comparable to those observed in bone, kidney and intestine (BORLE *et al.*, 1960; EGAWA and NEUMAN, 1963; BORLE *et al.*, 1963). In HeLa cells, a) PTH increased lactate production 28.5% from 32.2 ± 1.98 to 41.4 ± 1.16 μg/hr/10^6 cells ($p < 0.001$); b) PTH increased the cellular

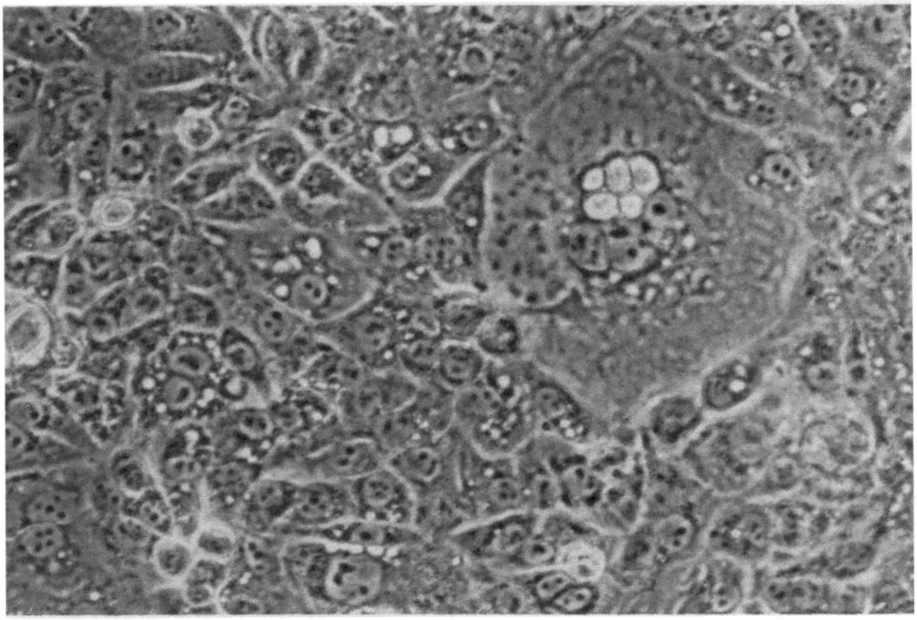

Fig. 2. Monkey kidney cells, 24 hrs after exposure to 1 U. PTH/ml.

P_i 21%; c) PTH increased ^{32}P incorporation into the lipid fraction of the cells 63% in one hour (relative specific activity 4.25×10^{-3} in control vs. 6.93×10^{-3} in the experimental group). In monkey kidney cells, PTH did not increase lactate production but increased the total cellular phosphate 30% from 26.1 to 34.0 μg P/mg cell protein ($p < 0.001$). Table 1 presents a summary of these changes and a comparison

Table 1. *Metabolic effects of PTH*

	Lactate Production	Cell P Uptake	^{32}P → lipid
HeLa Cells	+ 30%	(+ 21%)	+ 63%
Monkey kidney cells	0	+ 30%	—
Bone slices [1, 2] . . .	+ 34%	+ 38%	—
Kidney slices [2] . . .	—	+ 26%	+ 34%
Intestine [3]	+ 36%	+ 28%	—

[1] BORLE *et al.*, 1960. [2] EGAWA and NEUMAN, 1963. [3] BORLE *et al.*, 1963.

with the results previously obtained in bone, kidney and intestine. It appears from these studies, that PTH may enhance aerobic glycolysis, phosphate transport into the cell and probably the turnover of phospholipids. In view of the morphological observations reported above, it is of interest that very similar metabolic changes have been reported in phagocytosing leucocytes (SBARRA and KARNOVSKY, 1959, 1960).

The decreased adhesion of HeLa cells to the culture flask produced by PTH, which may suggest a change in membrane properties, was investigated. One unit of PTH/ml of medium increased the number of cells in suspension five fold from 62.0 ± 7.2 to 346.0 ± 9.1 μg cell protein in one hour ($p < 0.001$). To study whether these modifications were due to changes in calcium distribution between medium and cells, cultures were grown for 6 days in media containing ^{45}Ca and the decrease in specific activity of the medium analyzed at 2 hours, 3 and 6 days. Fig. 3 shows that cellular uptake of calcium is more than doubled in PTH treated cells. Whether this represents calcium binding to the membrane or calcium transport has not yet been determined, but viewed in the light of the observation that there is an optimal calcium concentration below and *above* which cell adhesion decreases (WEISS, 1960), the data may reflect a modification in the properties of the membrane. Since calcium increases membrane resistance in a variety of systems, the action of PTH on the electrical properties of the isolated toad bladder was investigated. Bladders of *Bufo Marinus* were mounted between lucite halfchambers. Membrane potential and short circuit current were determined and the resistance was calculated. One unit PTH/ml of Frog Ringer was added on the serosal side in the experimental group. Fig. 4 shows a drop in short circuit current and no significant change in potential. There was, therefore, a concomitant rise in membranes resistance. The results of 12 experiments summarized in Table 2 could be interpreted in terms of a shift of calcium from the extracellular fluid to the cell membrane induced by PTH and increasing membrane resistance.

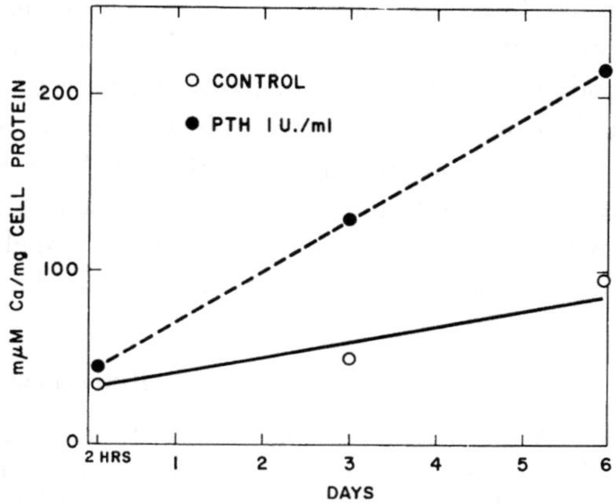

Fig. 3. Calcium exchange in HeLa cells

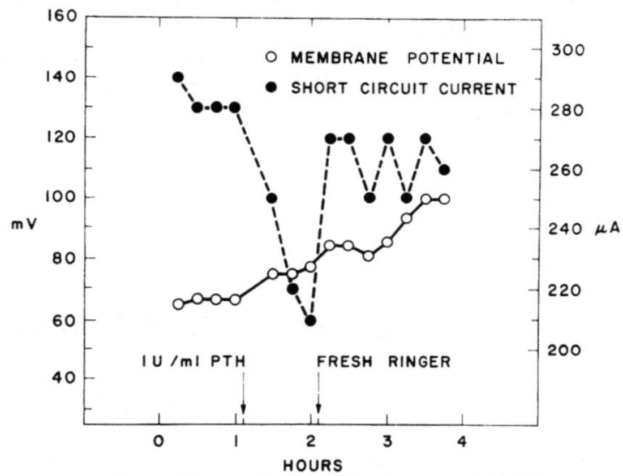

Fig. 4. Effects of 1 U. PTH/ml. on toad bladder

Table 2. *PTH on toad bladders*

	Control	PTH	p values
Potential (mV) . . .	32.2	33.0	N. S.
Short circuit current (uA)	58.2	41.3	0.001
Resistance (Ω) . . .	490	712	0.02

Summary

1. Morphological modifications by PTH have been observed in cell cultures, suggesting an effect on the cell membrane: microvilli, blebbing, decreased cellular adhesion, vacuolization and pinocytosis. 2. The changes in metabolism of these cells effected by PTH (increased lactate production, phosphate transport and ^{32}P incorporation into lipid phosphorus) are similar to those observed in bone, kidney and intestine. 3. Shifts of calcium from medium to cells were observed after PTH; these could explain the changes in cellular adhesion. 4. An increased membrane resistance was obtained in toad bladder after PTH, a finding consistent with an increased calcium binding to the membrane. 5. These results also suggest that PTH, beyond and above its role of increasing serum calcium, might play a further role in the distribution of calcium between the extracellular fluid and the cells.

References

BORLE, A. B., H. T. KEUTMANN, and W. F. NEUMAN: Role of parathyroid hormone in phosphate transport across rat duodenum. Amer. J. Physiol. **204**, 705 (1963).

—, and W. F. NEUMANN: Effects of parathyroid hormone on HeLa cell culture. J. Cell Biol. **24**, 316 (1965).

—, N. NICHOLS, and G. NICHOLS, JR.: Metabolic studies of bone *in vitro*. II. The metabolic patterns of accretion and resorption. J. biol. Chem. **235**, 1211 (1960).

EGAWA, J., and W. F. NEUMAN: Effects of parathyroid hormone on phosphate turnover in bone and kidney. Endocrinology **72**, 370 (1963).

SBARRA, A. J., and M. L. KARNOVSKY: The biochemical basis of phagocytosis. I. J. biol. Chem. **234**, 1355 (1959).

— — The biochemical basis of phagocytosis. II. J. biol. Chem. **235**, 2224 (1960).

WEISS, L.: Studies on cellular adhesion in tissue culture. III. Some effects of calcium. Exp. Cell Res. **21**, 71 (1960).

Vitamin D-ascorbic Acid Association in Bone Metabolism

P. A. THORNTON

Veterans Administration Hospital, Lexington, Kentucky, and the Departments of Physiology and Biophysics and Medicine, University of Kentucky, Lexington, Ky., U. S. A.

Previous results (THORNTON and BROWNRIGG, 1961) have indicated that ascorbic acid influenced the skeletal response of chicks to vitamin D_3 deficiency. Turnover of skeletal ^{45}Ca was enhanced in vitamin D_3 deficient individuals in the presence of ascorbic acid, suggesting a change in the bone metabolic rate. No specific role for vitamin D in bone cells has been evolved; however, investigations with cartilage have suggested a metabolic function in that tissue. It appears to be needed for normal formation and metabolism of citric acid (NEUMAN and NEUMAN, 1958).

Although no evidence has been presented linking ascorbic acid to bone cellular metabolism, it is accepted that this compound is involved in formation of the organic portion of bone. An increase in osteoclastic population (LEVY and GORLIN, 1953) and a decrease in bone alkaline phosphatase (GOULD and SCHWACHMAN, 1941) have also been shown in ascorbate deficiency. The present report concerns possible bone cellular roles for vitamin D and ascorbic acid and an attempt to relate these events to bone demineralization.

Methods

Male Leghorn chicks were given the experimental diets (Tab. 1) from one day until 15 and 16 days of age. Previous efforts (THORNTON *et al.*, 1959) attest to the adequacy of the control diet to support normal growth and to its rachitogenicity in the absence of vitamin D_3. At 15 and 16 days of age, an equal number of chicks from each group were sacrificed. The tibiae were quickly removed, freed of adhering tissue and placed in cold saline solution. Each were split lengthwise and the bone marrow removed. About 100 mg of compact bone tissue was placed in 2.8 ml of cold buffer solution and kept there until all samples were placed in the incubator. The medium, adjusted to a pH of 7.4, contained the following in μmoles: Tri-(hydroxymethyl)aminomethane (Tris) 20, $MgSO_4$ 15, glucose 10, NaCl 150, adenosine diphosphate (ADP) 10 and hexokinase at 0.5 mg per flask. Tissue from 6 animals from selected groups (Tab. 1) were incubated in the Warburg respirometer. All others were incubated in the Dubnoff metabolic shaker with air used as the gas phase in each case. All were incubated for 3 hours at 37 °C.

Table 1. *Dietary changes and bone response*

Dietary Treatment	NCN µg/100 mg Bone	Percent Bone Ash	O_2 uptake µl/mg NCN/hr.	Glucose uptake µg/mg NCN/hr.	Lactic Acid recovery µg/mg NCN/hr.
1. Control.	530 ± 17[1]	63.8 ± 0.3	22 ± 5[1]	859 ± 30	98 ± 9
2. Vitamin D_3 deficient	760 ± 31[aa]	58.4 ± 0.7[aa]	51 ± 10[aa]	451 ± 49[aa]	70 ± 9[a]
3. 2 + 44 mg ascorbic acid/kg diet . . .	849 ± 41[aa]	58.5 ± 0.5[aa]	—	470 ± 29[aa]	70 ± 8[a]
4. 2 + 220 mg ascorbic acid/kg diet . . .	564 ± 44[bb]	60.2 ± 0.4[aa,b]	31 ± 5	712 ± 54[bb,a]	93 ± 10

[1] Mean ± S. E.
a, *aa* — Different from the control at the 95 and 99% confidence levels respectively.
b, *bb* — Different from the vitamin D_3 deficient group at the 95 and 99% confidence levels respectively.

Chemical determinations of the media included glucose (HUGGETT and NIXON, 1957), lactic acid (BARKER and SUMMERSON, 1941), phosphate (FISKE and SUBBAROW, 1925) and calcium (WILLIS, 1961). Non-collagenous nitrogen (NCN) was measured, employing a modification of the LILIENTHAL *et al.* method (1950) as used by BORLE *et al.* (1960).

Compact bone tissue was ether extracted for 6 hours, dried to a constant weight at 105 °C and ashed 12—16 hours at 600 °C to determine percent ash.

Results and discussion

There was an apparent increase in NCN in the absence of vitamin D_3 (Tab. 1). Addition of ascorbic acid at the lower level augmented the response while the higher supplementation effected a value similar to the control. Whether these changes in bone NCN resulted from a shift in cell type or cell number cannot be elucidated since no histological data are available. Percent bone ash (Tab. 1) was reduced in all vitamin D deficient groups compared to controls. However, the reduced bone ash appeared to be partially corrected by the higher ascorbic acid addition.

Bone cellular activity (Tab. 1) indicated a metabolic shift in response to the vitamin D_3 deficiency. The increased oxygen uptake, reduced glucose utilization and diminished lactic acid production by bone from those individuals suggested a greater relative degree of oxidative metabolism. No explanation for this response or why dietary ascorbic acid appeared to reverse the effect can be given.

Both calcium and phosphate movement from bone to the incubating media were reduced by the vitamin D_3 deficiency (Tab. 2). This result probably reflects the fact

Table 2. *In vitro demineralization*

Dietary Treatment	Calcium release µg/100 mg bone/hr.	Phosphate release µg/100 mg bone/hr.	Calcium / Phosphate
1. Control	83 ± 11[1]	27 ± 7	3.6 ± 0.6
2. Vitamin D_3 deficient	63 ± 5	22 ± 12	3.7 ± 1.0
3. 2 + 44 mg ascorbic acid/kg diet . .	78 ± 5[b]	67 ± 10[aa,bb]	1.3 ± 0.2[aa,b]
4. 2 + 220 mg ascorbic acid/kg diet. .	104 ± 12[bb]	70 ± 12[aa,bb]	1.8 ± 0.3[aa]

[1], *a*, *aa*, *b*, *bb* — See Table 1.

that a reduced amount of these minerals were available for mobilization since the percent ash (Tab. 1) for this group was lower than controls. Mobilization of calcium was stimulated in vitamin D_3 deficient animals by dietary ascorbic acid (Tab. 2). More striking, however, were the results concerning phosphate release in response to this treatment. In spite of the three-fold increase in phosphate release and the elevation in calcium mobilization, the percent bone ash was not reduced by the ascorbic acid addition. In fact, bone ash was increased in vitamin D_3 deficient chicks given the higher level of ascorbic acid (Tab. 1). These results imply that the added ascorbate had a calcifying effect *in vivo* and a resorptive influence *in vitro*. From this, it may be surmised that the intact chick possessed an additional factor or factors which were involved.

The highly significant increase in phosphate mobilization induced by the ascorbic acid suggested that this vitamin was implicated in bone cellular activity. The phosphate values shown here are based on total phosphate of ashed media; therefore, the results do not differentiate between organic and inorganic fractions. Preliminary results (THORNTON, unpublished) have indicated that glucose-6-phosphate formation in bone tissue from vitamin D_3 deficient chicks fed ascorbic acid was 40—50 percent greater than either vitamin D_3 deficient or control animals. Thus, it seems probable that some of the increased phosphate mobilization could be attributed to its being bound in organic form. If this were true, it would suggest that ascorbate had an enhancing effect on energy transformation in the bone cell. To test this premise, calculations concerning the relationship between cell activity and phosphate recovery were made. The results (Tab. 3) show clearly that a highly significant direct relationship existed between both glucose and oxygen uptake and the release of phosphate in ascorbic acid groups. No interrelationships were found for the animals not given this compound.

COHN and FORSCHER (1962) presented evidence suggesting that lactic acid was the major end-product of glucose metabolism in bone tissue. GOLDHABER (1961) showed that oxidative metabolism was necessary for bone resorption while WALKER'S

Table 3. *Cellular activity and phosphate mobilization*

Dietary treatment	Glucose uptake and phosphate release	O_2 uptake and phosphate release
1. Control	0.001 [1]	0.356
2. Vitamin D_3 deficient	—0.249	—0.275
3. 2 + 44 mg ascorbic acid/kg diet . .	0.632 [2]	—
4. 2 + 220 mg ascorbic acid/kg diet. .	0.774 [2]	0.888 [2]

[1] Correlation value.
[2] Significant at the 99% confidence level.

results (1961) indicated operation of the Krebs cycle in the osteoclast and its inhibition in the osteoblast. These results point to the potential metabolic versatility of the bone cell. Thus, the increased oxidative metabolism exhibited by bone tissue from the vitamin D_3 deficient animals could be explained on a basis of an alteration in metabolic pathways. An explanation of this response and why dietary ascorbic acid appears to reverse the effect will be of interest in future investigations.

Summary

The results of this experiment suggested that both ascorbic acid and vitamin D_3 were involved in bone cellular metabolism. Little or no correlation was apparent between cell activity and *in vitro* bone demineralization in either control or vitamin D_3 deficient groups; however, the addition of dietary ascorbic acid was associated with a significant degree of relationship between these factors.

Acknowledgement

This investigation was supported by Public Health Research grant number: AM-07724-01 from the National Institutes of Health. The author was a member of the Endocrine Section, Colorado State University, Ft. Collins, Colorado, when the above work was conducted.

References

BARKER, S. B., and W. H. SUMMERSON: The colorimetric determination of lactic acid in biological material. J. biol. Chem. **138,** 535 (1941).

BORLE, A. B., N. NICHOLS, and G. NICHOLS, JR.: Metabolic studies of bone *in vitro*. I. Normal bone. J. biol. Chem. **235,** 1206 (1960).

COHN, D. V., and B. K. FORSCHER: Aerobic metabolism of glucose by bone. J. biol. Chem. **237,** 615 (1962).

FISKE, C. H., and Y. SUBBAROW: The colorimetric determination of phosphorus. J. biol. Chem. **66,** 375 (1925).

GOLDHABER, P.: Some factors affecting bone resorption in tissue culture. J. Bone Jt Surg. **43 B,** 180 (1961).

GOULD, B. S., and H. SCHWACHMAN: Bone and tissue phosphatase in experimental scurvy and studies on the source of serum phosphatase. Amer. J. Physiol. **135,** 485 (1941).

HUGGETT, A. S. C., and D. A. NIXON: Use of glucose oxidase, peroxidase and O-dianisdine in determination of blood and urinary glucose. Lancet, **273**, 368 (1957).
LEVY, B. M., and R. V. GORLIN: The temporomandibular joint in vitamin C deficiency. J. dent. Res. **32**, 622 (1953).
LILIENTHAL, J. L., JR., K. L. ZIERLER, B. P. FOLK, R. BUKA, and M. J. RILEY: A reference base and system for analysis of muscle constituents. J. biol. Chem. **182**, 501 (1950).
NEUMAN, W. F., and M. W. NEUMAN: The Chemical Dynamics of Bone. Chicago: The University of Chicago Press 1958.
THORNTON, P. A.: Unpublished.
—, and D. BROWNRIGG: Calcium utilization and skeletal development in chicks as influenced by parental dietary ascorbic acid. J. Nutr. **75**, 354 (1961).
—, C. W. WEBER, and R. E. MORENG: The effect of ascorbic acid in the diet of adult chickens on calcium utilization by the progeny. J. Nutr. **69**, 33 (1959).
WALKER, D. G.: Citric acid cycle in osteoblasts and osteoclasts. Bull. Johns Hopk. Hosp. **106**, 80 (1961).
WILLIS, J. B.: Determinations of calcium and magnesium in urine by atomic absorption spectroscopy. Analyt. Chem. **33**, 556 (1961).

Lysosomes and Cartilage Resorption in Organ Culture

C. B. SLEDGE

Strangeways Research Laboratory, Cambridge, England
and
Department of Orthopedics, Harvard Medical School, Massachusetts General Hospital, Boston, Mass., U.S.A.

The work of BASSETT and HERRMANN (1961) and BASSETT (1964) has shown that variations in environmental oxygen exert a modulating influence on skeletal tissues in culture. GOLDHABER (1963) has found that exposure of neo-natal mouse calvaria in organ culture to elevated partial pressures of oxygen results in bone resorption and increased osteoclasis. The mechanism of these interesting effects is unexplained.

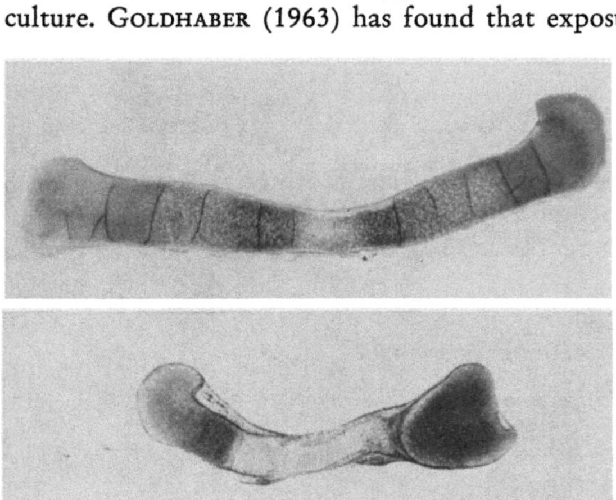

Fig. 1. Top: control rudiment exposed to 20% oxygen for 6 days. Toluidine blue. ×10. — Bottom: contralateral rudiment exposed to 85% oxygen for 6 days. Toluidine blue. ×10

In this work, the cartilaginous limb-bone rudiments of 8-day chick embryos have been exposed to elevated partial pressures of oxygen on a completely synthetic medium. This results in extensive loss of metachromatic material throughout the shaft of the rudiments (Fig. 1). This loss of metachromasis is accompanied by normal synthesis, but increased release of hexosamine into the medium. Thus, both the histological appearance and solubilization of mucopolysaccharide resemble the effect of excess of vitamin A. Since this vitamin has been shown to produce matrix degradation by increased release of a lysosomal acid protease (FELL and DINGLE, 1963), a similar mechanism was suspected for the hyperoxia effect.

Fig. 2 shows the growth of two groups of rudiments. One group of eight rudiments was exposed to 20% oxygen while the paired rudiments were exposed to 85% oxygen. At two-day intervals the amounts of acid protease and acid phosphatase in the medium were measured. The release of both of these lysosomal enzymes was increased in the group exposed to elevated oxygen.

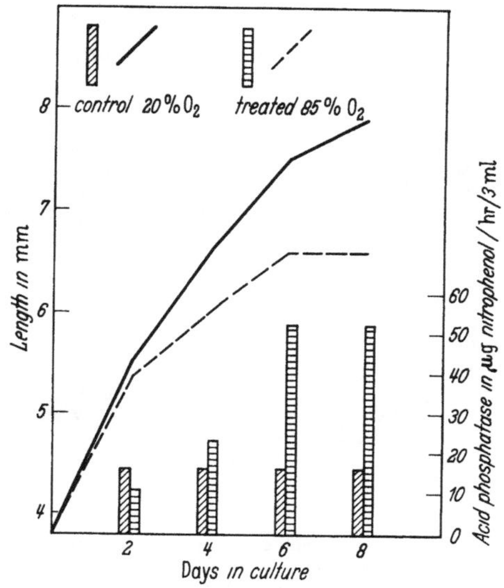

Fig. 2. Lengths of control and experimental rudiments shown in line graph. Release of acid phosphatase into medium shown in bar graph

The lysosome, a cytoplasmic body containing a variety of hydrolytic enzymes characterized by acid pH optima and structure-linked latency, was developed as a biochemical concept by DE DUVE *et al.* (1955), and DE DUVE (1963). The morphology of these single membrane limited structures has been described by NOVIKOFF (1963), and their presence in all mammalian cells except the erythrocyte and spermatocyte seems likely (DINGLE, personal communication). Alteration of the liproprotein membrane leads to activation of the enzymes, either by escape of enzyme or entrance of substrate. Many agents have been shown to produce such alteration of the membrane: acid pH, ultraviolet light, vitamin A, streptococcal endotoxin, antigen-antibody reactions, etc. Measurements of the free/bound ratio of the lysosomal enzymes in the rudiments showed that the fragility of the lysosomal membrane was increased in hyperoxia.

Since the membrane of the lysosome can be stabilized by cortisol in physiological doses (WEISSMANN and DINGLE, 1962), it was added to the cultures at 0.1 γ/ml. or 0.01 γ/ml. This steroid afforded complete protection from hyperoxia, by both histological and biochemical criteria.

In work with excess of vitamin A, FELL and DINGLE (1963) have shown that lysosomal acid protease is responsible for the degradation of matrix. ALI (1964) has shown that this protease is competitively inhibited by epsilon-amino-n-caproic acid (EACA), a synthetic amino acid which structurally resembles lysine. When EACA was added to our medium at 40 γ/ml. it, like cortisol, protected the rudiments from the effects of hyperoxia.

It appeared evident that excess oxygen was activating the lysosomes of the chondrocytes and releasing an acid protease which led to loss of matrix. What is the mechanism for this effect — acid pH, change in cell membrane permeability, or a direct effect on the lysosome? KENNY *et al.*, (1959) suggested a blockage in the Krebs cycle leading to accumulation of lactic and citric acids and a lowered pH as the mechanism of bone resorption in hyperoxia. I have not found this to be the case in our experiments. Citrate and lactate production, pH and glucose consumption are unchanged from control figures. What about the cell membrane? ALLISON (1965), working with cell cultures in 95% oxygen, found increased permeability of the lysosomes to the Gomori substrate 12 hrs. before the cell membrane became permeable to eosin. It was, therefore, suspected that the effect of hyperoxia was a direct one on the lysosomal membrane. Mr. DINGLE and I (SLEDGE and DINGLE, 1965) prepared lysosome-rich fractions from chick embryonic cartilage and incubated them with oxygen or nitrogen. Similar fractions from liver, kidney, spleen and brain were run as controls. Only in the case of lysosomes from cartilage was there activation by oxygen.

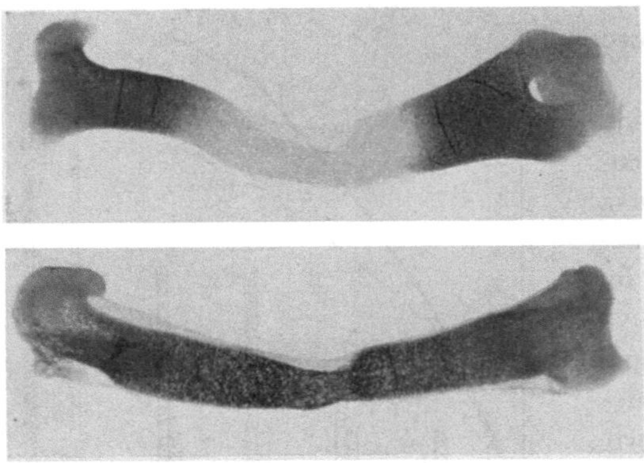

Fig. 3. Top: control rudiment exposed to 85% oxygen for 6 days. Toluidine blue. ×10. — Bottom: contralateral rudiment exposed to 85% oxygen for 6 days. 40 γ/ml. vitamin E added. Toluidine blue. ×10

When Vitamin E, a lipid soluble anti-oxidant, or vitamin C, a water-soluble anti-oxidant, were added to the culture medium, protection from hyperoxia was observed (Fig. 3). TAPPEL *et al.* (1963) have found increased lipid peroxidation in vitamin E deficiency. It therefore seems likely that the effect of hyperoxia is mediated through increased release of hydrolytic enzymes by lipid peroxidation of the lysosomal membrane. The protective effect of vitamin C is perhaps due to a re-cycling phenomenon whereby a membrane constituent, susceptible to oxidation, is protected by lipidsoluble reducing substance (perhaps vitamin E) which, in turn, is maintained in a reduced state by vitamin C in the cytoplasm.

The role of the osteoclast in these experiments has been most interesting. They are not normally seen in chick limb-bones in culture. However, in all of the rudiments exposed to hyperoxia alone, osteoclasts appear — never in great number and always after resorption is well underway. They are not due to hyperoxia, per se, as they are not seen in rudiments exposed to hyperoxia but protected from matrix degradation by cortisol, EACA, or vitamins E or C. From this it would appear that some product of matrix degradation is responsible for the induction of osteoclast formation. A possible scheme might be:

$$\text{oxygen} + \text{lysosome} \xrightarrow[\text{peroxidation}]{\text{lipid}} \text{acid protease}$$

$$\text{acid protease} + \text{protein-polysaccharide} \xrightarrow[\text{hydrolysis}]{\text{arginine bond}} \text{non-collagenous protein} + \text{polysaccharide}$$

$$\text{non-collagenous protein} + \text{undifferentiated mesenchymal cell} \xrightarrow{\text{fusion}} \text{osteoclast}$$

Using 85% oxygen and natural medium (plasma clot-embryo extract), a marrow cavity has been produced in chick limb bones in culture for the first time (Fig. 4). As no vessels were present at the time of explantation (8 days), this is a direct effect of oxygen on the tissues.

Indirect evidence for the role of lysosomes in skeletal morphogenesis is provided by the work of MOSCONA and KARNOFSKY (1959). Administration of cortisone to the chick embryo, in ovo, prevented the formation of the marrow cavity. In some species cortisone produces increased thickness of the epiphyseal plate due to failure of resorption on the metaphyseal side (HULTH and OLERUD, 1963). Both of these findings I would interpret as due to the stabilizing effect of cortisone on the membranes of cartilage lysosomes exposed to the relative hyperoxia of a highly vascularized region.

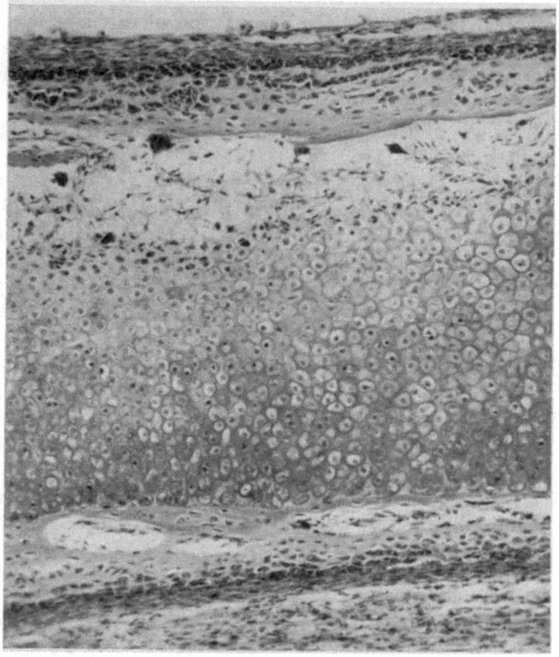

Fig. 4. 8-day rudiment on natural medium, exposed to 85% oxygen for 6 days. Osteoclasts can be seen participating in marrow cavity formation. Haematoxylin and Eosin. ×110

In conclusion, it is suggested that exposure of cartilage to elevated partial pressures of oxygen results in tissue degradation by enzymes released by lipid peroxidation of the lysosomal membrane. The often observed association between vascular invasion and degradation of skeletal tissues and susceptibility of cartilage to necrosis in hyperoxia may therefore be related. I would suggest that this phenomenon has important physiological as well as pathological implications. Cases in point would be the increased vascularity of the resorbing epiphyseal plate, the formation of the marrow cavity, the shedding of decidious teeth in humans and antlers in deer, and the erosion caused by the vascular pannus in rheumatoid arthritis.

Acknowledgements

The author is a Fellow of The Medical Foundation Inc. of Boston, Massachusetts.

I thank Dame Honor B. FELL, F. R. S. and Mr. J. T. DINGLE for their interest and advice. Certain aspects of this work were investigated in collaboration with Mr. DINGLE.

References

ALI, S. Y.: The degradation of cartilage matrix by an intracellular protease. Biochem. J. **93**, 611 (1964).

ALLISON, A. C.: Role of lysosomes in oxygen toxicity. Nature (Lond.) **205**, 141 (1965).

BASSETT, C. A. L.: Environmental and cellular factors regulating osteogenesis. In Bone Biodynamics. FROST, H. M. (ed.). Boston: Little, Brown 1964, p. 233.

—, and I. HERRMANN: Influence of oxygen concentration and mechanical factors on differentiation of connective tissues in vitro. Nature, (Lond.) **190**, 460 (1961).

Duve, C. de: The lysosome concept. In Lysosomes. de Reuck, A. V. S., and M. P. Cameron (eds.). London: Churchill 1963, p. 1.

—, B. C. Pressman, R. Gianetto, R. Wattiaux, and F. Appelmans: Tissue fractionation studies. 6. Intracellular distribution patterns of enzymes in rat-liver tissue. Biochem. J. **60**, 604 (1955).

Fell, H. B., and J. T. Dingle: Studies on the mode of action of excess of vitamin A. 6. Lysosomal protease and the degradation of cartilage matrix. Biochem. J. **87**, 403 (1963).

Goldhaber, P.: Some chemical factors influencing bone resorption in tissue culture. In Mechanisms of Hard Tissue Destruction. Sognnaes, R. (ed.). Washington: Amer. Acad. advanc. Sci. 1963, p. 609.

Hulth, A., and S. Olerud: The effect of cortisone on growing bone in the rat. Brit. J. exp. Path. **44**, 491 (1963).

Kenny, A. D., P. R. Draskoczy, and P. Goldhaber: Critic acid production by resorbing bone in tissue culture. Amer. J. Physiol. **197**, 502 (1959).

Moscona, M. H., and D. A. Karnofsky: Cortisone induced modifications in the development of the chick embryo. Endocrinology **66**, 533 (1959).

Novikoff, A.: Lysosomes in the physiology and pathology of cells. Contributions of staining methods. In Lysosomes. de Reuck, A. V. S., and M. P. Cameron (eds.). London: Churchill 1963, p. 36.

Sledge, C. B., and J. T. Dingle: Activation of lysosomes by oxygen: Oxygen-induced resorption of cartilage in organ culture. Nature, (Lond.) **205**, 140 (1965).

Tappel, A. L., P. L. Sawant, and S. Shibko: Lysosomes: Distribution in animals, hydrolytic capacity and other properties. In Lysosomes. de Reuck, A. V. S., and M. P. Cameron (eds.). London: Churchill 1963, p. 78.

Weissmann, G., and J. T. Dingle: Release of lysosomal protease by ultraviolet irradiation and inhibition by hydrocortisone. Exp. Cell Res. **25**, 207 (1962).

Acid Hydrolases, Lysosomes and Bone Resorption Induced by Parathyroid Hormone

G. Vaes

Laboratoire de Chimie Physiologique, Université de Louvain, Louvain, Belgique.

As pointed out elsewhere (Vaes, 1965; Vaes and Jacques, in press a), both mineral and organic matrix seem to be removed almost simultaneously in the process of bone resorption. Since organic acids produced and secreted by bone cells are thought to be the agents of the solubilization of bone mineral, the simultaneous hydrolysis of the organic matrix presumably occurs at an acid pH: the possibility that the acid hydrolases of bone cells may play a role in the digestion of the organic matrix was, therefore, considered.

So far, nine acid hydrolases have been demonstrated in homogenates of newborn rat calvaria (Vaes and Jacques, in press a): β-glucuronidase, β-N-acetylaminodeoxyglucosidase, acid deoxyribonuclease, acid ribonuclease, acid-β-glycerophosphatase and acid phenylphosphatase showing optimal activity around pH 5; cathepsin, β-galactosidase and hyaluronidase with an optimum around pH 3.6. The first eight hydrolases, and probably also hyaluronidase (Vaes, in preparation), have been shown by means of tissue fractionation techniques to be associated with a special group of cytoplasmic particles distinct both from mitochondria and from microsomes and similar to liver lysosomes (Vaes and Jacques, in press b). The acid hydrolases studied are largely latent in fresh untreated homogenates; they are released in a closely parallel fashion (with the possible exception of part of the acid phenylphosphatase) in preparations subjected to graded activating treatments, suggesting that they are associated either with the same particle, or with particles possessing similar properties (VAES, in press b). These experiments allow the conclusion that the acid hydrolases of bone cells are associated with particles having the main characteristics of lysosomes. No data have been obtained so far on the intracellular localization of the collagenase activity of bone cells, except for some preliminary experiments (with C. M. LAPIÈRE) showing that part of this activity could be associated with cytoplasmic particles; in liver, a collagenase activity has been located by others in the lysomoses (FRANKLAND and WYNN, 1962).

Further experiments have furnished evidence for an involvement of the acid hydrolases of bone cells in the process of bone resorption: they are reported here briefly; full details will be published elsewhere (see also as a preliminary note, VAES, in press a).

Experiments in a tissue-culture system of resorbing bone

Bone resorption was induced in cultures of calvaria from 18—19 day-old mouse embryos by the addition to the medium of 1 U.S.P. unit/ml. of parathyroid extract (PTE). Resorption lacunae first became macroscopically visible in the parietals after 1—2 days cultivation; they extended rapidly between the 2nd and the 4th day, forming actual holes in the parietals. Lacunae appeared in the frontals around the 3rd day and progressed slowly thereafter (Fig. 1 in VAES, in press a).

During the development of resorption increasing amounts of β-glucuronidase, β-galactosidase and β-N-acetylaminodeoxyglucosidase were released into the medium as compared to non-resorbing controls; this is true also for acid deoxyribonuclease and possibly for cathepsin. Two non-lysosomal enzymes, alkaline phenylphosphatase and catalase, were released in similar amounts in the medium of resorbing and of control calvaria during the first days of culture and thereafter appeared in smaller amounts in the medium of the resorbing calvaria (Fig. 2 in VAES, in press a). The medium of the resorbing calvaria was also found to be significantly more acid than

Table 1. *Balance of enzyme activies between the 2nd and 7th day of cultivation for control and resorbing (PTE) calvaria. Only means (mμmoles/minute per calvarium) and p values (for the difference between C and PTE) are presented*

Enzyme		In tissue day 2	Recovered from medium between day 2 and 7	In tissue day 7	Excess over day 2
β-Glucuronidase	C	0.34	0.15	0.39	0.20
	PTE	0.30 ($p < 0.01$)	0.48 ($p < 0.001$)	0.38 (N. S.)	0.56
Acetylamino-	C	3.40	1.40	3.60	1.60
deoxyglucosidase	PTE	3.00 ($p < 0.02$)	5.00 ($p < 0.001$)	4.80 ($p < 0.01$)	6.80
β-Galactosidase	C	0.62	0.06	0.52	—0.04
	PTE	0.60 (N. S.)	0.15 ($p < 0.001$)	0.63 ($p < 0.01$)	0.18
Alkaline	C	81	—	60	—21
phosphatase	PTE	62 ($p < 0.001$)	—	38 ($p < 0.01$)	—24

the medium of the control: this increased acidity was already detectable after 7—8 hours cultivation (VAES, in press a).

The average activities present in one calvarium on the 2nd and on the 7th day of cultivation and those recovered from its cultivation medium between these 2 days, are shown in Table 1. It is apparent from these data that both resorbing and control calvaria synthesize acid hydrolases during this interval of time; but this synthesis is considerably higher in the resorbing calvaria than in the controls. This is not true for alkaline phenylphosphatase, a nonlysosomal enzyme, which is progressively lost by both control and resorbing calvaria, but more rapidly by resorbing calvaria. In this tissue culture system, PTE thus appears to stimulate both the release (or excretion) and the synthesis of lysosomal acid hydrolases. It stimulates also the excretion of acid into the extracellular spaces.

Experiments with rats treated with parathyroid extract

An increased activity of various acid hydrolases (but not of the mitochondrial cytochrome oxidase) (Table 2, A) was observed in the calvaria of newborn rats

Table 2. *Rats treated with PTE. A) Enzyme activities in homogenates of calvaria; B) Free activities of enzymes in cytoplasmic extracts of calvaria. — All results expressed as percentage (mean ± S.D.; N = 6 or 7) of the activities found for paired controls taken as 100%. For absolute values in controls, see* Vaes *and* Jacques *(1965 a) and* Vaes *(1965 c)*

Enzyme	A	B
β-Glucuronidase	124 ± 17 ($p < 0.02$)	119 ± 11 ($p < 0.01$)
β-N-Acetylaminodeoxyglucosidase	111 ± 16 (N. S.)	135 ± 29 ($p < 0.05$)
β-Galactosidase	110 ± 6 ($p = 0.01$)	109 ± 8 ($p < 0.05$)
Hyaluronidase (in cytoplasmic extract)	114 ± 13 ($p < 0.05$)	—
Cathepsin	126 ± 10 ($p < 0.01$)	95 ± 5 (N. S.)
Acid Deoxyribonuclease	138 ± 24 ($p < 0.02$)	114 ± 7 ($p < 0.01$)
Acid Phenylphosphatase	146 ± 22 ($p < 0.01$)	110 ± 16 (N. S.)
Acid β-Glycerophosphatase	—	108 ± 12 (N. S.)
Cytochrome Oxidase	99 ± 11 (N. S.)	—

treated during 3 days with PTE. This increased concentration of enzymes may be compared with the increased synthesis of acid hydrolases observed in tissue culture under the action of PTE: it suggests that the same phenomenon occurs *in vivo* and *in vitro*. Moreover, a larger proportion of the activity found for the acid hydrolases in homogenates of calvaria of rats treated with PTE was found to be in the free state (Table 2, B). This is to be expected if the release of acid hydrolases observed in culture also occurs in vivo, since more soluble enzyme should then be present in the extracellular spaces of the calvaria.

Conclusions

The results reported suggest that parathyroid hormone induces a specific release of lysosomal acid hydrolases by bone cells (osteoclasts?). This could be a critical step of the mechanism whereby the hormone causes bone resorption. Presumably, all lysosomal hydrolases are excreted together in concentrated form at the level of the resorption lacunae, where they exert a concerted eroding action on the matrix before slowly diffusing passively into medium. The same interpretation probably applies to the excretion of hydrogen ions responsible for the acidification of the medium of resorbing calvaria: the local pH shift at the resorption sites is probably much greater than that observed in the medium. It could be sufficient to cause a solubilization of bone mineral, leaving the organic matrix uncovered and directly accessible to the digestive action of the lysosomal hydrolases, simultaneously creating a suitable environment for the action of these enzymes. This environment could be limited to the small area underlying the excretory pole of the cells active in resorption, since the excreted acid will be rapidly buffered by the bone mineral itself when it is diffusing away from the resorption lacunae. Such a buffering would limit considerably the extension of the resorption process and confine it to minute areas under direct control of the cells.

This extracellular function of the lysosomal hydrolases in the digestion of bone matrix could possibly be completed by an intracellular function in the digestion of fragments of matrix taken up in the cells by pinocytosis. Lysosomes are indeed known to be involved in the intracellular digestion of exogenous material engulfed by phagocytosis or pinocytosis in other cell types. Evidence of active pinocytosis in osteoclasts has been shown repeatedly by others.

Acknowledgements

Supported by the Fonds de la Recherche Scientifique Fondamentale Collective and the U.S. Public Health Service Research Grant n° MG-08705. The author is Chercheur Qualifié du F.N.R.S. He is indebted to Professor C. de Duve for his critical suggestions and for his help in the preparation of the manuscript.

The tissue culture work was done at the laboratory of Cell Biology and Histology of the University of Leiden thanks to the courtesy of Professor P. J. Gaillard and to a travelling fellowship of the Fondation Universitaire. Useful advices for the tissue culture technique from Professor P. J. Gaillard and Dr. W. A. de Voogd van der Straaten are gratefully acknowledged.

References

More details and complete bibliography may be found in the following papers:

Frankland, D. M., and C. H. Wynn: The degradation of acid soluble collagen by rat liver preparations. Biochem. J. **85**, 276 (1962).

Vaes, G.: Hydrolytic enzymes and lysosomes in bone cells. In Calcified Tissues. Richelle, L. J., and M. J. Dallemagne (eds.). Liège: L'Université de Liège 1965, p. 51.

— Excretion of acid and of lysosomal hydrolytic enzymes during bone resorption induced in tissue culture by parathyroid extract. Exp. Cell Res. (a. in press).

— Studies on bone enzymes. 3. The activation and release of latent acid hydrolases and catalase in bone tissue homogenates. Biochem. J. (b. in press).

—, and P. Jacques: Studies on bone enzymes. 1. The assay of acid hydrolases and other enzymes in bone tissue. Biochem. J. (a. in press).

—, and P. Jacques: Studies on bone enzymes. 1. The assay of acid hydrolases and other phenylphosphatase, cytochrome oxidase and catalase in fractionations of bone tissue homogenates. Biochem. J. (b. in press).

Le forage des canaux de Havers

A. Dhem

Laboratoire de Chirurgie Orthopédique et Traumatologie, Université de Louvain, Louvain, Belgique.

Nous nous sommes proposé d'étudier le creusement des canaux de Havers en faisant appel à l'histologie et à la microscopie de fluorescence.

Pour bien faire comprendre nos documents, rappelons brièvement l'aspect que présente, en coupe transversale, un ostéone en voie de dépôt.

La Fig. 1 provient d'une coupe transversale de la partie moyenne de la diaphyse tibiale d'un chien adulte. Le tissu non décalcifié a été enrobé dans le méthacrylate de méthyle et débité à la scie. Les coupes ont été amincies par usure, puis, toujours incluses dans leur milieu d'enrobage, colorées au bleu de méthylène à 1% tamponné par le biphtalate à pH 4,8.

Les détails de la figure sont indiqués par des lettres dont la signification est définie dans la légende.

Pour essayer de saisir la phase négative du remaniement, le forage du tunnel, nous avons utilisé des coupes longitudinales passant par le centre de la Fig. 1 et perpendiculaire au plan de cette photographie.

La Fig. 2 reproduit une telle coupe. La flèche désigne, au fond d'un cul-de-sac, un gros ostéoclaste multinucléé. Comme les études récentes au microscope électronique permettent d'y voir l'agent actif de la résorption (Hancox et Boothroyd 1964), cet ostéoclaste peut être considéré comme le trépan qui fore le canal de Havers. Seules donc, on le constate, des coupes longitudinales sont susceptibles de faire observer convenablement le phénomène.

Ce qui se passe dans le sillage de la résorption est partiellement décelable dans la Fig. 2. On y discerne un gros capillaire sinueux (*a*) et des ostéoblastes (*b*) qui, dès que la destruction est terminée, tapissent les parois du canal et amorcent aussitôt la reconstruction (*c* et *d*).

La Fig. 2 ne permet pas de mesurer l'allure de la résorption. Pour y parvenir, il fallait recourir à la microscopie de fluorescence.

Un chien adulte a reçu, par voie intrapéritonéale, une dose unique de tétracycline correspondant à 50 mg par kilogramme. Dix-sept jours plus tard, on lui a injecté, par la même voie, de l'alizarine (sulfonate sodique) à raison de 65 mg par kilogramme, quelques heures avant le sacrifice.

La diaphyse radiale a été débitée en coupes longitudinales et ce sont les documents ainsi obtenus que nous allons maintenant commenter.

La Fig. 3 représente, en lumière normale, un canal de Havers en voie d'extension. Elle montre, à son extrémité inférieure, la région de résorption et, dans son sillage, le liseré préosseux, d'épaisseur remarquablement constante. La Fig. 4 traduit la même image en fluorescence. C'est elle qui va nous permettre de mesurer l'allure de la résorption.

Le liseré préosseux, tel qu'il existait au moment du sacrifice, tel qu'on le voit en lumière normale dans la Fig. 3, est maintenant illuminé en fluorescence par la dose terminale d'alizarine. Les deux autres bandes fluorescentes de la partie supérieure de l'illustration marquent les stratifications qui se sont déposées depuis le jour de

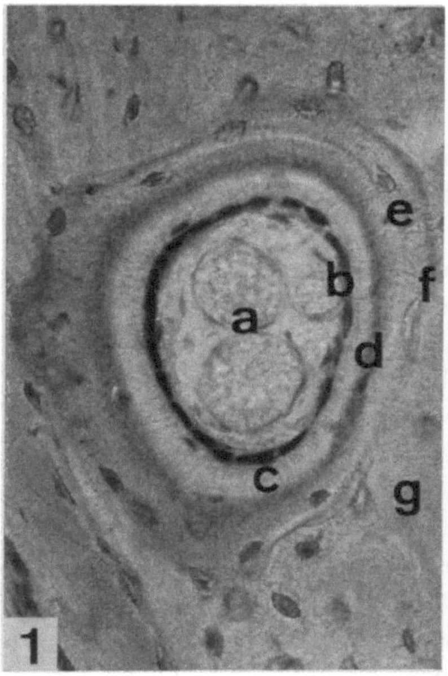

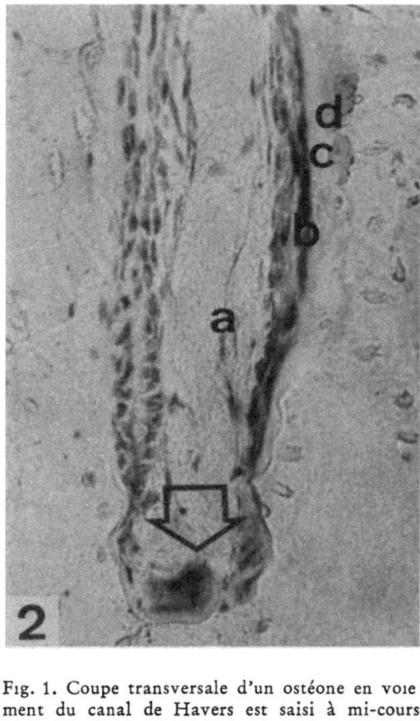

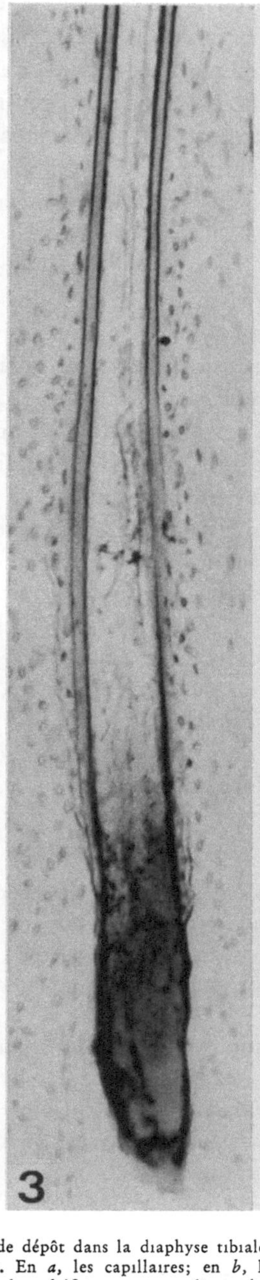

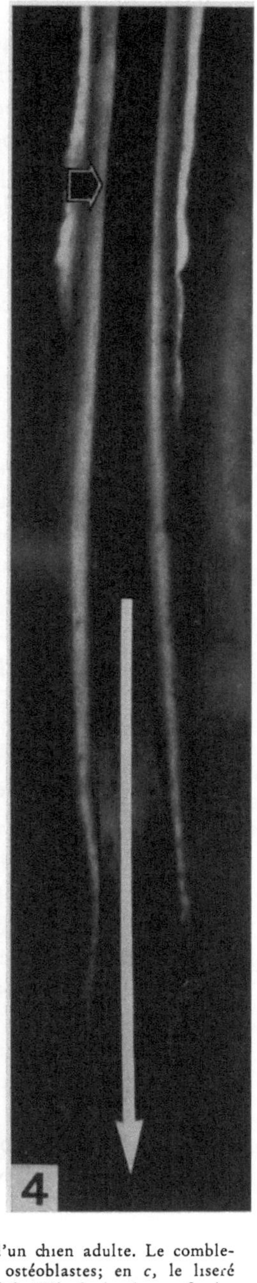

Fig. 1. Coupe transversale d'un ostéone en voie de dépôt dans la diaphyse tibiale d'un chien adulte. Le comblement du canal de Havers est saisi à mi-course. En *a*, les capillaires; en *b*, les ostéoblastes; en *c*, le liseré préosseux; en *d*, la ligne-frontière où commence la calcification; en *e*, l'os calcifié à 75% de la charge finale; en *f*, la ligne cimentante et, en *g*, l'os ancien au sein duquel s'était creusé le canal par les processus que vont étudier les figures suivantes. (×347)

Fig. 2. Coupe longitudinale passant par l'extrémité d'un canal de Havers en voie d'extension. Diaphyse tibiale d'un chien adulte. La flèche désigne un gros ostéoclaste, les lettres correspondent à celles de la figure précédente. (×222)

Fig. 3. Coupe longitudinale de la diaphyse radiale d'un chien adulte intéressant un canal de Havers qui s'étend à son extrémité inférieure et qui se comble dans les trois quarts supérieurs de l'image. L'orientation rigoureusement axiale de la coupe est attestée par l'épaisseur uniforme de liseré préosseux. (×107)

Fig. 4. Région identique à celle de la figure précédente, mais photographiée en lumière ultra-violette. La flèche noire indique l'épaisseur du tissu nouveau déposé en dix-sept jours. Pendant ce temps, la résorption a progressé d'une distance au moins égale à la longueur de la flèche blanche. (×107)

l'injection jusqu'au jour où la tétracycline a disparu du sang. L'une de ces deux bandes, celle de droite, se prolonge vers le bas par une ligne grêle qui, d'après les corrélations, n'est autre que la ligne cimentante. Celle-ci s'est donc constitutée à cet endroit pendant les tout premiers jours de l'expérience.

Il s'agit de superposer à cette Fig. 4 la situation du trépan au jour de l'injection de tétracycline, dix-sept jours avant le sacrifice.

Il est vraisemblable, d'après ce que nous venons de dire de la portion fluorescente de la ligne cimentante, que le trépan se trouvait alors à un niveau très proche de celui de l'extrémité inférieure de la ligne grêle, illuminant la ligne cimentante. Toutefois, afin d'écarter d'avance toute surestimation possible de l'allure, certainement rapide, de la résorption, nous plaçons délibérément ce niveau bien au-dessous.

En dix-sept jours, la résorption a progressé d'une distance au moins égale à la longueur de la flèche blanche.

Quelle est la mesure correspondante de l'apposition? Au maximum, la distance qui va de la surface extérieure à la surface intérieure des deux fourreaux fluorescents, distance indiquée par une grosse flèche noire.

Compte tenu du parallélisme des quatre bandes fluorescentes du haut de la Fig. 4, compte tenu de l'épaisseur uniforme du liseré dans les Fig. 3 et 4, on est certain d'avoir sous les yeux une image privilégiée, parfaitement radiaire, permettant une lecture correcte.

Mesurons, sur la photographie, les distances qui nous intéressent, et nous constatons que l'allure linéaire de la résorption est, au moins, seize fois plus rapide que l'allure linéaire de l'apposition.

Cette estimation nous a paru compatible avec d'autres observations recueillies de façon analogue, chez le chien adulte.

Summary

1. The boring of Haversian canals has been studied in the diaphyseal compact bone of adult dog, by fluorescence microscopy.

2. Longitudinal sections are more useful than transverse serial sections. They show that the reconstruction process follows immediately in the wake of the destruction process (Fig. 2 to 4).

3. The linear destruction rate is much faster than the linear reconstruction rate (sixteen times faster in the example illustrated by Figs. 3 and 4).

4. It follows that, in a given sample of bone tissue, where destruction and reconstruction are in equilibrium, surfaces covered with osteoblasts are much more extensive than surfaces covered with osteoclasts.

Bibliographie

HANCOX, N. M., and B. BOOTHROYD: Ultrastructure of bone formation and resorption. In Modern Trends in Orthopaedics. CLARK, J. M. P. (ed.). London: Butterworths 1964, p. 26.

Experimental Studies of the Non-inflammatory Vascular Pannus

E. RUTISHAUSER, W. TAILLARD, B. FRIEDLI

Institut de Pathologie, Université de Genève, Genève, Suisse.

Ischemia produces a profound transformation of the vascularization of the osteo-articular tissue. A vascular bud of tissue sprouts from the articular capsule and becomes adherent to the cartilaginous surface (the surface or articular pannus). There is stasis and arterial ischemia in the bone marrow, particularly pronounced at the epiphyseal extremities, and the articular plate is invaded by histiocytic and vascular buds which constitute the internal pannus. This phenomenon has already been recognized in human pathology (RUTISHAUSER, 1963), and the present paper is an experimental contribution to its study.

Material

Series I: In 50 young adult rabbits, ischemia of the femoral bone marrow was produced by injection of a carbon suspension into the femoral nutrient artery or by intramedullary injection of a thrombin solution. The techniques used, and the diaphyseal and metaphyseal lesions observed in these animals have been described (RUTISHAUSER *et al.*, 1960).

Series II: In 14 young adult rabbits, the lateral vascular connections of the patella were severed along with the insertions of the vasti lateralis and medialis (HUGUENIN-VIRCHAUX, to be published).

Series III: The neck of the right femur and the sciatic nerve of 17 young adult rabbits were severed.

Results

Series I: Both methods used in this series yielded identical results. In 35 of the animals, the circulatory disturbances produced by the injection did not affect the epiphyseal regions, and the joints remained normal. In the other 15, alterations in the epiphyseal circulation were noted, and the joints also showed discrete but definite changes. One animal (033), after 23 days, presented some of the most marked articular effects. There was a deepening of the coxo-femoral recesses, and the synovial villi were characterized by congestion, edema, and proliferation of the synovial cells. The congested periosteum invaded the cartilage, which presented a fuso-cellular metaplasia of chondrocytes. The terminal plate was partially destroyed (Fig. 1 a).

This same rabbit also presented alterations in the distal femoral epiphysis. The epiphyseal marrow and the cruciate ligaments were congested. From the bases of the ligaments there were fibro-capillary expansions into the cartilage (Fig. 1 b).

Fig. 2 a (103, 5 days) is an example of more discrete, though clearly noticeable, articular alterations. Near the cruciate ligaments, vessels penetrated the terminal plate, reached the cartilage, and provoked a fuso-cellular metaplasia. The edges of the femoral cartilage were reduced by a border of fuso-cellular tissue which contained small vessels.

Series II: The patella was the site of vascular congestion and of active peri- and endosteal resorption. The cartilage was eroded from the periphery by periosteal vascular buds and showed, at some distance from these buds, a chondrocytic multiplication and fuso-cellular metaplasia. The cortical bone showed a few foci of

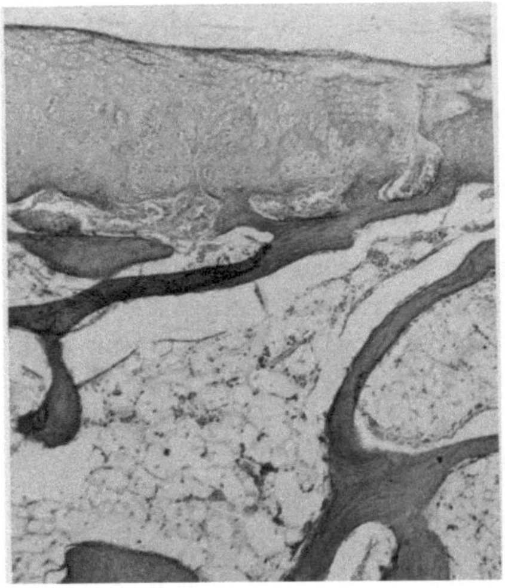

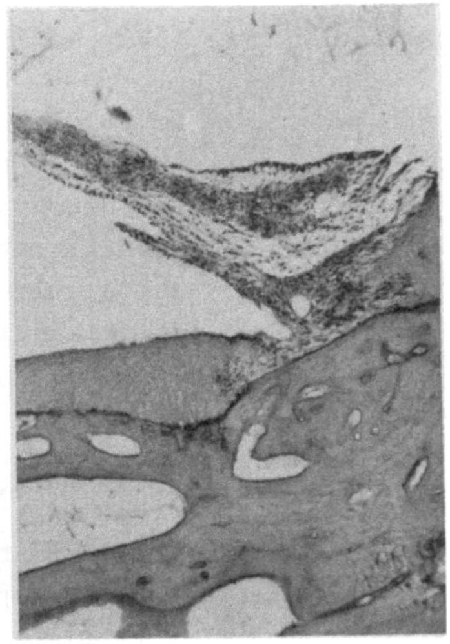

Fig. 1a. Series I. Rabbit no. 033; 23 days. Van Gieson. ×57.5. Internal border of the articular margin of the femoral head. Epiphyseal congestion; the modification of the osseous plate is very marked. A pannus slides over the cartilage, at the same time as the latter is partially destroyed by the medullary pannus

Fig. 1b. Series I. Rabbit no. 033; 23 days. Van Gieson. ×47.5. Cellular hyperplasia; congestion and edema of cruciate ligament. Erosion of the cartilage

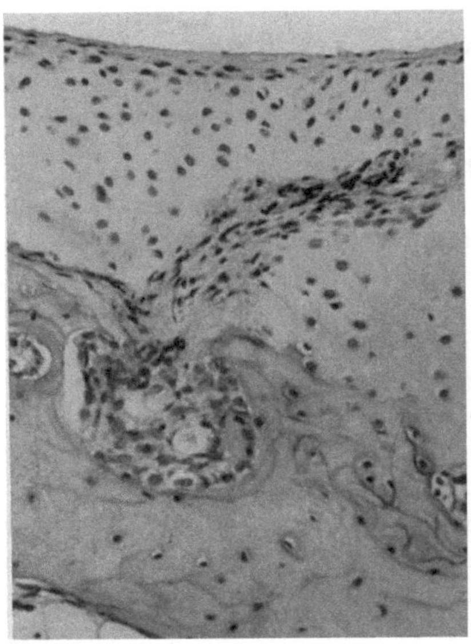

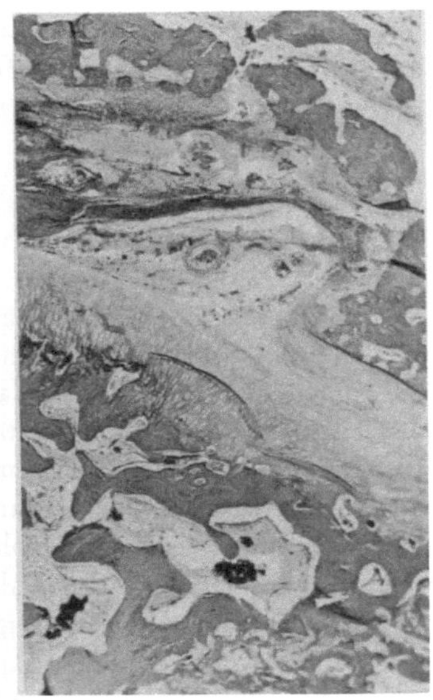

Fig. 2a. Series II. Rabbit no. 103; 5 days. Hem.-Eosin. ×128. Knee, femoral epiphysis. The articular plate (near the cruciate ligament) presents a focus of modification from which departs a growth of fusocellular metaplasia of the cartilage without capillary contact

Fig. 2b. Series III. Rabbit no. 11; 56 days. Van Gieson. ×20. Articular pannus in activity, splitting the cartilaginous plate

resorption by fibrovascular sprouts from its medullary side. These transformations were greatest after about 3 or 4 weeks and then regressed.

Series III: Fig. 3 illustrates the case of an animal (11) sacrificed 56 days after low cervical osteotomy. The fracture had healed spontaneously with external tilting of the head. In the metaphyseal marrow, which was poorly vascularized, a few enlarged veins were visible. Hemopoietic tissue was absent, and the internal part of the cortex had become spongy. The articular space was greatly enlarged. The territory of the artery of the ligamentum teres formed a triangle of densified bone, and the ligament and its insertion in the socket were enlarged. From it, as well as from the articular capsule, fibrovascular growths (vascular pannus) emerged. This pannus war irregularly developed and hyalinized over 2/3 of its course. The action of the internal pannus upon the modification of the external table of the socket is especially visible at this magnification.

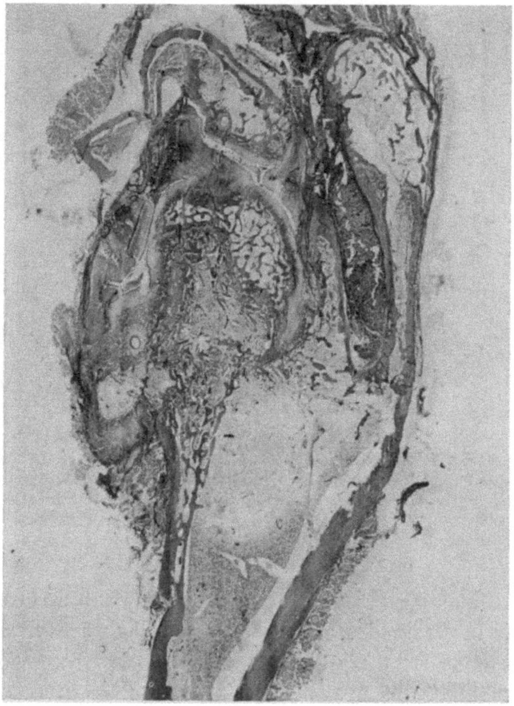

Fig. 3. Series III. Rabbit no. 11; 56 days. Van Gieson. ×2. Topographical view (see text)

The internal extremity of the coxo-femoral articulation was obliterated by a congested external capsular pannus (Fig. 2 b) in front of which the cartilage underwent a lysis and was split longitudinally into two sheets of equal thickness. The marrow was markedly congested and showed fibro-vascular sprouts eroding the terminal plate and reaching the cartilage (internal pannus).

Fig. 4 (rabbit 5) shows the effect of the operation after 28 days. A well limited medullary territory showed congestion, plasmostasis, and reticular hyperplasia as well as absence of hematopoiesis. An avascular layer of cuboidal cells covered the cartilage of the femoral head; the latter showed zones of chondrocytic activation and chondrolysis which, in 2 foci, had formed cysts. Serial sections showed these cysts to have no topographical relation to the articular surface or to the blood vessels.

The results of Series I, II, and III show that a local reduction of circulation modifies the different tissues of an articulation. The consequent stasis is accompanied by a fibro-vascular expansion originating in the synovial membrane and in the vascularized ligaments of the knee (Series I: Fig. 1 a, 1 b) and of the hip (Series III: Fig. 2 b); also a medullary pannus arises in the marrow. These external and internal pannuses constitute the elements responsible for the modification of the osteo-cartilaginous plate of the articulation. Certain modifications of the cartilage cannot be accounted for by direct contact with the pannus; this suggests that the action of the latter is perhaps mediated by the diffusion of some humoral factor.

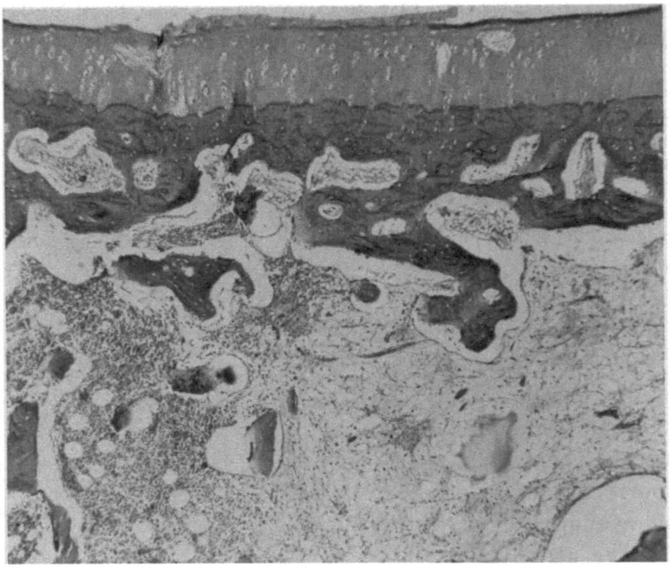

Fig. 4. Series III. Rabbit no. 5; 28 days. Hem.-Eosin. ×52.5. Socket in the region of the insertion of the ligamentum teres. To the left, marrow hardly altered, active hemopoiesis. To the right, ischemic alterations of the marrow (reticulosis). An avascular surface pannus. Alterations of the cartilage due to humoral derangement. 2 cartilaginous cysts are visible

Discussion

The aim of reproducing relatively simple examples of vascular pannuses was only partly attained in the experiments of Series I and II. The involvement of the articular regions in the circulatory disturbances produced by the injection methods (Series I) is inconstant. When the patella is isolated from its lateral vascular connections (Series II), an effective collateral circulation develops and starts to normalize the local condition after 4 weeks. However, this technique seems to us to be the most satisfactory. The operation is simple and does not entail a direct interference with articular function. The division of the femoral neck initiates a pathological condition which resembles that described by Rokkanen (1962) in his excellent monograph. Experiments of immobilization and remobilization have been carried out by Mastromarino and Maiotti (1956) on the rabbit and by Evans *et al.* (1960) on the rat. Here again the histopathological picture resembles that which we have described; however, these authors reach more limited conclusions than those to which our findings have led us. In any case, their method is even more complicated than ours.

Conclusions

Articular ischemia achieved in the rabbit by different experimental procedures resulted in a typical transformation of the joints concerned. The terminal plate was simultaneously eroded by outgrowths of periosteal and synovial tissue (surface or intra-articular pannuses) and by sprouts of vasculo-reticular tissue from the marrow spaces (internal or medullary pannuses).

These findings parallel closely certain aspects observed in posttraumatic or gerontologic joint pathology. It is suggested that local ischemia is an essential factor in the pathogenesis of degenerative and postinflammatory arthroses.

References

Evans, E. B., G. W. N. Eggers, J. K. Butler, and J. Blumel: Experimental immobilization and remobilization of rat knee joints. J. Bone Jt Surg. **42 A**, 737 (1960).

Mastromarino R., e A. Maiotti: Ricerche sperimentali sugli effetti dell'immobilizzazione e sulla ripresa funzionale in articolazioni normali. Riv. Ortop. Traumatol. **24**, 173 (1956).

Rokkanen, P.: Rôle of surgical intervention of the hip joint in the aetiology of aseptic necrosis of the femoral head. Acta orthop. scand. Suppl. **58** (1962).

Rutishauser, E.: Kreislaufstörungen im Knochensystem. Verh. dtsch. path. Ges. **47**, 91 (1963).

—, A. Rohner und D. Held: Experimentelle Untersuchungen über die Wirkung der Ischämie auf den Knochen und das Mark. Virchows Arch. path. Anat. **333**, 101 (1960).

Urinary Pyrophosphate in Disorders of Bone Metabolism

L. V. Avioli, Ph. H. Henneman

Division of Endocrinology, Department of Medicine,
New Jersey College of Medicine and Dentistry, Jersey City, N. J., U.S.A.

The identification of pyrophosphate in bone by Perkins and Walker (1958) and its inhibitory role in hydroxyapatite precipitation noted by Fleisch and Bisaz (1962) suggested that pyrophosphate played an important role in bone formation and remodeling processes. The present study was undertaken to investigate urinary pyrophosphate excretion in patients with diseases characterized by accelerated rates of bone turnover. Concomitant measurements were also made of urinary hydroxyproline and total inorganic phosphorus.

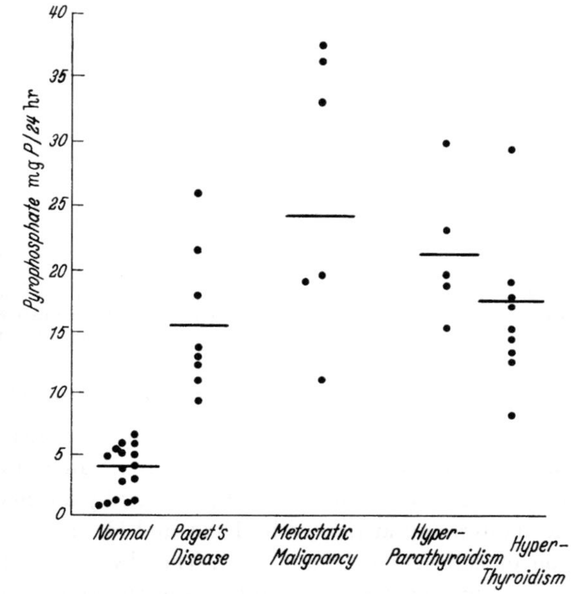

Fig. 1. Pyrophosphate excretion in normal adults and in patients with bone disease. Black circles represent the average pyrophosphate values of two consecutive 24-hr urinary collections; horizontal bar in each group represents calculated mean values

Methods

Pyrophosphate was isolated from duplicate 1.0 ml aliquots of cold homogenized 24-hour urine samples by a modification of the differential acid elution methods of Fleisch and Bisaz (1962). The completeness of orthophosphate-pyrophosphate recovery was substantiated by the recovery of known amounts of stable and radioactive ortho- and pyrophosphate from human urine and the completeness of separation was demonstrated by thin layer chromatographic techniques. Total urinary hydroxyproline was measured in hydrolyzed urine samples by the method of Prockop and Udenfriend (1960) and inorganic phosphate according to the method of Fiske and Subbarow (1925). Microphosphate determinations on hydrolyzed pyrophosphate eluates were made by a modification of the method of Chen *et al.* (1956).

Results

Urinary pyrophosphate excretion in normal adult subjects and in patients with increased bone turnover are illustrated in Fig. 1. The normal mean pyrophosphate excretion of 3.99 mg P/24 hr. (S.E. ± 0.45) was much lower than that observed in Paget's disease (15.48 ± 1.76), metastatic bone disease (24.33 ± 4.61), hyperparathyroidism (21.31 ± 4.78), and hyperthyroidism (20.79 ± 2.09). The elevated mean values in subjects with increased bone turnover differed significantly from normal with $P < .001$ in each case. Urinary hydroxyproline excretion was also elevated in the subjects with bone disease and paralleled the observed pyrophosphaturia in each group (Fig. 2). Despite the marked increments in urinary pyrophosphate in disorders of bone metabolism, no correlated changes were noted in orthophosphate excretion.

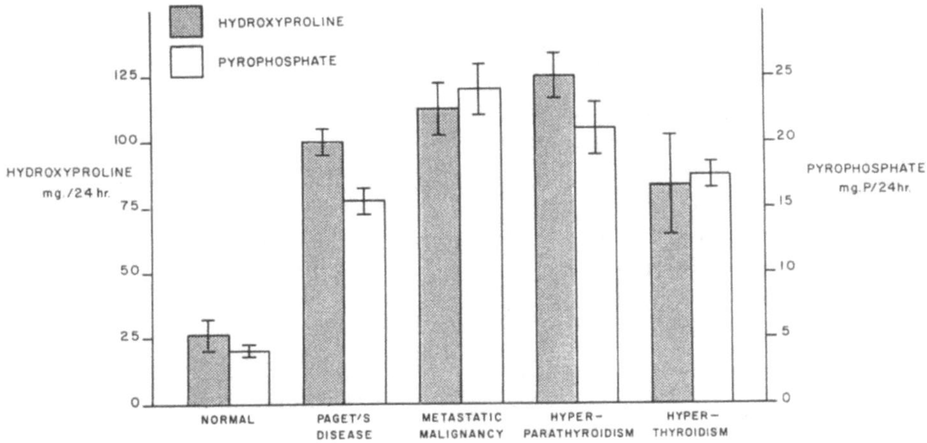

Fig. 2. Urinary pyrophosphate and total hydroxyproline in normals and in patients with bone disease. The height of the horizontal bar in each group represents the respective mean values; I-bars represent twice the standard error about the mean

Comments and conclusions

Recent observations by Fleisch (1964) suggest that the normal 24-hour pyrophosphate excretion corresponds approximately to the amount of bone resorbed daily. Hydroxyprolinuria has been repeatedly documented in clinical disorders of bone metabolism and attributed by Dull and Henneman (1963) to an accelerated resorption of collagenous bone matrix. The observation of parallel increments in urinary hydroxyproline and pyrophosphate in the present study suggests that urinary pyrophosphate is derived primarily from bone dissolution. The significant elevations of urinary pyrophosphate observed in Paget's disease, hyperparathyroidism, metastatic bone disease and hyperthyroidism suggest that pyrophosphate excretion may be as useful an index of bone resorption as is serum alkaline phosphatase for bone formation in patients with accelerated bone turnover.

Acknowledgements

These studies were supported in part by AEC Contract AT(30-1) 3174, USPHS grants AM-5211-05, AM-06404-03, USPHS Clinical Research Center Grant FR-41 and a National Institutes of Medical Science Career Research Development Award (6-K3-GM-22, 676-01A1).

References

CHEN, P. S., T. Y. TORIBARA, and H. WARREN: Microdetermination of phosphorus. Analyt. Chem. **28**, 1756 (1956).

DULL, T. A., and P. H. HENNEMAN: Urinary hydroxyproline as an index of collagen turnover in bone. New Engl. J. Med. **268**, 132 (1963).

FISKE, C. H., and Y. SUBBAROW: The colorimetric determination of phosphorus. J. biol. Chem. **66**, 375 (1925).

FLEISCH, H., and S. BISAZ: Isolation from urine of pyrophosphate, a calcification inhibitor. Amer. J. Physiol. **203**, 671 (1962).

— — Role of collagen, pyrophosphate and pyrophosphatase in calcification. In Bone and Tooth. BLACKWOOD, H. J. J. (ed.). Oxford: Pergamon Press 1964, p. 249.

PERKINS, H. R., and P. G. WALKER: The occurrence of pyrophosphate in bone. J. Bone Jt Surg. **40 B**, 333 (1958).

PROCKOP, D. J., and S. UDENFRIEND: A specific method for the analysis of hydroxyproline in tissues and urine. Analyt. Biochem. **1**, 228 (1960).

Bone Formation and Resorption in Bone Disorders

J. JOWSEY

Mayo Clinic, Rochester, Minn. U.S.A.

The recognition of the majority of disorders of skeletal bone depends largely upon their radiological appearance. The various pathological processes may then be further differentiated by alteration in such biochemical parameters as the plasma calcium and phosphorus levels.

The gross changes demonstrated by x-ray examination represent a change in the balance between formation and resorption of tissue but do not measure either of these two processes independently; it was in order to define the relative contribution of formation and resorption to bone structure that the method of quantitative microradiography of bone was developed and applied to the study of skeletal disorders.

This brief report compares bone turnover, that is, formation and resorption, in a number of normal individuals with values obtained from subjects suffering from the more common disorders of the skeleton.

Method

The technique of quantitative microradiography (JOWSEY, 1960; JOWSEY *et al.*, 1965) depends on the analysis of formation and resorption of bone seen on a micro-x-ray of a thin slice of calcified bone taken from a biopsy. These two processes are recognised by the distribution of mineral seen in the microradiograph. Extensive correlative studies (JOWSEY *et al.*, 1965) have demonstrated the validity of this method in measuring only formation and resorption and not other processes occurring simultaneously in this tissue. Formation and resorption take place on the surfaces of the bone and the results presented in this report are based on quantitation of the length of surface undergoing either formation or resorption expressed as a percentage of the total surface examined.

Hyperparathyroidism and hypoparathyroidism

Radiological evidence of bone disease is present only in some cases of primary hyperparathyroidism; more frequently renal stones and invariably an elevated blood calcium and lowered phosphorus level are the presenting features of this disorder. In this communication a series of twenty-seven patients were studied of whom seven had bone disease visible on x-ray while the remainder did not. Quantitative microradiography demonstrated that resorption is elevated in all cases, the average value for this group being +5.7 standard deviations. Bone formation levels were normal in two thirds and elevated in one third of the cases.

It would seem, therefore, that increased resorption is characteristic of all cases of primary hyperparathyroidism and that the x-ray appearance recognises only instances where resorption is extensive or has been going on for some time. The increased formation in a third of the cases tends to mask any increase in porosity of the bone produced by the high level of resorption.

Hypoparathyroidism can result from either accidental removal of the parathyroid glands in thyroidectomy or, less frequently, from idiopathic lack of function of the parathyreoid tissue. The blood and urine calcium levels are low but the x-ray appears normal. The five cases reported here include two surgical parathyroidectomies and three individuals with idiopathic hypoparathyroidism. Quantitation of bone formation and resorption demonstrated both to be reduced, resorption to a significantly lower level with formation in the low normal range.

Osteoporosis

The x-ray picture of osteoporosis is typical of an extensive loss of bone tissue from the skeleton, this being particularly evident in the spine where crush fractures of the vertebrae and ballooning of the intervertebral spaces follow from the loss of bone.

The diagnosis of osteoporosis in the present study has been based on the radiological examination, the blood calcium and phosphorus levels being normal and other causes of osteoporosis, such as multiple myeloma, being excluded. Direct measurements of formation and resorption in seventy-two cases of idiopathic or senile osteoporosis by the method of quantitative microradiography demonstrate an increase in the amount of bone resorption while the level of formation falls within normal limits. It appears therefore that an increase in the level of resorption is the prime factor in the loss of bone tissue in this disorder.

Cushing's disease

Generalised decreased density on x-ray is found in Cushing's syndrome; prolonged therapy with cortisone will also produce loss of bone mass, particularly in the spine and often in a few months. The fourteen cases presented here showed osteoporosis as the result of either exogenous or endogenous hypercortisonism. Resorption was elevated, often considerably, in all but four cases. Formation was reduced in all cases, values in nine cases falling below two standard deviations from the normal. The osteoporosis of hypercortisonism, therefore, differs from idiopathic or senile osteoporosis in that, as well as the increased resorption which contributes most importantly to the loss of bone, there is a decrease in bone formation.

Bed-rest

Immobilization has been shown to result in decreased density of the skeleton (HEANEY, 1962); therefore any individuals who had more than four days of bed-rest were excluded from the main part of the study.

Such individuals fell into two groups, namely "normal" individuals who had no bone disorder and osteoporotic individuals who had been in bed from four to seventeen days. The results of measurements of formation and resorption in fourteen

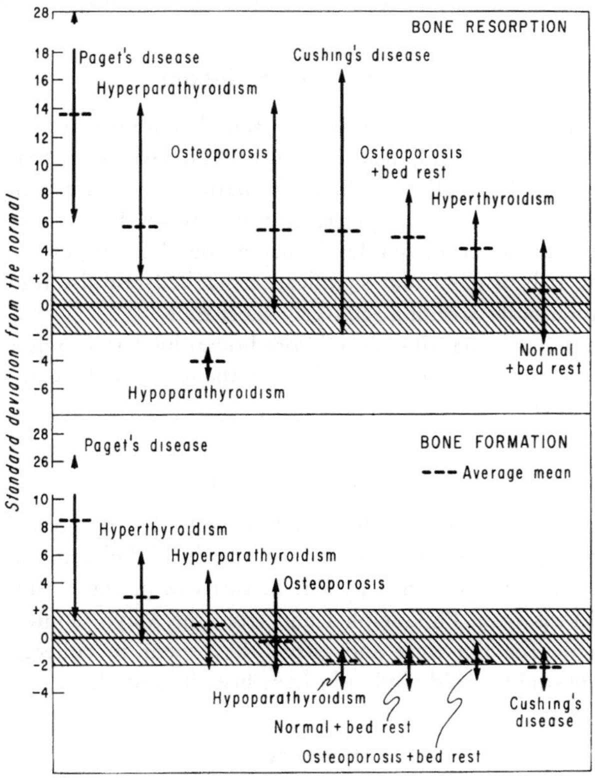

Fig. 1. Bone resorption and formation in some disorders of the skeleton

individuals from each of these groups suggested that the result of bed-rest was to depress bone formation. Bone resorption was within normal levels in the group with no bone disease and characteristically elevated in the osteoporotic individuals.

Hyperthyroidism

Osteoporosis or decreased density of the skeleton on x-ray is frequently associated with hyperthyroidism. The five cases reported here show an increase in the level of the resorption of bone in all but one case, and two of the five also demonstrate an increase in the level of bone formation. The values are similar to those seen in osteoporotic bone but the levels of formation appear to be higher.

Paget's disease

Paget's disease differs from other conditions discussed in this report in that it is a localised lesion and is not considered as a metabolic abnormality. The x-ray changes seen in this disease are dramatic and are characterised by an increase in the volume of localised areas of bone accompanied by a decrease in the density. Histology demonstrates many cement lines associated with a great deal of formation and resorption of bone. Quantitative microradiography has not really added much to our knowledge; the study of fourteen specimens show the very high levels of both resorption and formation that are to be predicted from the histological picture.

Summary and conclusions

Decreased skeletal density is a frequently found radiological appearance in most bone disorders and can be explained, in terms of turnover measurements, by an increased resorption of bone (Fig. 1). Bone formation levels are increased in a percentage of subjects suffering from hyperparathyroidism and hyperthyroidism and in all cases of Paget's disease, decreased levels being found in hypoparathyroidism and hypercortisonism. It is of particular significance that bed-rest also results in a decrease in bone formation usually within a relatively short time.

The introduction of quantitative microradiography has provided a measure of bone turnover, which can explain radiological changes and further characterise the various bone disorders.

Acknowledgements

A large part of this study has depended on collection of normal material from different institutions, in particular the city morgues in Philadelphia and Minneapolis; pathological material was provided by Dr. L. Lutwak of the National Institutes of Health, Dr. S. Lewis from Philadelphia and from the Mayo Clinic. I would like to thank these people for the time and effort they spent in collecting the material without which the study would obviously have been impossible.

References

Heaney, R. P.: Radiocalcium metabolism in disuse osteoporosis in man. Amer. J. Med. **33**, 188 (1962).

Jowsey, J.: Age changes in human bone. Clin. Orthop. **17**, 210 (1960).

—, P. J. Kelly, B. L. Riggs, A. J. Bianco, D. A. Scholz, and J. Gershon-Cohen: Quantitative microradiographic studies of normal and osteoporotic bone. J. Bone Jt Surg. **47-A**, 785; 872 (1965).

Studies of Iliac Crest Bone from Controls and Patients with Bone Disease by Means of Chemical Analysis, Tetracycline Labelling and Histology

J. C. Birkenhäger, J. van der Sluys Veer, R. O. van der Heul, D. Smeenk

Department for Clinical Endocrinology and Metabolism and Department for Pathology, Academisch Ziekenhuis, Leiden, Nederland.

1. Introduction

In 1964 van der Sluys Veer *et al.*, showed that in hyperparathyroidism tetracycline labelling of iliac crest bone is increased in the majority of cases.

In Cushing's syndrome tetracycline uptake by bone was found to vary from values below to values definitively above the normal range even among cases with the same degree of osteoporosis as measured histologically (van der Heul *et al.*, 1964).

In the present study of bone from cases of hyperparathyroidism or hyperadrenocorticism we have tried to correlate the degree of mineralization assessed by chemical methods with the degree of tetracycline labelling.

2. Material and methods

The study comprised iliac crest bone biopsy material from eighteen patients with hyperparathyroidism, eleven patients with Cushing's syndrome, three patients who were treated with high doses of prednisone and thirteen controls. The material from the controls was not submitted to a tetracycline uptake study.

The method of measurement of tetracycline uptake and the histological methods have been described earlier (van der Sluys Veer *et al.*, 1964). For chemical analysis a small part of cancellous bone was ground and washed with distilled water. After defatting and powdering the bone was freed of water by drying to a constant weight over anhydrous potassium carbonate (Birkenhäger-Frenkel *et al.*, 1961). The bone was hydrolysed for five hours at 140 °C with 6 N hydrochloric acid. Phosphorus (Fiske and Subbarow, 1925, modified) and hydroxyproline (Kivirikko and Liesmaa, 1959) were estimated after neutralization with sodium hydroxide.

3. Results

A. Hyperparathyroidism

In the cases of hyperparathyroidism a high percentage of tetracycline labelled bone surface (average 32%, range 16—49%) was found. This confirms the results of earlier studies when an average of 25% was found in eighteen cases of hyperparathyroidism and an average of 12% in seventeen controls (van der Sluys Veer *et al.*, 1964). Histologically in nearly all cases an increase in the number of osteoblasts, osteoclasts, osteoid seams and fibrosis was seen.

The results of the chemical analysis in hyperparathyroidism and in the control group are shown in Fig. 1. The phosphorus content averaged 92.4 (range 80.8 to 100.9) μg per mg (hydrated) bone in hyperparathyroidism and 100.7 (range 97.3 to 103.3) μg per mg bone in the controls.

In hyperparathyroidism the average hydroxyproline content of bone was about the same as that of the controls, but in the former group the range was considerably wider, 29.5—40.2 as compared to 31.6—35.7 μg per mg bone. The average phosphorus-hydroxyproline ratio (P/PH) was significantly lower in hyperparathyroidism than in the controls.

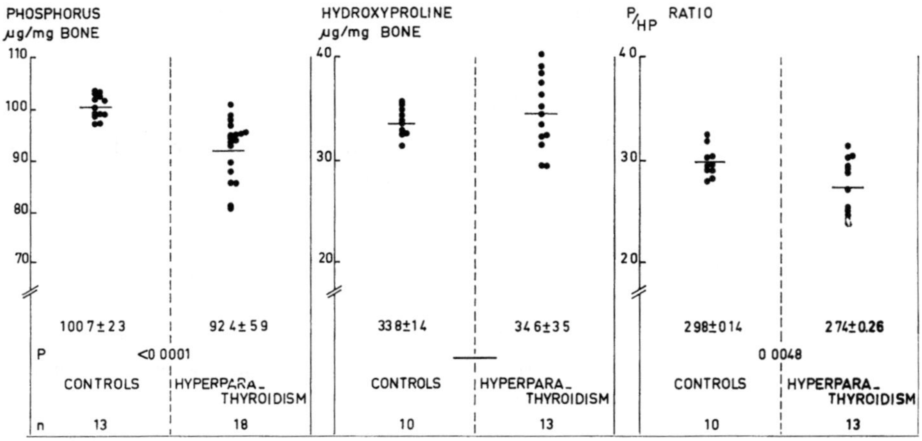

Fig. 1. Phosphorus and hydroxyproline content (and their ratio) of iliac crest bone from controls and patients with hyperparathyroidism. Averages ± S.D.

B. Hyperadrenocorticism

In the bone from seven cases of Cushing's syndrome and from two patients treated with prednisone the percentage of tetracycline labelled surface varied from

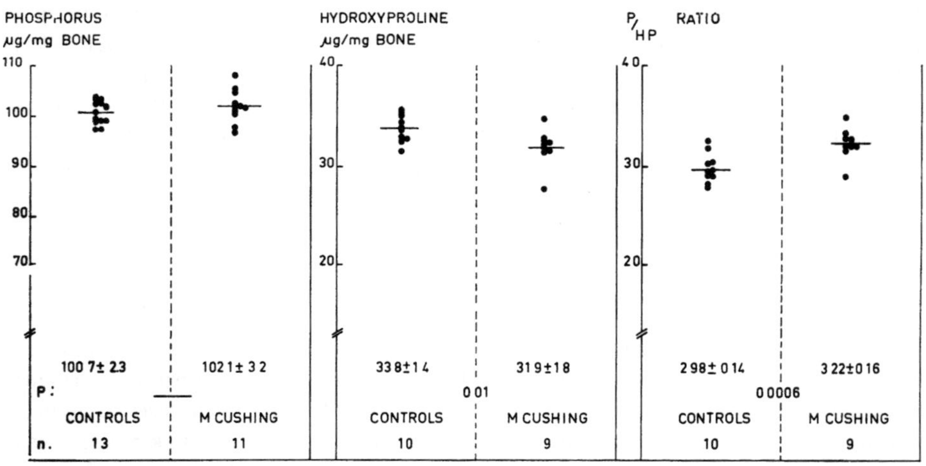

Fig. 2. Phosphorus and hydroxyproline content (and their ratio) of iliac crest bone from controls and patients with Cushing's syndrome or under prednisone treatment. Averages ± S.D.

2—25% with an average of 14%. The average phosphorus content of bone in Cushing's syndrome or cases under prednisone treatment did not differ statistically from that in the control group, whereas the average hydroxyproline content appeared to be significantly lower than normal (Fig. 2). Consequently the P/HP ratio was found to be significantly higher than normal.

The nine cases of hyperadrenocorticism for which a P/HP ratio is given, showed histologically a decreased amount of trabecular bone (13%, range 6—18%), as compared with the controls (20%, range 18—24%, van der Heul *et al.*, 1964).

4. Discussion

The degree of variability of the results of the chemical analysis is illustrated by the data in Table 1, in which bone from the left and right iliac crest is compared.

Table 1. *Chemical analysis of human iliac crest bone*

Subject	Phosphorus µg/mg bone		Hydroxyproline µg/mg bone		P/HP	
	left	right	left	right	left	right
1	97.6	101.4	34.7	36.2	2.81	2.80
2	95.7	98.9	32.3	32.3	2.96	2.94
3	104.1	103.7	32.3	33.1	3.22	3.13

The low phosphorus content which was found in most cases of hyperparathyroidism is in agreement with the abnormally low mineral content found by microradiography (Smeenk, 1961). To eliminate the expression of one variable (the mineral or collagen content) in another dependent one (the weight of the bone) (Arnold, 1960), we have used the phosphorus-hydroxyproline ratio.

Changes in the P/HP ratio, however, leave the question open whether they are due to a change in the phosphorus or the hydroxyproline content. In hyperparathyroidism the relative decrease of the P/HP ratio is less conspicuous than that of the phosphorus content per mg bone. This suggests that there is an increased water content of bone in addition to the subnormal degree of mineralization which exists in hyperparathyroidism. Concerning the high P/HP ratio (and the decreased hydroxyproline content per mg bone) in bone in Cushing's syndrome it is not possible to decide from our data alone whether the alteration is caused by an abnormally high bone salt content or an abnormally low collagen content per unit of bone volume.

This is due to the fact that bone salt constitutes such an important part of the weight of bone that an abnormally high bone salt content per unit of volume is not so easily reflected in a high bone salt content per unit of weight, whereas it may entail an abnormally low hydroxyproline content per unit of weight. However, in osteoporosis in elderly people Mrs. Birkenhäger-Frenkel (in press) has recently found a low hydroxyproline content of iliac crest bone, both per unit of volume and of weight, with a high P/HP ratio. The normal values she found for phosphorus and hydroxyproline per unit of bone weight agree reasonably well with ours. These findings in osteoporosis of hyperadrenocorticism and in osteoporosis of elderly people suggest the existence of "collagen-deficient" bone in developing or established osteoporosis. In using hydroxyproline as representative of collagen we are conscious of the fact that it is not known whether in pathologic conditions the collagen molecule still contains the normal amount of hydroxyproline (13.6% of weight).

It has been shown in different cases of Cushing's syndrome but with the same degree of osteoporosis that osteoblastic activity and tetracycline uptake may vary from subnormal to higher than normal (van der Heul *et al.*, 1964). This suggests that in this condition bone disease is initiated by an increase of bone resorption. This view is supported by the finding of a normal (Sissons, 1956) or sometimes increased (van der Heul *et al.*, 1964) osteoclasis in histologic studies, and of the primary catabolic effect of corticoids in kinetic studies with a bone-seeking tracer (Gordan and Eisenberg, 1963).

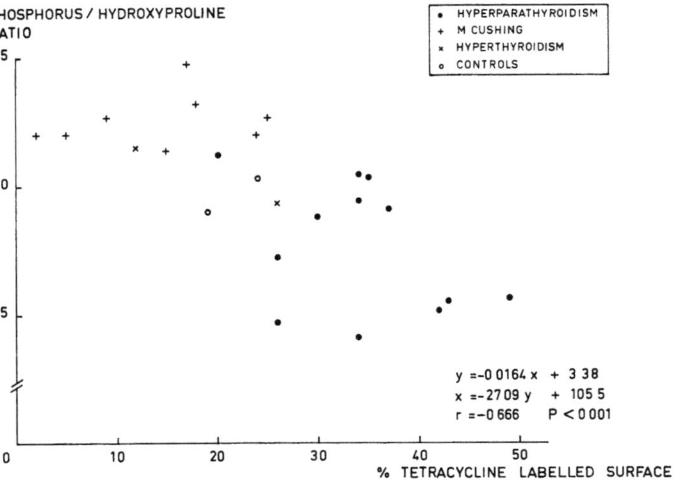

Fig. 3. Correlation between the phosphorus-hydroxyproline ratio and percentage tetracycline labelled bone surface in iliac crest bone

In Fig. 3 a negative correlation is shown between the percentage tetracycline-labelled bone surface and the P/HP ratio of bone from the groups of patients with hyperparathyroidism or hyperadrenocorticism, from two patients with hyperthyroidism and from two controls. As the P/HP ratio reflects the average degree of mineralization it could be expected that bone with a low P/HP ratio contains a relatively large amount of bone with a very low degree of mineralization and consequently will show a high tetracycline uptake. The P/HP ratio appears to be independent of age in the three groups studied (hyperparathyroidism, hyperadrenocorticism and control group) as can be seen in Fig. 4.

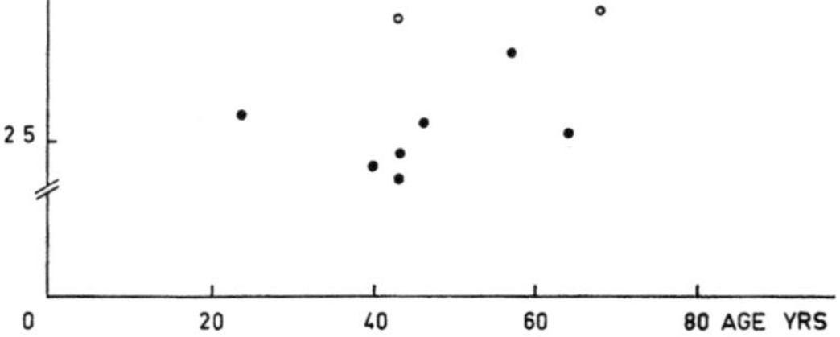

Fig. 4. Phosphorus-hydroxyproline ratio of iliac crest bone plotted against age

Summary

1. Iliac crest bone from patients suffering from hyperparathyroidism and hyperadrenocorticism was studied chemically (phosphorus and hydroxyproline content), histologically and by means of tetracyline labelling.

2. In hyperparathyroidism a low phosphorus content, a low phosphorus-hydroxyproline ratio and a high percentage of tetracycline labelling was found; histologically the bone showed the signs of a high turnover rate.

3. In hyperadrenocorticism the bone (which was shown to be porotic) contained a normal amount of phosphorus and a subnormal amount of hydroxyproline per mg bone, resulting in a higher than normal phosphorus-hydroxyproline ratio. Tetracycline labelling varied from subnormal to higher than normal.

4. There was a negative correlation between the percentage tetracycline labelled bone surface and the phosphorus-hydroxyproline ratio when the data from the various groups of patients were combined.

Acknowledgement

The authors are very grateful to Miss INGEBORG B. A. M. VAN DER BRAND for expert technical assistance.

References

ARNOLD, J. S.: Quantitation of mineralization of bone as an organ and tissue in osteoporosis. Clin. Orthop. **17**, 167 (1960).

BIRKENHÄGER-FRENKEL, D. H.: Hydroxyproline and mineral content of osteoporotic bone. (in press).

—, J. J. GROEN, J. A. BÉDIER DE PRAIRIE, and F. G. J. OFFERIJNS: A simple physico-chemical method of assessment of osteoporosis. Voeding **22**, 634 (1961).

FISKE, C. H., and Y. SUBBAROW: The colorimetric determination of phosphorus. J. biol. Chem. **66**, 375 (1925).

GORDAN, G. S., and E. EISENBERG: The effect of oestrogens, androgens and corticoids on skeletal kinetics in man. Proc. roy. Soc. Med. **56**, 31 (1963).

HEUL, R. O. VAN DER, J. VAN DER SLUYS VEER, and D. SMEENK: Histological aspects of osteoporosis. In L'Ostéoporose. HIOCO, D. J. (ed.). Paris: Masson 1964, p. 25.

KIVIRIKKO, K. I., and M. LIESMAA: A colorimetric method for determination of hydroxyproline in tissue hydrolysates. Scand. J. clin. Lab. Invest. **11**, 128 (1959).

SISSONS, H. A.: The osteoporosis of Cushing's syndrome. J. Bone Jt Surg. **38 B**, 418 (1956).

SLUYS VEER, J. VAN DER, D. SMEENK, and R. O. VAN DER HEUL: Tetracycline labelling of bone in hyperparathyroidism. In Bone and Tooth. BLACKWOOD, H. J. J. (ed.). Oxford: Pergamon Press 1964, p. 85.

SMEENK, D.: Studies of bone of patients with hyperparathyroidism by means of phosphate exchange experiments in vitro and quantitative microradiography. J. clin. Invest. **40**, 433 (1961).

Electro-mechanical Factors Regulating Bone Architecture*

C. A. L. Bassett**

The Orthopaedic Research Laboratories, Columbia University, College of Physicians and Surgeons and the New York Orthopaedic Hospital, Columbia Presbyterian Medical Center, New York, N. Y., U.S.A.

Bone has been defined as a hard substance, a mineralized connective tissue, the structural material upon which muscles and ligaments are hung. From early childhood, when man becomes conscious of the meaning of a skeleton, he is aware of the permanence of bone. The surgeon saws it, drills it, screws it, nails it and otherwise treats it very much as he would a piece of oak or pine in his workshop. In fact, its desirable physical properties, such as hardness, elasticity and durability, have prompted men to employ bone in the construction of many diverse items. It has been used in the hunt, as arrowheads and corset stays, and in the pleasures of the parlor, as dice and toothpicks. Truly, bone is a most remarkable substance! Its enduring behavior as an inanimate material, however, is not matched by its conduct in the animate state, for living bone is changing bone.

The capacity of living bone to adapt its structure to meet mechanical demands has been a source of wonder through much of recorded history and forms the basis of many tribal customs. Centuries ago, the concept that skeletal growth could be shaped by properly applied external forces was incorporated in the practice of orthopaedics by men such as Andry (1741). The famous etching, included in his text of 1741, epitomizes this concept; as the twig is bent, so grows the tree — as the bone is bent, so grows the bone. In more recent times, the close relationship between bone architecture and mechanical principles has stimulated much analysis and speculation. Of the many writings on the subject, those of Wolff (1892) are most universally known and are referred to as Wolff's law. Most simply stated by Jansen (1920), this law holds that, "The form of the bone being given, the bone elements place or displace themselves in the direction of the functional pressure". As pointed out by Thompson (1963), the placement and displacement of bone elements is such that they are best oriented to resist compressive and tensile stresses, while being out of the line of shearing stresses. This adaptive mechanism permits the organism to achieve harmony with its surroundings so that it is not limited to a skeletal shape or size pre-determined by inflexible genetic and hormonal factors. Furthermore, in order to meet the challenge of a changing environment, a vertebrate must have the capacity not only to reorient bony elements but also to alter their mass (Wunder *et al.*, 1960). In view of this latter statement, Wolff's law might be improved if amended to state "The form of the bone being given, the bone elements place or displace themselves in the direction of the functional pressure and increase or decrease their mass to reflect the amount of functional pressure". The purpose of this paper is to consider new data that may help clarify the mechanisms by which bone meets the functional demands of mechanical stress. It is hoped that the speculations based upon these data will stimulate a new approach to certain aspects of bone physiology and pathology.

* Supported in part by grants from the U.S. Public Health Service, TI AM 5408, and AM 07822, and the Easter Seal Research Foundation.

** Career Investigator, Health Research Council of the City of New York.

During recent years, the principle of negative feedback (closed loop) control systems, commonly used in the electronics industry, have been applied in biology. In this application, such a system requires an environmental signal, a sensor to detect and convert the signal to a meaningful biologic response (a transducer), and a sensor to translate this response to action which will stop or correct the original environmental signal. McLEAN (1958) has suggested that the serum calcium is regulated by such a five-part mechanism. A low serum calcium is the signal which triggers the parathyroid gland (transducer # 1) to produce parathormone which, in turn, activates osteoclasts (transducer # 2) to release calcium, thereby raising serum calcium and cutting off the original signal. It now is apparent that WOLFF's law probably is another example of a negative feedback control system. In this case, the environmental signal and final correcting response have been known for many years. They are, respectively, a deforming force and a change in bone structure, appropriate to resist the applied force. The mechanisms by which one lead to the other, however, could not be known until the character of the transducers and their responses had been identified.

Since bone is a multicrystalline material, it was postulated in 1951 that it might possess piezo-electric properties (JOHNSON, personal communication). If such were the case, bone would convert a mechanical signal directly to an electrical signal. This type of transducer response is analogous to that of a crystal in the tone arm of a phonograph. In the mid-fifties, the postulate was confirmed independently in Japan and America by the demonstration that electrical potentials were developed by bone when it is deformed (FUKADA and YASUDA, 1957; BASSETT, in press). Although additional evidence has been reported recently to substantiate the fact that mechanical stress evokes an electrical response from bone (BASSETT and BECKER, 1962; SHAMOS *et al.*, 1963), the origin of this response remains obscure. It is evident, however, that the stress-generated potentials are not dependent upon cell viability, are not related directly to membrane potentials and arise, most probably, in the extracellular osseous matrix.

Potential differences are generated in certain types of crystal lattices when charges are separated by pressure on the crystal (MASON, 1950). Similar activity results when thin film p-n junctions[1] are deformed (HUBER, 1963). Furthermore, displacement potentials are generated by bending rod-like polyelectrolytes, such as potassium hyaluronate (CHRISTIANSEN *et al.*, 1961). If each of these charge separation phenomena is classified as piezo-electric, there seems little doubt that the electric potentials produced by stress in bone are also piezo-electric in nature.

While it may be possible to classify pressure-induced charge generation in the crystal lattices of diverse materials as piezo-electric, it is likely that signals generated by different materials will have different characteristics. For example, the internal resistance and capacitance of the crystal can determine the pattern of electrical pulse for a given deforming force. Furthermore, if the signal is produced by a semiconductor, p-n junction device, rectification may possible occur in it or in other devices in the circuit, since current flow across the device is more efficient in forward than in reverse bias. Therefore, it is important not only to demonstrate that electric potentials

[1] A p-n junction is formed in a monocrystalline lattice, such as purified germanium, when impurity atoms with an excess of holes, i.e., a deficit of electrons (p-type doping agents) occupy lattice positions on one side of the crystal and atoms with an excess of electrons (n-type doping agents) the other.

are generated in bone by piezo-electric phenomena, but also to determine the electrical properties of osseous tissue. Extensive studies of these properties have led BECKER (BECKER and BROWN, 1965) to the conclusion that bone possesses most of the known solidstate or semiconductor properties of p-n junctions diodes. Non-living bone demonstrates rectification, photoconductivity and photovoltaic effects suggesting that the crystals of calcium hydroxyapatite have p-type characteristics and the crystals of collagen have n-type. The action spectrum, measured by emission spectroscopy and recombination radiation, is composed of three distinct peaks which suggests further that two different semiconductors are associated. This being the case, bone possesses broader electric capabilities than it would if it were composed only of crystals with simple, classic piezo-electric properties, such as quartz. Under such circumstances, substances such as vitamins, hormones and trace elements, active in minute quantities, may function by changing the electrical properties of bone at the interface between the semiconductors and their bathing electrolytes, as has been demonstrated for cupric ion and germanium crystals (BODDY and BRATTAIN, 1962). These substances also might accomplish similar modifications in behavior by being incorporated into crystal lattices as impurities (doping agents) or by providing for charge transfer (BECKER *et al.*, 1964). Furthermore, it is conceivable that byproducts of aberrant metabolism may alter the electric properties or environment of bone and result in pathologic changes in mass or histologic appearance.

Returning to the concept that WOLFF's law is an example of a negative feedback system, it is possible, on the basis of the foregoing, to identify four of the five steps involved in the mechanism (Fig. 1). The initial, environmental signal is a deforming force. It activates multitudinous, piezo-electric transducers, located in thn extracellular osseous matrix, which generate electric potentials proportional to the applied force. The potentials then stimulate a second transducer mechanism to alter osseous architecture, in a manner which will best resist the applied force. If the force is directed along the axes of preexisting bone structures, the alterations may involve only an increase in bone mass, while, if the force producers shear, the modifications will involve realignment.

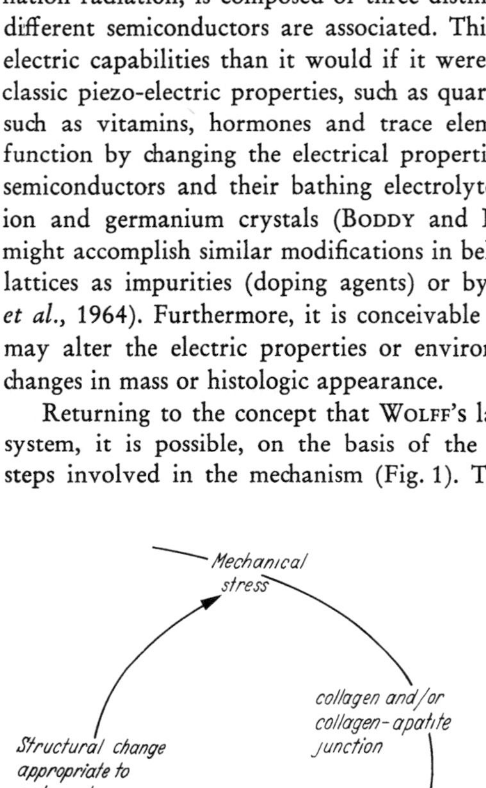

Fig. 1. Representation of proposed negative feedback control system controlling the orientation and mass of bone structures

Before presenting details of data indicating that the second transducer involves the response of cells and their byproducts to electric fields, additional factors relating to the generation of the electric potentials should be considered. At the present time, two different concepts about the identity of the electric generator have developed. On the one hand, SHAMOS and LAVINE (1964) believe that the demonstration of piezo-electric properties in tendon by FUKADA *et al.* (1959), coupled with earlier observations on bone (FUKUDA and YASUDA, 1957; SHAMOS *et al.*, 1963) indicates that collagen fibrils are the most likely source of stress-induced potentials. On the other hand, BASSETT and BECKER postulated in 1962 that bone has solid-state, semiconductor properties, associated most probably with the collagen-apatite units (BECKER *et al.*, 1964) and that these units may form piezo-electric p-n junctions responsible for electrogenesis in bone. The generator units are so small, however, that it is quite impossible to determine directly their electrical properties. Therefore, both opinions about their nature are based on indirect evidence derived from the behavior of sizeable masses of whole bone. Although both views are necessarily speculative, it does not follow that both are equally valid. For example, it should be noted that the investigations of FUKADA and YASUDA (1957), FUKADA *et al.* (1959) and SHAMOS *et al.* (1964) have been conducted with dry bone and dry tendon. Since collagen exists *in vivo* in a hydrated, rather than dry, state, BASSETT and BECKER (1962) employed wet tendon and wet collagen from decalcified bone as controls for their studies of the electrical responses of bone to deformation. With this type of hydrated preparation, no electrical activity was detected in response to bending. Recent studies in these laboratories have yielded additional data that may be helpful in understanding the apparent differences in the electrical behavior of dry and wet collagen, aside from the obvious alterations in resistance, possibly, capacitance.

Electrical output from hydrated bone strips, mounted and deformed as cantilevers, was measured and found to be nearly a linear function of the amount of deformation (Fig. 2) (COCHRAN *et al.*, unpublished). The plots resembled the classic, stress-strain relationship only until the plastic range was reached; thereafter, there was a diminution in the rate of increase of electric output. The roll off was most marked, however, in thicker specimens, since they reached the plastic range with significantly less deformation.

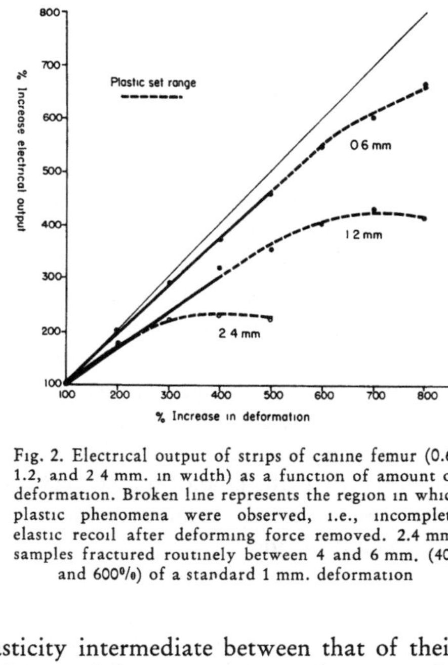

Fig. 2. Electrical output of strips of canine femur (0.6, 1.2, and 2 4 mm. in width) as a function of amount of deformation. Broken line represents the region in which plastic phenomena were observed, i.e., incomplete elastic recoil after deforming force removed. 2.4 mm. samples fractured routinely between 4 and 6 mm. (400 and 600%) of a standard 1 mm. deformation

Bone has been classed as a two-phase material by CURREY (1964). As he points out, this class of materials, of which fiberglass is an excellent example, has a of elasticity intermediate between that of their two components. In bone, collagen is the low modulus component and apatite, the high. While each collagen fibril is encrusted in mineral, the individual units probably are held together by a third material acting as a cement, so that in actuality, bone is a three-phase material. On the basis of this concept and the known ultrastructural features of osseous matrix, it seems reasonable that significant stress will develop at the junctional zone between the flabby collagen and the rigid amalgam of encrusting minearl-cement, whenever bone is subjected to any deforming force (Fig. 3). Such a system is admirably fitted for electrogenesis if the generator unit is postulated to be a collagen-apatite, p-n junction with piezo-electric properties. Its operation is assured, although there may be a limited range of deformation, under normal, physiologic conditinns.

This argument has not been advanced to reject the concept that unmineralized collagen may develop electric potentials in response to mechanical stress. In fact, it

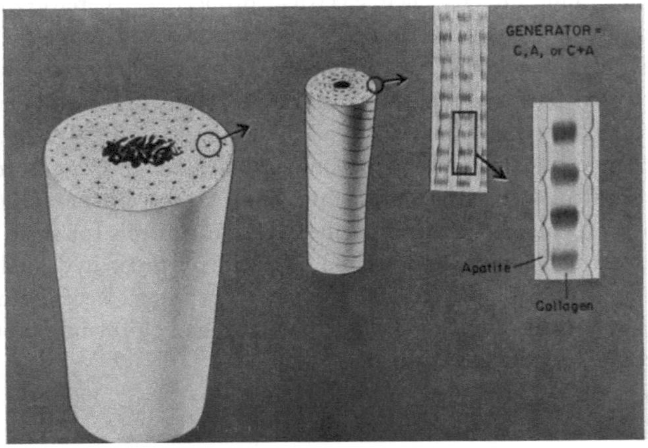

Fig. 3. Diagram of proposed electro-generator unit in bone, most probably the apatite-collagen (C+A) junction, rather than collagen (C) or apatite (A) alone. Whole bone at left, osteone in center, mineralized-collagen at right

seems reasonable to assume that this long-chain, cross-linked, crystalline polymer may have piezo-electric properties, too, or may develop displacement potentials of the type described by CHRISTIANSEN *et al.* (1961). Once this assumption has been made, however, it is important to consider again the fact that the rigid mineral component of bone limits the deformation of the elastic collagen and, thereby, limits also the capacity of collagen to produce stress generated potentials by itself. On the other hand, unsupported collagen in soft tissues, such as tendon, periodontal membrane and SHARPEY's fibers, generally is subjected to tensile deformation which is concentrated and may approach the elastic limits, resulting in significant stress. It is possible, therefore, that these and similar collagenous structures may generate electricity. Bone is not the only connective tissue that adapts its alignment and mass to meet functional demands!

Before leaving the subject of electro-mechanical properties of bone, TISCHENDORF's studies (1951) should be considered briefly. This investigator demonstrated that the major microscopic units of bone, such as osteones and lamellae, slid on one another, in response to a deforming force. When the force was removed, the structures returned to their normal relationships, probably through elastic recoil. More recently, SMITH and WALMSLEY (1959) concluded that the deformation of bone under stress varied with stress duration. From these studies and others (COCHRAN *et al.*, unpublished), it is reasonable to assume that, although bone may exhibit visco-elastic flow or creep, the rate at which stress is developed in the skeleton *in vivo* probably is rapid enough to deform individual collagen-apatite junctions.

Thus far, a proposed negative-feedback control system and the nature of the first transducer which converts mechanical signals to electrical potentials have been considered. Now, the mechanisms by which stress-generated electrical potentials might effect changes in osseous architecture will be discussed. In 1962, Bassett and Becker postulated "it is probable that these (electrical) potentials influence the activity of osseous cells directly. Furthermore, it is conceivable that they may direct, in some manner, the aggregation pattern of the macromolecules of the extracellular matrix." Investigations in these laboratories since 1962 have demonstrated that these postulates may be true. Osteogenesis *in vivo* was found to be affected by weak, artifically induced, direct currents and alignment of collagen fibers was affected *in vitro* by similar means. The amount of current employed in these studies was comparable to that calculated to occur in fresh bone in response to deformation. While it was not surprising that collagen, a charged molecule, would migrate in an electric field, it was notable that it moved so rapidly and into such an orderly pattern at current values as low as those employed. Drops of soluble collagen, derived from acetic acid extraction of rat tail tendons, and icthyocol were subjected to currents of 0.2 to 1 μ amps. for periods ranging from 1—30 minutes. Within 1—5 minutes, a birefringent band of collagen was formed at right angles to the electric field and near the cathode. Collagen fibrils in the drop could be reconstituted in this band by the addition of salts of proper ionic strength. Once reconstituted, the fibrils remained stationary after the current was stopped and were found to be well oriented, parallel to one another, and perpendicular to the lines of the electric field in which they were developed. Alteration of the current pattern from continuous to intermittent did not change the result. In fact, collagen drops wired with a multivibrator in the circuit to produce an on-off square-wave cycle at intervals of 1—2 seconds seemed to produce uniform bands somewhat faster than drops in which continuous current was employed (Becker *et al.*, 1964; Bassett, in press).

On the basis of these *in vitro* results, it seems possible that molecules, having a net charge, may migrate and align themselves under the influence of currents of the magnitude found *in vivo*. In view of this likelihood, the nature of the electrical signal being produced is of utmost importance. If the signal or pulse is biphasic, with equal positive and negative components, similar to that produced by a classic piezoelectric crystal such as quartz, a charged molecule would be moved equally in opposite directions, thereby resulting in no change in position. One exception to this behavior, however, might occur. Should the time constants of the signal and the rate of molecular migration fall within a certain range, it is possible that the molecule might be involved in a chemical reaction, such as polymerization, during a half cycle of the biphasic pulse. During the reverse phase of the pulse, the molecule would be unable to migrate. On the other hand, if the signal is purely or essentially uniphasic, it is not necessary to invoke such an exception.

Is it possible that extracellular macromolecules, by generating electrical potentials in response to stress, possess an "auto-control" mechanism which can direct not only their size and orientation, but influence others in their neighborhood? Certainly the high degree of orientation evident in the collagen fibers of osteones and lamellae of bone and in basement lamellae of adult lamprey skin, implies that a very precise control mechanism must exist. Perhaps the orientation of extracellular molecules may be cell-mediated, as suggested by Porter (1964) or mechanically mediated (Bassett, 1964). Certainly, it seems likely that there may be a close interrelationship between the electrical characteristics of a cell's membranes, organelles and macromolecules and its external electrical environment. On the other hand, the paucity of cells and the relatively large amount of extracellular material in many connective tissues might make a cellular control system unwieldy. If, as WEISS (1960) has proposed, action potentials in peripheral nerves may cause reorientation of molecules in the axonal membrane, why is it not possible that stress-induced potentials in macromolecules may not accomplish similar results? Such a system would permit finite regulation of extracellular material without specific cellular intervention and may well have been the major control mechanism for eons before the evolution of a nervous system. Certainly, the cellulose fibers in wood (another two phase material) have, without neural regulation, a highly ordered structure similar in many respects to collagen in bone (BASSETT, in press), Finally, it seems possible that the electrical activity of mechanically stressed organic macromolecules may influence directly their chemical reactivity (e.g., "mineralizability"), particularly if, as has been suggested recently (LITTLE, 1964), the macromolecules behave as superconductors.

Studies cited previously (BASSETT and BECKER, 1962; BECKER *et al.*, 1964; COCHRAN *et al.*, unpublished) have demonstrated that the amplitude and decay characteristics of the electrical pulse, from bone, vary significantly, depending upon the rate, magnitude and duration of deformation. The orientation of vessels, osteones, lamellae or mineralized collagen bundles, in relation to the direction of the applied force, also may affect the character of the pulse. Furthermore, it is probable that the relative degree of mineralization and the state of hydration of any given region in the osseous matrix will determine, in part, its electrical behavior (BECKER *et al.*, 1964). As pointed out earlier in this report, it is impossible to measure the activity of individual generators with dimensions in the Ångstrom unit range. Therefore, the pulses recorded in these studies represent a summation of billions of individual events (some additive, some subtractive, some simultaneous, others not) occurring within the specimen under investigation. Both equally and unequally biphasic signals have been recorded. Truly uniphasic signals, however, have not been observed. The statement by SHAMOS and LAVINE (1964), "the reverse pulse is an electrical artifact caused by . . . capacitane", ignores the fact that, on release, piezo-electric materials normally produce a reverse pulse, if the initial, pressure-induced charge separation is permitted to leak off while the material is still deformed. How, then, does an unequally biphasic signal result? Three of many possible explanations can be advanced. First, the generator seems to be a p-n junction which, in itself, may rectify the signal, since current passes in forward bias more efficiently than it does in reverse bias. Second, the rate and duration of loading (deformation) in the living vertebrate is such that the signal may not decay fully before the next cycle begins (Fig. 4). Third, although a specimen, gradually loaded, produces little or no detectable signal, a uniphasic spike of normal magnitude results when it is rapidly unloaded (BASSETT, in press; COCHRAN *et al.*, unpublished).

Although signal magnitude and decay time vary considerably, as a function of different bone specimen characteristics, there is much greater uniformity in signal polarity. Regions under compression, generally concave surfaces, are routinely negative with respect to regions under tension, generally convex. It is known clinically and experimentally that the concave aspects of a bone will be buttressed with new bone and the convex removed (MURRAY, 1936). These two observations lead teleologically to the prediction that regions of negativity may be associated with osteogenesis, while regions of positivity may be characterized by osteolysis. It was interesting, therefore, to observe the effects on living bone of artificially induced, continuous, direct currents (BASSETT *et al.*, 1964). These experiments involved the

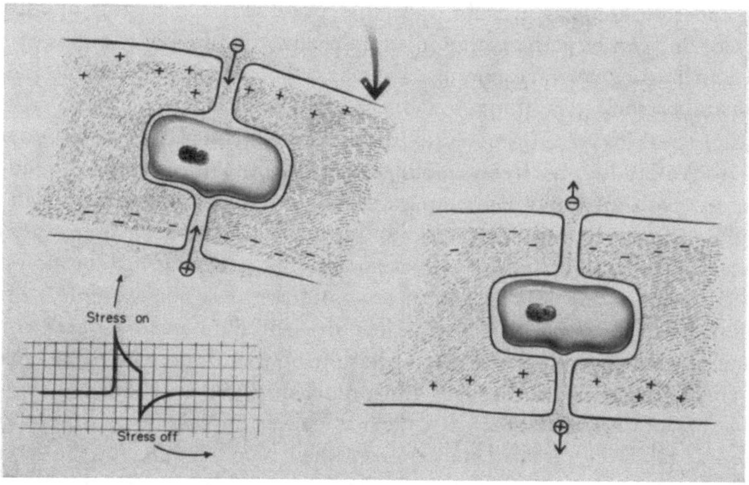

Fig. 4. Scheme of possible effects of stress-generated potentials in aiding the ebb and flow of charged molecules and ions about an osteocyte. Note pulse pattern — it is unequally biphasic since deforming force removed before signal had decayed

implantation of small, active and inactive-control, silicone-coated battery packs in canine thighs, so that two platinum electrodes projected through the lateral mid-femoral cortex into the medullary canal. The active packs delivered currents ranging from 0.7 to 3.4 μ amps. *in vivo.* Control specimens developed small masses of new, reactive bone around each inactive electrode where it projected into the marrow space. When 2 to 3 μ amps. were flowing, the mass of newly formed bone was increased markedly about the cathode, but not the anode. The larger bone mass near the negative pole seemed to result from an increased cellularity which was most marked at 14 days after operation and which decreased by 21 days. From the pattern of deposition, both at the cathodes and anodes, it was unlikely that the results could be ascribed to an electrophoretic action of the current on precursors of osseous matrix.

There was no evidence that an anticipated increase in osteoclastic activity had occurred in the anodal region. In seeking an explanation for this result, it is important to note that the animals were active during the post-operative period and developed, most probably, significant stress concentrations in the region of both holes in the cortex. Such stress concentrations could result in increased electrical activity which might have overridden the local effects of the anode. On the other hand, osteoclasis may not be related to anodal activity.

This experiment, employing unphysiologic, continuous, direct currents, demonstrates that osteogenesis is increased in regions of electronegativity. Although suggestive, it does not establish conclusively a link between stress-induced potential and the activity of bone cells. For example, all of the evidence so far indicates that the intermittant electrical signals measured on bone surfaces usually are biphasic, although under certain circumstances they may be predominantly uniphasic. In the light of this observation, it seems reasonable to ask whether a cell can discriminate between the positive and negative phases of the signal and act accordingly? Or, does it react to the greater or lesser electrical activity, produced by greater or lesser stress? Although concrete answers are not available presently, a working hypothesis has been devised. Such an hypothesis should explain how, despite the stimulus of systemic hormonal and nutritional factors, mesenchymal cells can specialize simultaneously as osteoblasts and osteoclasts within a few micra of one another.

Generally speaking, when a potential difference is measured between two surfaces, the relative availability of freely mobile electrons is being detected. Under these circumstances, positivity may be comparable to cold, i.e., cold represents an absence of heat, while positivity represents a lack of electrons. If this definition is permissible, then osteoclasis may result when electrical activity is diminished or non-existant. This line of reasoning can lead in any of several directions. For example, diffusion of extracellular fluids in bone probably is less efficient than in any other connective tissue. Bone substance is relatively incompressible, so that fluids cannot be "massaged" back and forth. Canaliculae, through which nutrient fluids must diffuse, comprise, at most, only 3% of the total area of a lacunar space. Furthermore, many osteocytes are situated at relatively great distances from their blood supply. In the face of such an inefficient supply line, it might be expected that most osteocytes would be on the brink of starvation or, at least, of anaerobic glycolysis. Under the impetus of minor, physiologic skeletal deformations, however, an alternating signal could aid electrophoretically in the ebb and flow of charged molecules and ions, thereby aiding greatly in the nutrition of these cells (Fig. 4) (Bassett, in press). If the locus for electrogenesis proves to be collagen-apatite junction, then the average osteocyte is surrounded by more than 1.1×10^9 generating loci!

If electrogenesis were increased above maintenance levels in a given region, local cells might be activated to produce bone to stabilize the regions. Conversely, diminished electrical activity might be followed by osteocyte death through starvation. It should be re-emphasized here that the stress generated potentials apparently are not dependent upon cell viability and, therefore, dead bone may continue to generate potentials if subjected to intermittant deformation and if it remains electrically competent. Should electrical activity cease in a region, osteoclasis would result. This hypothesis seems to fit well with the observed behavior of teeth in orthodontia. Normally, a tooth is suspended in its socket by a periodontal membrane comprised of collagen bundles that penetrate the surrounding bone, much as Sharpey's fibers would (Fig. 5). When orthodontists move a tooth with 1—2 grams of steady, lateral pressure, the periodontal fibers become taut on the trailing edge of the root, where osteoblasts appear to deposit layers of appositional bone. On the leading edge, where the fibers are slack, osteoclasts are active, removing bone. Similar osteoblastic behavior has been observed during regeneration of bone in Millipore-isolated defects in dog radii (Bassett *et al.*, 1961). Unless stimulated by major instability, these defects fill rapidly with fibrous tissue which gradually is converted directly to bone in a centripetal manner. The interface between bone and fibrous tissue is spanned by many collagen bundles that are oriented along major lines of stress. At the point where they emerge from the osseous tissue, rows of active osteoblasts are found (Rüedi and Bassett, unpublished). This picture is not greatly different from that in ossifying turkey tendon (JOHNSON, 1964), and suggests that osteogenic "induction" has a major physical facet. In fact, it has long been recognized that tension above usual limits may lead to ossification of tendon (MURRAY, 1936).

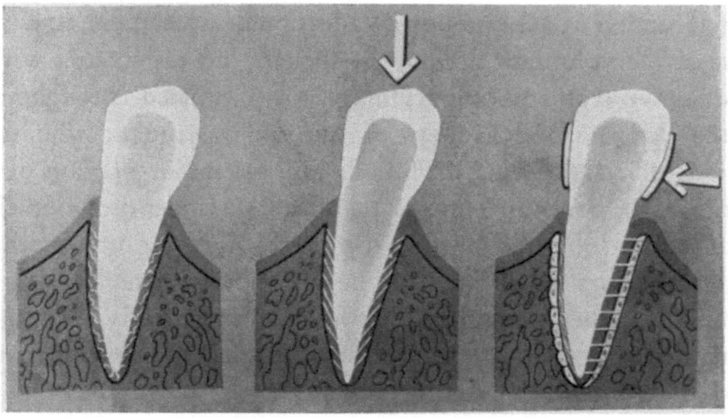

Fig. 5. Diagram of relationship of periodontal fibers and tooth; at left fibers are relaxed with no pressure on tooth. Center sketch depicts biting, fibers are taut. At right, tooth is being moved by force which tightens periodontal fibers at trailing surface of root where osteoblastic activity occurs and slackens fibers at leading surface, where osteoclasts are removing bone

If osteoclasts occur in regions where the electrical signal is diminished or absent, it should be possible to find a common electrical link between factors known to cause osteolysis. For example, although it has been stated that bone removal depends on vascular changes (GEISER and TRUETA, 1958), it is not entirely clear yet whether they are attendant upon or responsible for the removal. If, as JOHNSON (1964) believes, active hyperemia causes bone destruction, it might do so by providing more electron "sinks" through hyperoxia or streaming potentials. Arterial walls are positively charged on the adventitial surface and negatively charged on the endothelial (SAWYER and PATE, 1953). It is conceivable, therefore, that the erosion of bone by an aneurysm may be electrically mediated, since the vessel wall could conduct away more electrons than were generated by deformation.

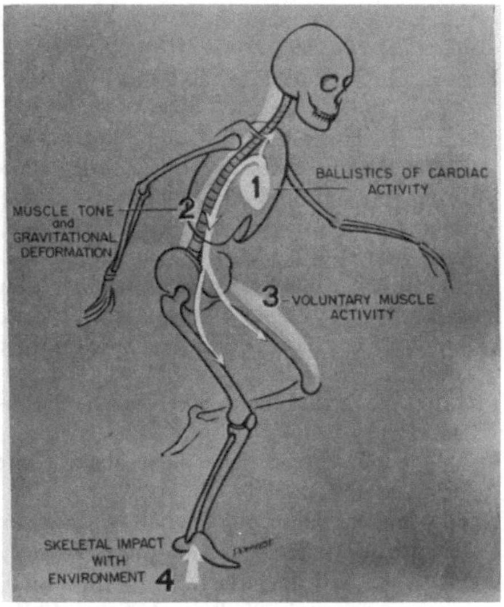

Fig. 6. Four main sources of mechanical input to normal skeleton

Finally, since it appears likely that bone mass and orientation may be controlled by stress-generated electrical potentials, the origin of mechanical stresses in the skeleton deserve brief attention. Actually, bone may function in a manner similar to an exquisitely sensitive, piezoelectric accelerometer, responding to the slightest jar or deformation. There are four main sources of mechanical input for the skeleton (Fig. 6). The cardiovascular system provides a continual deforming force (GEBHARDT, 1905) through hydrostatics in the vessels and, quite possibly, through the ballistics of cardia action. Gravity causes not only direct distortion of the skeleton, but is major impetus for the muscle tone which stabilizes the body against its effect. Trough aponeurotic origins and insertions, this muscle tone intermittently deforms the underlying bone. When voluntary muscle action is superimposed, additional mechanical stress is developed. If in the course of the voluntary action, the skeleton makes contact with its environment, the shock wave from the impact may be transmitted throughout the skeletal system. Pity the skeleton and kidneys of the poor astronaut who is subjected to prolonged periods of weightlessness! He will lose the major portion of the last three mechanical stimuli to bone and must, therefore, become osteoporotic at a more rapid rate than those subjected only to bed rest. A better understanding of these electro-mechanical factors may lead, in time, to improved methods for combating a loss of bone mass, whether generalized as the result of inactivity, weightlessness, or metabolic aberration, or whether localized as the result of rigid, internal fixation or loss of function.

References

Andry, N.: L'Orthopédie. Paris: Lambert et Durant 1741.

Bassett, C. A. L.: Environmental and cellular factors regulating osteogenesis. In Bone Biodynamics. Frost, H. (ed.). Boston: Little, Brown 1964, p. 233.

— In minimum ecological systems for man. Trans. N. Y. Acad. Sci. (in press).

—, and R. O. Becker: Generation of electric potentials by bone in response to mechanical stress. Science **137**, 1063 (1962).

—, D. K. Creighton, and F. E. Stinchfield: Contributions of endosteum, cortex, and soft tissues to osteogenesis. Surg. Gynec. Obstet. **112**, 145 (1961).

—, R. J. Pawluk, and R. O. Becker: Effects of electric currents on bone in vivo. Nature (Lond.) **204**, 652 (1964).

Becker, R. O., and F. M. Brown: Photoelectric effects in human bone. Nature (Lond.) **206**, 1325 (1965).

—, C. A. L. Bassett, and C. H. Bachman: Bioelectric factors controlling bone structure. In Bone Biodynamics. Frost, H. (ed.). Boston: Little, Brown 1964, p. 209.

Boddy, P. J., and W. H. Brattain: Effect of cupric ion on electrical properties of the germanium-aqueous electrolyte interface. J. electrochem. Soc. **109**, 812 (1962).

Christiansen, J. A., C. E. Jensen, and Th. Vilstrup: Displacement potentials and bending of rod-like polyelectrolytes. Nature (Lond.) **191**, 484 (1961).

Cochran, G. V. B., R. J. Pawluk, and C. A. L. Bassett: Unpublished.

Currey, J. D.: Three analogies to explain the mechanical properties of bone. Biorheol. **2**, 1 (1964).

Fukada, E., and I. Yasuda: On the piezo-electric effect of bone. J. phys. Soc. Japan **12**, 1158 (1957).

— —, and R. Goto: The piezo-electric effect in collagen. Reports on Progress in Polymer Physics in Japan, **2**, 101 (1959).

Gebhardt, F.: Über funktionell wichtige Anordnungsweise der gröberen und feineren Bauelemente des Wirbeltierknochens. Arch. Entwickl.-Mech. Org. **20**, 1901 (1905).

Geiser, M., and J. Trueta: Muscle action, bone rarefaction and bone formation: An experimental study. J. Bone Jt Surg. **40 B**, 282 (1958) .

Huber, F.: Piezo-effect in P-N junctions of semi-conducting titanium oxide film. Appl. Phys. Letters **2**, 76 (1963).

Jansen, M.: On Bone Formation, Its Relation to Tension and Pressure. London: Longmans, Green 1920.

Johnson, L. C.: Morphologic analysis in pathology: The kinetics of diseases and general biology of bone. In Bone Biodynamics. Frost, H. (ed.). Boston: Little, Brown 1964, p. 543.

LITTLE, W. A.: Possibility of synthesizing an organic superconductor. Phys. Rev. **134 A,** 1416 (1964).
MCLEAN, F. C.: The ultrastructure and function of bone. Science **127,** 451 (1958).
MASON, W. P.: Piezo-electric Crystals and Their Application to Ultrasound. New York: D. Van Nostrand 1950.
MURRAY, P. D. F.: Bones. New York: Cambridge University Press 1936.
PORTER, K. R.: Cell fine structure and biosynthesis of intercellular macromolecules. In Connective Tissue: Intercellular Macromolecules. Boston: Little, Brown 1964, p. 167.
RÜEDI, T., and C. A. L. BASSETT: Unpublished.
SAWYER, P. N., and J. W. PATE: Bioelectric phenomena as an etiologic factor in intravascular thrombosis. Amer. J. Phys. **175,** 103 (1953).
SHAMOS, M. H., and L. S. LAVINE: Physiological basis for bioelectric effects in mineralized tissues. Clin. Orthop. **35,** 177 (1964).
— —, and M. I. SHAMOS: Piezo-electric effect in bone. Nature (Lond.) **197,** 81 (1963).
SMITH, J. W., and R. WALMSLEY: Factors affecting the elasticity of bone. J. Anat. **96,** 503 (1959).
THOMPSON, D'ARCY W.: On Growth and Form. Cambridge: University Press 1963.
TISCHENDORF, F.: Das Verhalten der Haversschen Systeme bei Belastung. Arch. Entwickl.-Mech. Org. **145,** 318 (1951).
WEISS, P.: Molecular reorientation as unifying principle underlying cellular reactivity. Proc. nat. Acad. Sci. **46,** 993 (1960).
WOLFF, J.: Das Gesetz der Transformation der Knochen. Berlin: A. Hirschwald 1892.
WUNDER, C. C., S. R. BRINEY, M. KRAL, and C. SKAUGSTAD: Growth of mouse femurs during continual centrifugation. Nature (Lond.) **188,** 151 (1960).

Topographic-quantitative Study of Bone Tissue Formation and Reconstruction in Inert Bones

G. MAROTTI, F. MAROTTI *

Istituto di Anatomia Umana, Universitá di Bari, Bari, Italia

A quantitative estimation of the amount of new bone tissue formed in the shafts of bones was carried out on bones rendered mechanically inert for various periods of time.

The left anterior limbs of young immature and adult dogs were freed of skin and fixed to the thoracic wall in a cutaneous pouch after division of the brachial plexus. The animals were sacrificed from 20 days to several months after the operation; ten days before sacrifice, 20 to 30 mg of Acromycin/Kg of body weight was administered daily for three successive days.

The area occupied by newly formed acromycin labelled bone (*NB*) and by unlabelled bone present before (*PB*) the administration of the antibiotic, was computed using an automatic point counter on photomicrographs made with U.V. light (color reversal film). Entire cross-sections taken from various levels of the unloaded and denervated bones, as well as from corresponding levels of the homotypic bones of the opposite mobile leg were examined. The relative amount of bone tissue laid down during acromycin treatment was expressed as % NB/(PB + NB) and is shown in Figs. 1 to 4.

* Staff member of the Orthopaedic Clinic, University of Padova; Holder of a scholarship of the italian C.N.R.

The data relating to 4 dogs operated when two-month old and sacrificed 20, 60, 180 and 360 days after the operation are shown in Fig. 1. On the left in Fig. 2, are shown the results obtained from two dogs operated when four months old and sacri-

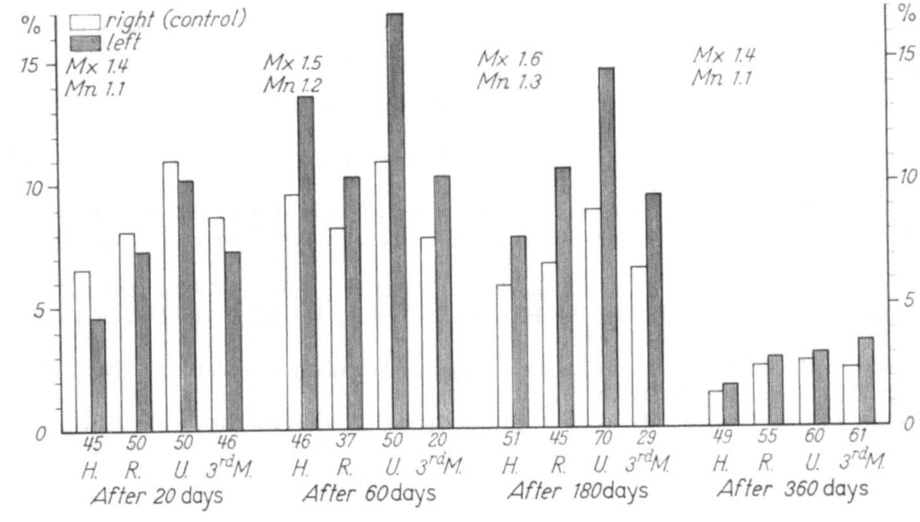

Fig. 1

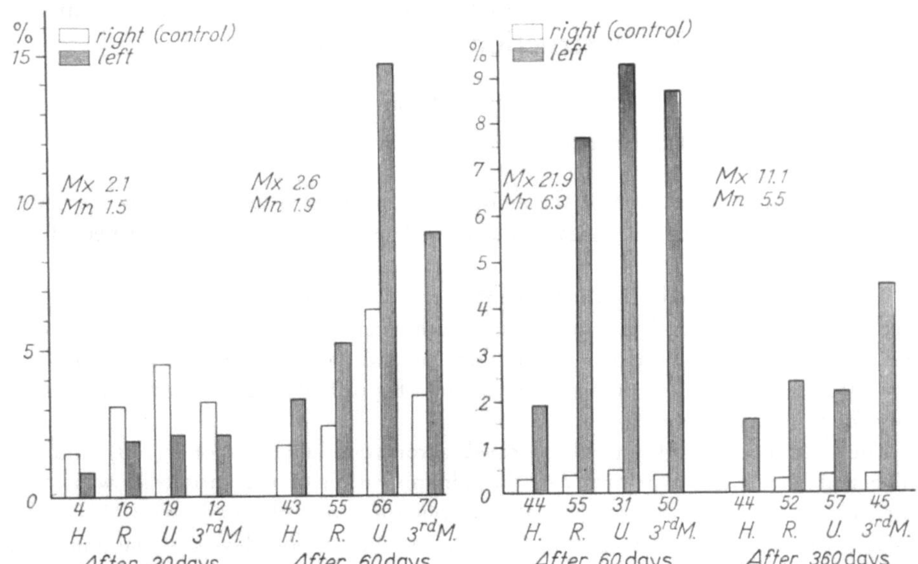

Fig. 2

ficed after 20 and 60 days respectively. On the right in Fig. 2, are shown the data from two other dogs operated when 3 years old and sacrificed at 60 and 360 days. In all the diagrams, the various pairs of bones studied in the inert (left) and mobile (right) bones, namely humerus (H.), radius (R.), ulna (U.) and 3rd metacarpal bone (3rd M.), are indicated on the x axis; recorded on the y axis are the means of the values % NB/(PB + NB) of three consecutive cross sections of the mid-shaft taken serially at 1 mm intervals. The numbers at the base of each couple of bars indicate the mean percent reduction of the amount of osseous tissue (PB + NB) recorded in the three mid-shaft cross sections of the inert bone compared to the contralateral mobile bone taken as unity (= 100). The maximum (Mx) and minimum (Mn) values of the ratio between the relative amounts of labelled newly formed osseous tissue, recorded for the left and right sides of the various pairs of bones studied, are reported for each subject above the groups of bars.

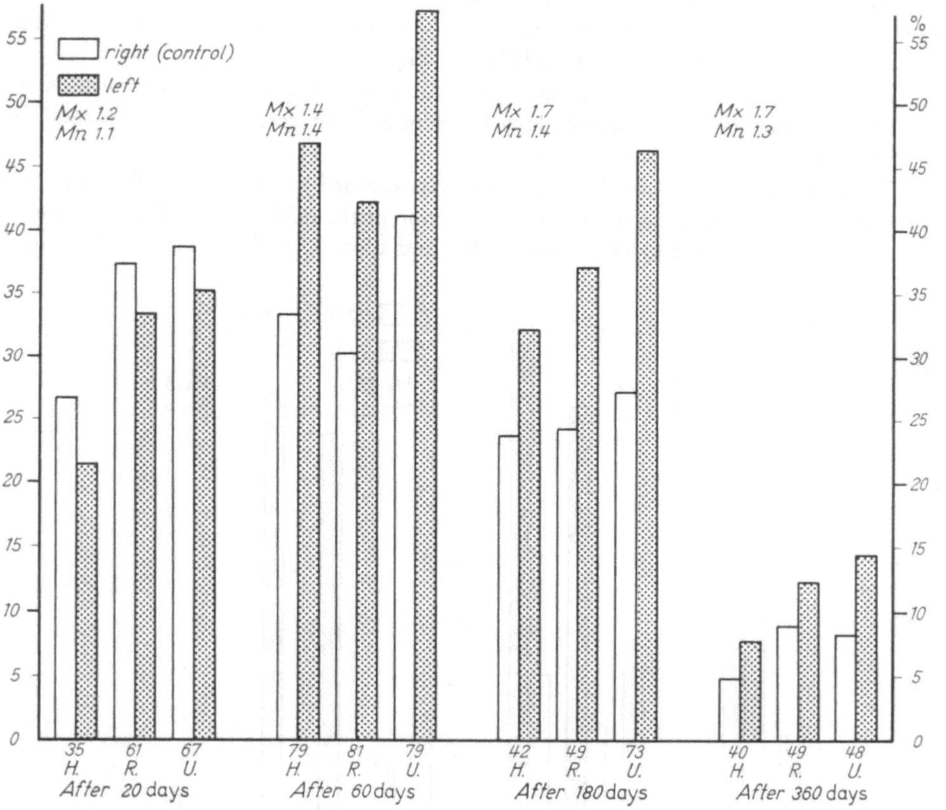

Fig. 3

Fig. 3

It is concluded that:

1. A remarkable loss of osseous tissue takes place in the cortex of inert and denervated bones in comparison to the mobile homotypic bones. The degree of this reduction varies in the shaft bones of each subject, and in each bone in subjects sacrificed at different time intervals after operation. In general, the ulna undergoes the greatest reduction. For equal periods of immobilisation, the degree of bone tissue reduction is greater the younger the subject at the time of limb suspension and

denervation. In groups of dogs operated at the same age, the reduction of bone tissue appears, in general, to be more marked in subjects sacrificed 60 and 180 days after limb immobilisation. Obviously, two concurrent factors play a part in this reduction in the growing animals: namely, a decrease in appositional growth in the shaft and an increase in resorption which is not fully compensated by deposition of newly formed bone.

2. A relatively greater amount of osseous tissue is laid down in the inert than in the contralateral mobile bones during the period of acromycin administration. This is more marked in the two dogs operated upon in adult life: the relative amount of newly formed osseous tissue is from 5 to 20 times greater in the inactive than in the mobile bones in these subjects (Fig. 2, *right*). In the two dogs sacrificed 20 days after operation, such a difference in osteogenic activity in the inactive compared with the control mobile bones was not observed (Fig. 1; Fig. 2, *left*).

3. The amount of bone tissue undergoing reconstruction in the inert as well as in the mobile bones varies in different long bones in each subject: relatively it is smaller in the humerus and much greater in the ulna.

The percentage values of the ratio of newly apposed acromycin labelled bone to the total bone, estimated on an entire cross section at the middle level of the proximal metaphysis of the humerus (H.), radius (R.) and ulna (U.) of the inert and mobile

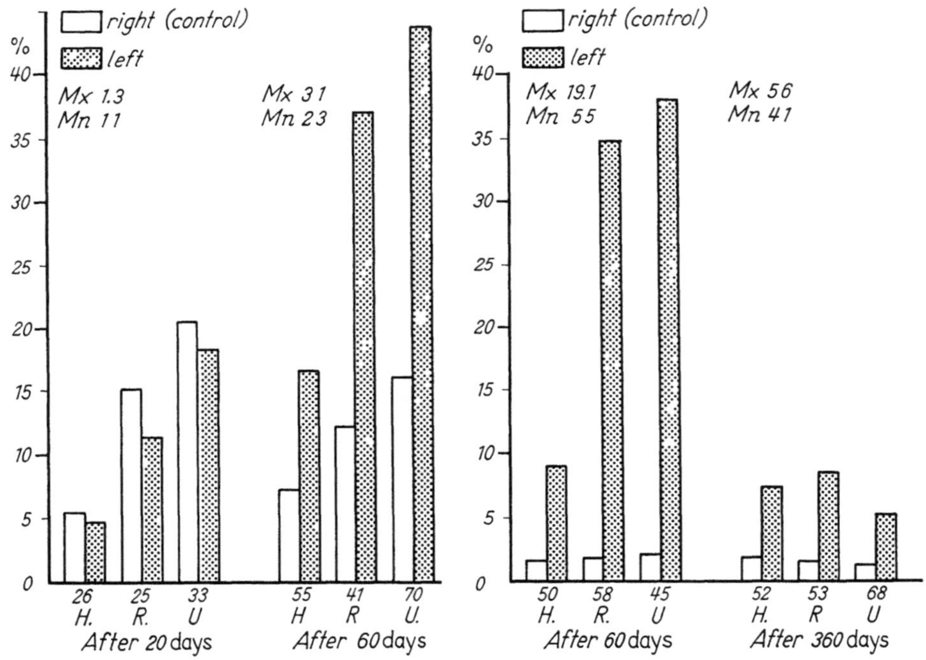

Fig. 4

limbs of all the dogs studied are shown in Fig. 3 (operation at 2-month old) and in Fig. 4 (*left*, operation at 4-month of age; *right*, operation at 3 years of age).

The results obtained at the level of the metaphysis are similar to those of the same bones at the mid-shaft level. However, bone turnover, during the period of acromycin administration, is three to five times greater at the metaphysis than at the diaphyseal level in both the inert and the loaded bones.

As previously observed by VIGLIANI (1955 a, b) in the dog, and in the rat by LANDRY and FLEISCH (1962, 1964), three successive stages can be distinguished in the response of shaft bones to unloading and/or denervation. We observed an *initial stage*, characterised by increased resorption and temporary decrease of bone tissue deposition; a *second stage*, in which both resorption and apposition of new bone are increased. During this period, the difference in the relative amount of new formed bone in the homotypic bones of the inert and mobile limb are greatest; a *third stage*, in which both bone resorption and deposition are greater in the inert than in the mobile bones, but a decrease of bone turnover occurs in comparison to the second stage.

These quantitative changes in bone apposition and bone turnover due to unloading and denervation are not paralleled by qualitative changes in structures of the 2nd and 3rd order. AMPRINO (1938) has shown in man and VIGLIANI (1955 b) in the dog that normally structured osteones are formed and renewed in the cortex of bones rendered mechanically inert for long periods of time. Hence, the stresses normally undergone by skeletal components at rest and in motion do not appear to be strictly necessary for the formation of normally structured and normally arranged bone tissue, once the general pattern of bone architecture has been laid down.

It may, therefore, be claimed that bones, which no longer serve their normal mechanical function, can participate to a greater extent than normally loaded and innervated bones in the mineral metabolism of the organism, acting as stores of inorganic and organic materials and undergoing continuous turnover.

References

AMPRINO, R.: La struttura delle ossa dell'uomo sottratte alle sollecitazioni meccaniche. Arch. Entwickl.-Mech. Org. **138**, 305 (1938).

LANDRY M., and H. FLEISCH: Influence de l'immobilisation sur la formation et la destruction osseuse évaluées par l'incorporation des tétracyclines dans l'os. Helv. physiol. pharmacol. Acta **20**, C 69 (1962).

— — The influence of immobilisation on bone formation as evaluated by osseous incorporation of tetracyclines. J. Bone Jt Surg. **46 B**, 764 (1964).

VIGLIANI, F.: Accrescimento e rinnovamento strutturale della compatta in ossa sottratte alle sollecitazioni meccaniche. Nota I. Z. Zellforsch. **42**, 59 (1955 a).

— Accrescimento e rinnovamento strutturale della compatta in ossa sottratte alle sollecitazioni meccaniche. Nota II. Z. Zellforsch. **43**, 17 (1955 b).

Structure and Healing of Bone as a Response to Continuous and Discontinuous Strain and Stress

H. WAGNER

Orthopädische Universitätsklinik Münster, Deutschland

The structure of bone tissue is a response to the forces of stress and strain, these control the disposition of the trabeculae in cancellous bone as well as the orientation of the Haversian systems in compact bone. A change of the direction of force causes an alteration of the bone structure.

The influence of mechanical factors upon the weight-bearing skeleton has been well known for a long time. The first investigator, who published on this subject, was probably GALILEO GALILEI in 1638. However, the biomechanic relations seem to be much more complicated, as we already know.

In the experiment we have studied the reaction of bone tissue to weight-bearing metal implants, especially metal screws, such as we are using in orthopaedic surgery. We have tested screws of a new type, being developed by the AO-Group in Switzerland (MÜLLER *et al.*, 1963). The fundamental characteristics of these screws are:

1. the wide and spacious threads,

2. the fact that the weight-bearing side of the thread is standing at right angles to the direction of force,

3. the electrolytically polished surface, which gives the implants a high corrosion resistance in the body fluids.

Histological examination shows a tight embedding of the screws in bone tissue during periods of years without any foreign-body reaction. Also two years after implantation we see a close contact between the metal and the bone tissue without a fibrotic reaction in the marrow.

But what is going on, when a screw is exposed to mechanical pressure?

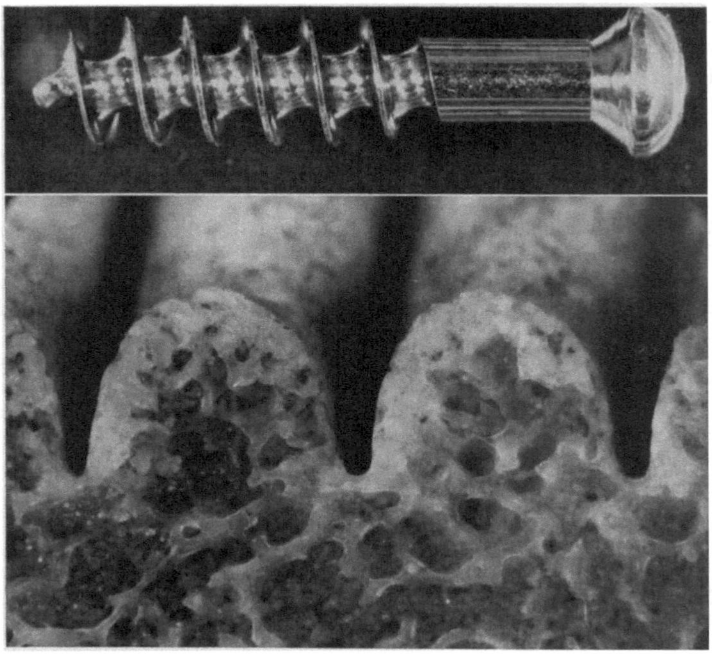

Fig. 1. Screw inserted into the femur condyle across the growth cartilage. 6 months after implantation appositional ossification on the weight-bearing (left) side of the corresponding bone thread, as a biomechanic adaptation of bone tissue to mechanical pressure

In animal experiments it is difficult to keep a screw under continuous weight-bearing, because fractures and osteotomies in animals heal very quickly. Therefore we inserted the screws into the condyle of the femur across the epiphyseal line, by this means the screws were exposed to the constant growing pressure of the epiphyseal cartilage. As a result we see in the corresponding bone thread on the weight-bearing side an appositional ossification, as an adaptation of bone tissue to mechanical pressure (Fig. 1). This adaptation does not occur in cancellous bone only, but also in compact bone, where the osteons change their direction according to the stress-lines of the screws.

The primary stability of metal implantation into bone tissue and a continuous mechanical pressure between the screw and the bone are the basic conditions for this biomechanic adaptation. A primary instability leads to fibrotic bone resorption.

In another experiment a screw was inserted between radius and ulna of a dog (Fig. 2). The slight movement between both bones produced a discontinuous pressure and a movement between bone and metal surface and led to an osteolytic reaction.

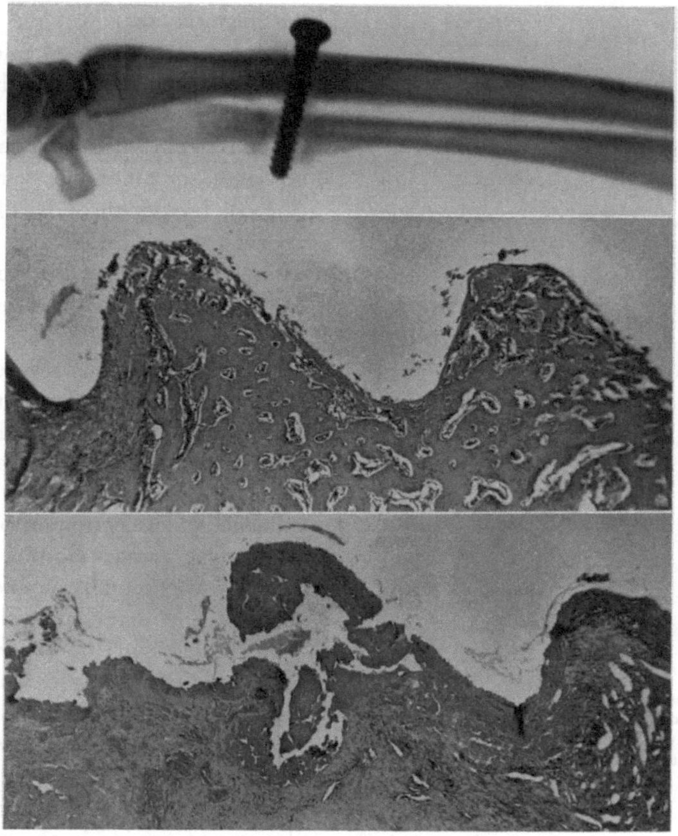

Fig. 2. Screw inserted across radius and ulna in the dog. The slight movement produced fibrotic and osteolytic reaction. Because of the lesser diameter the instability was relatively greater in the ulna, as well as the bone resorption (histolog. section below)

Under the influence of rigid fixation fractures and osteotomies heal by primary ossification without chondro-fibrotic callus. At the ends of the fragments the HAVERSIAN cavities are reorganized by the so-called "creeping substitution", and the HAVERsian vessels are recanalized across the fracture line, producing immediately mature lamellar bone in concentric layers.

This phenomenon led to the opinion, that the reduction of bone fragments in cases of internal fixation is so perfectly possible, that no tissue from the periosteum and the endosteum can invade the bone fissure and the healing is maintained by the Haversian vessels alone.

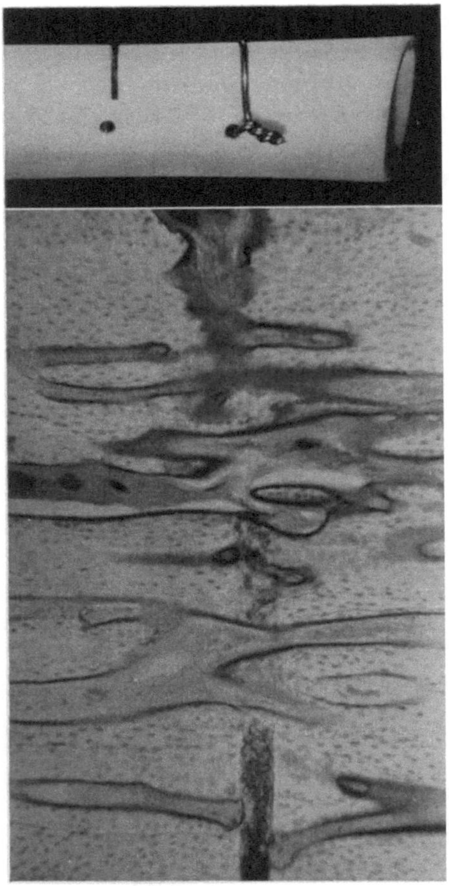

Fig. 3. Transverse saw-section in the femoral shaft of the dog, without opening the marrow-cavity. After 23 days recanalisation of Haversian vessels, without any difference, whether the bone defect was closed by hemicerelage or not

This explanation is not satisfactory, because we find a primary ossification also in cases of rigid fixation without anatomical reduction. Other factors, mechanical ones, must therefore be responsible for this phenomenon.

In a further experiment we cut into the femoral shaft of the dog small transverse saw-slots of 60 micron width, without opening the medullary cavity. A number of the slots were closed to the periosteum with a wire-suture (hemicerclage), the other ones were left upon (Fig. 3). Twenty-three days later we see a primary ossification and a recanalization of the Haversian vessels, without any difference between the two groups.

Now we modified the experiment: we cut the saw-slot deep into the marrowcavity until we got a slight movement in the slot when bending the bone. We now expected to find, under the influence of discontinuous pressure and traction, a chondro-fibrotic callus formation. We actually found bone resorption and chondrofibrotic callus, as we expected, but the experiment gave us an additional result, which we had not expected namely, at the ends of the slot there appeared also a primary ossification (Fig. 4).

This finding can be explained by the rate of motion in the bone-gap: in the centre of the slot, where the amplitude of movement is high, we find bone resorption and chondro-fibrotic callus, at the ends of the slot, where the amplitude is low, almost zero, there appears a primary ossification.

These biomechanic relations are of great practical importance in bone surgery: the primary stability of metal implantation is the basic condition for the rigid fixation of bone fragments. The primary instability leads to bone resorption and delayed healing.

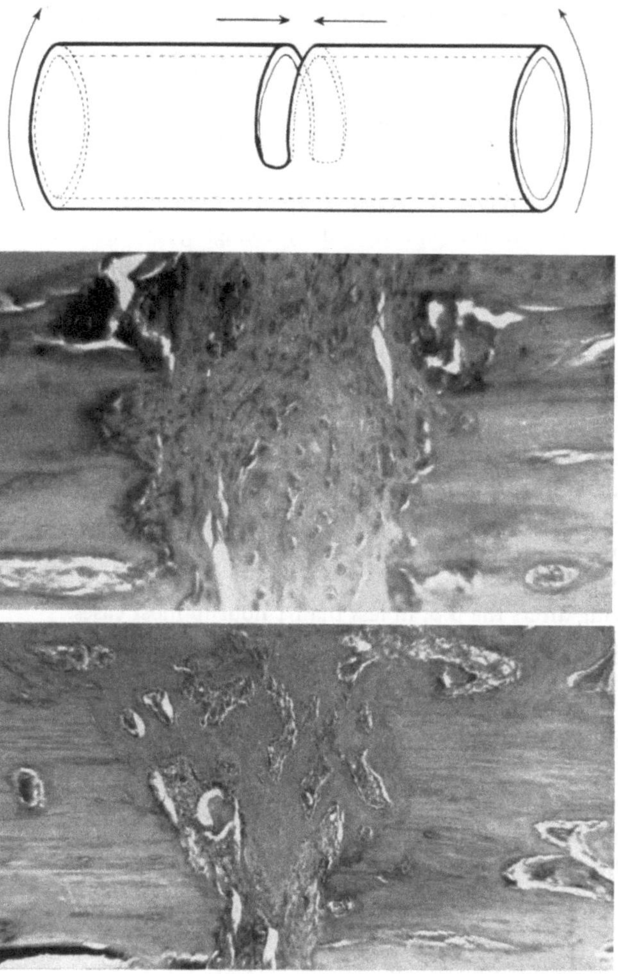

Fig. 4. Deep transverse saw-section in the femoral shaft of the dog, with slight movement in the gap, when bending the bone. Chondrofibrotic callus formation in the centre of the saw-slot by the influence of discontinuous pressure and traction (histolog. section above). Primary bone formation at the ends of the saw-slot, where the amplitude of movement is low (histolog. section below)

References

Galilei, G.: Mechanic, Dialog I (1638). Cited by Koch, J. C.: The laws of bone architecture. Amer. J. Anat. **21**, 177 (1917).

Krompecher, St.: Die Knochenneubildung. Jena: Fischer 1937.

Müller M. E., M. Allgower und H. Willeneger: Technik der operativen Frakturenbehandlung. Berlin - Göttingen - Heidelberg: Springer 1963.

Rheological Considerations in the Physical Properties of Bone*

E. D. SEDLIN **, L. SONNERUP ***

The Biomechanics Laboratory, Department of Orthopaedic Surgery, University of Göteborg, Göteborg, Sweden

Our studies of the physical properties (p.p.) of bone have concerned three general questions. (1). How are the p.p. altered by changing the method of testing, storage, and preparation? (2) How may one account for the variations that are noted? (3) How is bone to be classified in the general realm of physical bodies insofar as its mechanical behavior? A complete description of all of our findings and methods is beyond the scope of this presentation, and is presented elsewhere (SEDLIN and HIRSCH, in press). Some of the findings relative to questions 1 and 2 are noted below. These are based upon compression, bending, and tension tests on more than 500 samples of femoral cortical bone obtained from 20 autopsy subjects. The tests were performed wet, usually at body temperature, on an Instron Tensile Test Machine.

a. There is no significant effect of temperature on maximum stress (σ_M) and energy absorption, in the range from 21 °C to 37 °C. The modulus of elasticity (E) may increase slightly at 21 °C.

b. Air drying alters the p.p. in less than 1 hour in most cases.

c. Freezing of specimens prior to testing increases σ_M slightly, but does not change any other p.p.

d. Fixation in formalin does not appear to alter E.

e. In small sample testing, size of specimen does not contibute to the variation noted in ranges tested. (1 mm $\times$ 2 mm to 3 mm $\times$ 3 mm)

f. Repeated loading of the same specimen does not change E, if loads of the order of 35% of the failure load are used, and one minute or more be allowed for recovery between loads.

g. In bending tests, E can be significantly changed by changing the distance between supports.

h. It is important to measure specimen size before testing.

i. There are significant differences in σ_M and E in specimens from different quadrants of the mid-femur, the lateral ranking highest, with posterior lowest in regard to these variates.

The volume occupied by the Haversian canals in these specimens did not correlate well with the p.p. in the majority of instances.

k. Significant differences exist in the p.p. of bone from different individuals that are not accounted for by age.

l. An high correlation exists between σ_M and E in bending.

m. Testing of small samples appears to be a reliable method for the demonstration of differences in p.p. between individuals.

During conduct of the experiments indicated above, some information became available that provided insight into the third question posed. Some background is necessary before considering this question.

---

* Work supported in part by U.S. National Institutes of Health and Swedish Medical Research Council.

** Special Research Fellow, U.S. National Institutes of Health.

*** University Lecturer, Dept. of Strength of Materials, Chalmers Tekniska Högskola, Göteborg.

Bone has long been known to be an anisotropic material. As such, the laws and formulae that are utilized in determining p.p. should be applied with caution. Our use of the standard formulae has been for the sole purpose of comparing the effects of methods of handling, or differences in individuals. An example of this would be the use of the straightest portion of the stress-strain curve in determining E, when, in fact, only a rare curve in our series possessed a truly linear component. To account for this phenomenon, and to reconcile it and other findings with statements that bone is an elastic material, visco-elastic material, two or three phase material, we were lead into the field of rheology, which in the broadest sense is the study of the deformation of all materials (REINER, 1958).

There are four fundamental properties of materials, all others being reducible to definitions in terms of these. They are elasticity, plasticity, viscosity, and strength (REINER, 1958). We will consider the first three of these at this time, the fourth being beyond the limits set for discussion. To better understand what is meant by the terms, one can use idealized models, as are presented in Fig. 1. Thus, we can speak of the

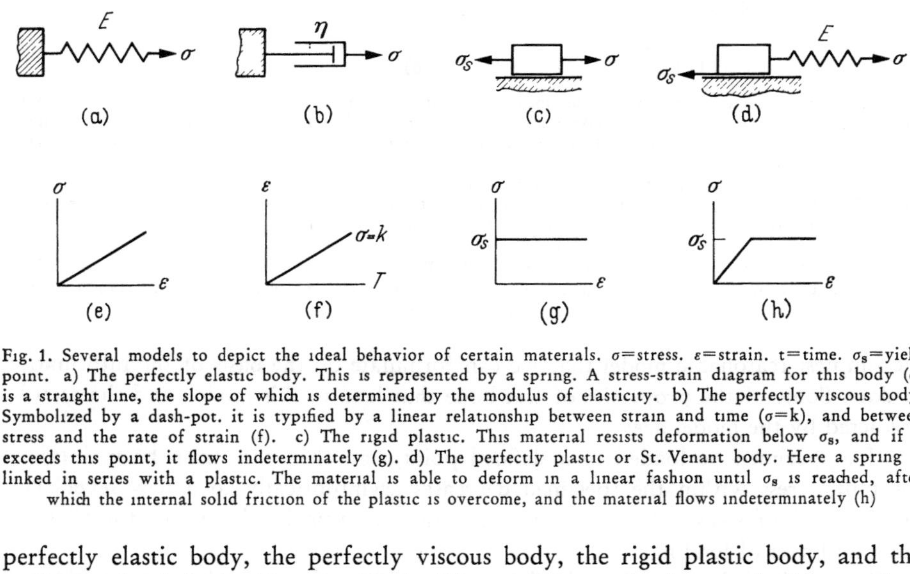

Fig. 1. Several models to depict the ideal behavior of certain materials. σ=stress. ε=strain. t=time. σ_s=yield point. a) The perfectly elastic body. This is represented by a spring. A stress-strain diagram for this body (e) is a straight line, the slope of which is determined by the modulus of elasticity. b) The perfectly viscous body. Symbolized by a dash-pot. it is typified by a linear relationship between strain and time (σ=k), and between stress and the rate of strain (f). c) The rigid plastic. This material resists deformation below σ_s, and if σ exceeds this point, it flows indeterminately (g). d) The perfectly plastic or St. Venant body. Here a spring is linked in series with a plastic. The material is able to deform in a linear fashion until σ_s is reached, after which the internal solid friction of the plastic is overcome, and the material flows indeterminately (h)

perfectly elastic body, the perfectly viscous body, the rigid plastic body, and the perfectly plastic body (JAEGER, 1956). All materials can be characterized by various combinations of these basic elements. In the perfectly elastic body, σ is proportional to strain (ε) and is related by the constant E. If this material be loaded, it is immediately strained, and if unloaded, the strain is instantaneously recovered, so that no deformation remains when $\sigma = 0$. In the viscous body, the rate of strain ($\mathring{\varepsilon}$) is proportional to σ, and is related by a constant η. These are statements of HOOKE's and NEWTON's laws. In the rigid plastic body, no deformation whatsoever takes place below the yield point (σ_S), and if $\sigma = \sigma_S$, the material flows indeterminately. In the perfectly plastic body, $\sigma = E\,\varepsilon$ for $\sigma < \sigma_S$, and when $\sigma = \sigma_S$ the material flows indeterminately. Our stress-strain curves for all axes of testing show that bone is a more complex material than can be typified by the ideal bodies cited. Other types of testing, in addition to the ones cited have lead us to formulate a model for the behavior of bone under moderate load (Fig. 2). This is a model of a HOOKE body linked in series to a

HOOKE and NEWTON body linked in parallel. (Kelvin body). The rationale for eliminating other model types is too lengthy for presentation here. It is not claimed that the model is a complete rheological formulation for the behavior of bone, but it is

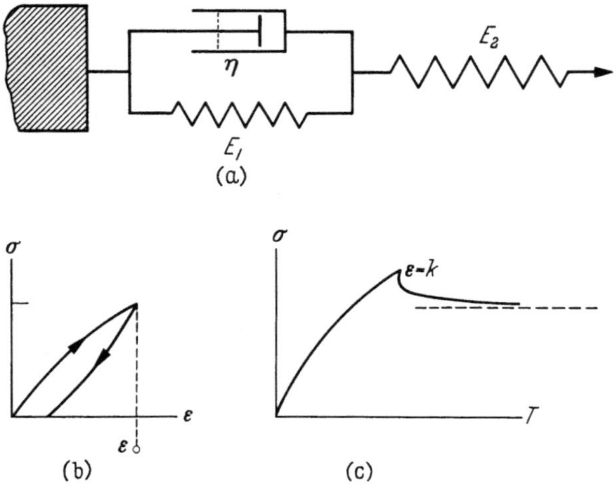

Fig. 2. A rheological model to explain some mechanical features of bone. Notation is as in Fig. 1, and in the text. a) The model consisting of a Hooke body linked in series with a Kelvin body. The independent spring has its E_2 as does the spring in the Kelvin element, E_1. The E for the material is a result of the combination of the two separate E's combined with the damping effect of the dash-pot. If a load be applied very slowly or very rapidly, the damping effect of the dash-pot is minimized, and the stress-strain curve is more nearly linear. For intermediate cases, the slope of the curve is determined by relations of the various constants for the components. The constitutional equation for the model can be written:

$$\mathring{\sigma} + a\sigma = b\mathring{\varepsilon} + cE$$

where $\mathring{\sigma}$ = rate of stress, $\mathring{\varepsilon}$ = rate of strain, $a = \eta\ (E_1+E_2)$, $b = E_2$ and $c = \eta\ E_1E_2$. The behavior of the model under the conditions of loading and unloading at a constant rate, and under a constant strain are shown in diagrams (b) and (c)

the simplest reasonable model that we can formulate on the basis of the information to date. Some of the properties of wet bone that lead to this model, and that can be predicted by the model are:

If a specimen be loaded to a defined point, and then the strain be maintained constant, stress within the specimen decreases asymptotically to a new level. This phenomenon of stress relaxation under a constant strain has been true for all sizes, rates, and axes of loading.

If a specimen be progressively deformed at a constant rate, the stress strain diagram is a curve with asymptote determined by the rate of loading. If the rate of deformation be made extremely slow or extremely fast, then a more nearly linear relation of stress to strain is obtained. The obvious conclusion is that a straight line on a stress-strain curve does not necessarily mean a perfectly elastic substance.

If a specimen is loaded up to some predetermined load, and then unloaded at the same rate, then when the load returns to zero, some residual deformation is present. The amount of residual deformation can be altered by changing the rate and size of the load.

The residual deformation of the unload cycle described above will be recovered, if the load is less than 40% of the ultimate breaking load. If more, some permanent deformation remains. In other words, while being loaded, bone is capable of conserving a certain amount of energy, a limit which can be exceeded.

If a constant moderate load be applied to bone, the final deformation is usually obtained within 10 minutes, with no further deformation appearing to occur after this time. We have only studied this phenomenon for periods up to 30′, this time limit being used since it appeared to be the biological ultimate for substained load. It can thus be stated that primary creep does not appear to exist in bone.

As bone is dried, a more nearly linear response is obtained on a stress-strain curve. In terms of the model, the damping effect of the dash-pot is reduced, and two springs are left in series, tending to approximate a single spring, or perfect elastic.

The modulus of elasticity is significantly changed by altering the rate of deformation. The more rapid σ, the higher E becomes.

As stated, the model is not complete. Qualitatively, it explains, fairly well, the behavior of bone under various types of load approximating 50% of the breaking strength or less. To account for the behavior of bone near the failure point, a rigid plastic or a series of rigid plastics will probably have to be inserted. In addition, in order to predict quantitatively the behavior under all conditions of loading, constants for the springs, dashpot, and plastic that may be added must be derived. This task is currently underway.

The use of a model system such as the one described, while old in theoretical mechanics, is new to bone. Its advantages are many, but one of the chief ones is that it enables one to predict behavior under complex circumstances which cannot be tested in the laboratory.

Summary

Findings relative to the physical properties of femoral cortical bone tested in the fresh, wet state have been described. A rheological model that explains the behavior of bone under certain conditions has been presented.

References

Jaeger, J. O.: Elasticity, Fracture and Flow. London: Methuen 1956.

Reiner, M.: Rheology. In Encyclopedia of Physics. Vol. VI, Flügge, S. (ed.). Berlin: Springer 1958, p. 434.

Sedlin, E. D., and C. Hirsch: Factors affecting the determination of the physical properties of femoral cortical bone. Acta orthop. scand. (in press).

Haemodynamic Data on the Osseous Circulation

M. Brookes

Department of Anatomy, Guy's Hospital, Medical School, London, England

The physical constants of the blood in the osseous circulation are likely to be significant factors in the regulation of calcification and bone growth. This paper describes a method for estimating some formerly unknown data, including flow rates, pertaining to a variety of subcompartments of the femoral circulation in the rat.

Materials and methods

Female albino rats, mean weight 140 gm were used. All investigations were carried out under ether anaesthesia. Results are given on the middle third of the femoral cortex, the marrow core inside it, the superior and inferior metaphyses and the inferior epiphysis.

Blood Volume. A red cell dilution technique was employed. Rat red cells were labelled with ^{51}Cr, washed in saline and centrifuged. The labelled cells were prepared and used on the same day. Each rat was given 0.3 ml i.v. packed labelled cells. After 15 minutes to allow complete mixing of the label, the tail of the animal was swiftly amputated and a drop of blood caught on a glass slide. The anaesthetised rat was then dropped into acetone at $-50\ ^{\circ}C$, and the circulation thereby suddenly stopped. The femora were fixed in ice-cold formalin. All extra-osseous soft tissue including cartilage was removed from the bone. It was then broken down into the various samples to be investigated. The weight of each sample was taken and its radioactivity measured as also that of a 0.005 ml sample of tail blood collected in a micropipette.

From these readings, the blood volume/100 gm selected tissue was calculated in terms of ml tail blood. The red cell volume was also arrived at knowing the haematocrit of rat tail blood (43.4%).

Rate of flow

The above procedure was modified as follows. Each rat was weighed and a 0.005 ml sample was taken of the measured volume of labelled blood given to the rat. The rats were killed by freezing at known intervals varying from 5—45 sec. after injection i.v. of the label. The radioactive concentration of the tissue was calculated and appropriate corrections made for variation in rat weight, dose volume of label, radioactive decay, and radioactive concentration of the dose given to each rat. Graphs were then constructed relating measured radioactive concentration to time in seconds after injection. From the graphs, it was possible to estimate the rate of flow through individual tissues in ml packed red cells/100 gm/min, or in terms of peripheral whole blood applying an arbitrary haemotocrit of 43.4%.

Circulation time and velocity

The former is given by Vol/Flow. A comparative estimate of the velocity of the cells through the tissue is given by the reciprocal of the circulation time.

Results

Blood volume

Tables 1 and 2 summarize the findings on 21 rats.

Flow, circulation time, and velocity

These are derived from flow curves (Figs. 1, 2) constructed from the mean readings of 61 rats. The area A under the initial wave divided by T, the transit time, gives a measure of the bolus of label traversing 1 gm tissue in time T. The radioactivity of 0.005 ml label is known. Hence the flow rate F can be calculated. V/F then yields the circulation time C.T. Velocity is given by I/C.T. (Tables 3 and 4).

Table 1. *Raw data work sheet for volume estimation*

Rat No. 12	Rat wt. 110 gm	Date 27. 11. 1963 Haematocrit 43.4		Count/0.005 ml. Blood = 2571 Count less Background = 2406 (Real Count)		Background Count = 165
Tissue	Count	Real Count	Tissue wts	Radioactive Concentration Counts/gm	Red Cell Mass ml/100 gm	Whole Blood Vol ml/100 mg
Superior metaphysis . .	413	248	0.0194	12783	1.151	2.65
Cortex	745	580	0.0718	8077	0.729	1.68
Marrow	469	304	0.0240	12666	1.142	2.63
Inferior metaphysis . .	1335	1170	0.0686	17050	1.538	3.54
Inferior epiphysis . . .	1237	1072	0.1166	9193	0.829	1.91

Table 2. *Blood volumes in rat femur*

Tissue	Number of rats	Red Cell Vol ml/100 gm $P < 0.05$	s. e.	Whole Blood Vol ml/100 gm
Superior metaphysis	21	1.203	0.053 (4.4%)	2.77
Cortex	15	0.937	0.029 (3.1%)	2.16
Inferior metaphysis	21	1.874	0.082 (4.4%)	4.32
Marrow	21	1.587	0.088 (5.5%)	3.66
Inferior epiphysis	21	1.124	0.066 (5.9%)	2.59

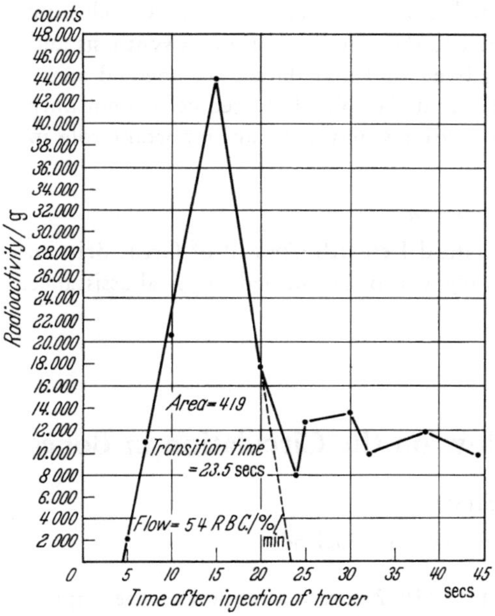

Fig. 1. Flow curve for superior metaphysis constructed from mean readings of 61 rats

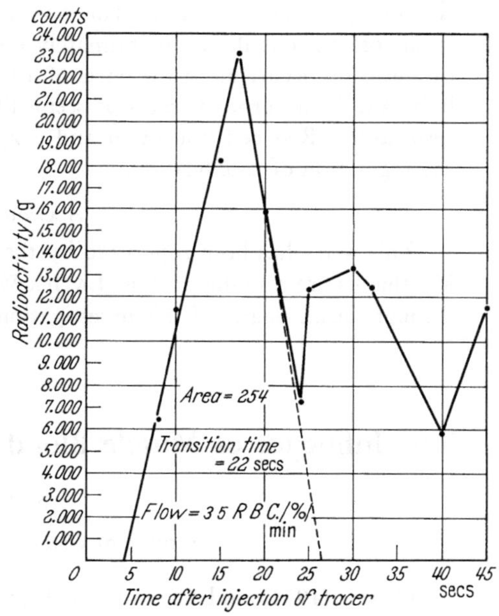

Fig. 2. Flow curve for diaphyseal cortex constructed from mean readings of 61 rats

Table 3. *Haemodynamic constants for rat femoral tissues*

	Flows ml % min		Vols ml %		Circulation Time in secs	Velocity (1/C. T.)
	Whole blood	RBC	Whole blood	RBC		
Inferior metaphysis	22.7	9.9	4.32	1.874	11.4	0.0877
Marrow	12.8	5.5	3.66	1.587	17.3	0.0578
Superior metaphysis	12.3	5.4	2.77	1.203	13.4	0.0746
Cortex	8.0	3.5	2.16	0.937	16.1	0.0621
Inferior epiphysis	6.7	2.9	2.59	1.124	23.3	0.0429

Table 4. *Relative haemodynamic data (inferior metaphysis = 100%)*

	Flow	Volume	Velocity
Inferior metaphysis	100%	100%	100%
Marrow	56%	85%	66%
Superior metaphysis	55%	64%	86%
Cortex	35%	50%	71%
Inferior epiphysis	29%	60%	49%

Discussion

The investigation has yielded a comprehensive set of haemodynamic data for the femur of the 140 gm rat under ether anaesthesia. Attention is drawn to the following:

1. Flow, volume, and velocity of red cells are not necessarily correlated. Presumably haematocrit values differ considerably from tissue to tissue within bone.

2. The 3 : 1 predominance of flow in the "growing" metaphysis over that of the adjacent epiphysis is in striking contrast to recent and opposite opinion.

3. The highest flow is in the growing metaphysis and is roughly double that in the non-growing metaphysis. This flow-growth correlation suggests that red cell flow in the osseous circulation is intimately related to the amount of protein synthesis and calcification occurring in the parts of a long bone, and that these have unequal metabolic and bone turnover rates. It seems likely that the role of the red cells is not only respiratory. Red cell potassium and enzyme systems may play an important role in the regulation of calcification.

Acknowledgement

This work has been supported by the Medical Research Council of Great Britain. My thanks are also due to Miss LATIFA WAFAQUANI for her skilled technical assistance throughout all phases of this investigation.

The Influence of Muscle Blood-flow on the Circulation in Bones

N. E. SHAW

Institute of Orthopaedics, London, England

HEALD (1951) and CECCHI and FIUMICELLI (1952) drew attention to the importance of the osseomuscular circulation. Examination of bone and muscle blood-flow using the heated thermocouple technique (SHAW, 1963) showed that studies could be carried out under physiologically normal conditions providing that careful dissection was performed. Studies on different tissues in the same limb were also shown to be possible and the dependence of blood-flow in one tissue on the blood-flow in another could be investigated. The present studies have been designed to examine the relation between the circulation in bone and in the overlying muscle.

Materials and methods

Experiments were conducted on 15 adult cats anaesthetized with chloralose (80 mg. per kg.). Tracheotomy was performed. Heparin was given to prevent coagulation around the probes and cannulae. In 5 experiments the animal was fixed in a frame to prevent movement of the hind limb in spite of muscle contraction. The right tibia was transfixed at the upper and lower ends by a Kirschner wire held rigidly in a frame and the pelvis was similarly fixed; the femur and its overlying muscles which were to be examined remained undisturbed.

Pressure was measured by Statham pressure transducers; arterial blood pressure from a carotid artery and femoral intramedullary pressure from a cannula in the upper third of the right femur. Saline was used as a conducting medium.

Bloodflow was recorded in ten experiments using the heated thermocouple technique (Shaw, 1963) and in five using the temperature compensated flow velocity probe (Shaw, 1964); one probe was placed in the medulla of the upper third of the right femur and another in the adjacent quadriceps muscle. In the studies using the heated thermocouple the output was fed into Pye D.C. amplifiers and recorded by a Siemens-Ediswan Pen recorder. The output from the temperature compensated flow velocity probe was fed into an A.C. Amplifier (Cybernetics Laboratories) and the records transcribed by a U.V. Recorder (S.E. Laboratories). In some animals estimation of the hind-limb venous return was made with an electronic drop-counter sampling from the femoral vein in the femoral triangle and simultaneous records of muscle blood-flow were made with the temperature compensated flow velocity probe. The output from the drop-counter was fed directly into the U.V. recorder. Similarity in flow changes recorded by the drop-counter and probe were considered to validate the latter method as a means of estimating rate of change of muscle blood-flow.

The right femoral nerve was exposed in the femoral triangle and isolated and divided in a paraffin pool. Platinum electrodes were used for nerve stimulation and square wave stimuli through an R.F. probe were used. Stimulus parameters were varied from 2—8 volts; 250 μsec. to 1 m.sec. duration and 10 per min. to 100 per sec. frequency. The size of this stimulus is sufficient to stimulate all components of the nerve.

Decamethonium iodide was given to examine the effect of peripheral nerve stimulation on bone blood-flow when the surrounding muscles are paralysed.

Results

Stimulation of the proximal cut end of the femoral nerve caused a rise in arterial blood-pressure which was reflected in the rise in femoral intramedullary pressure and bone and muscle blood-flow.

Stimulation of the peripheral cut end of the femoral nerve was also carried out:

(1) Continuous stimulation caused an initial fall in muscle blood-flow, but during sustained muscle contraction the blood flow increased above the resting level until

stimulation stopped. Muscle relaxation was accompanied by a further increase in muscle blood-flow which returned to its resting level after about three minutes. There was an initial fall in medullary pressure and blood flow followed by a rise until nerve stimulation ceased when there was a sudden fall followed by a marked rise in both these characteristics of the circulation in bone (Fig. 1).

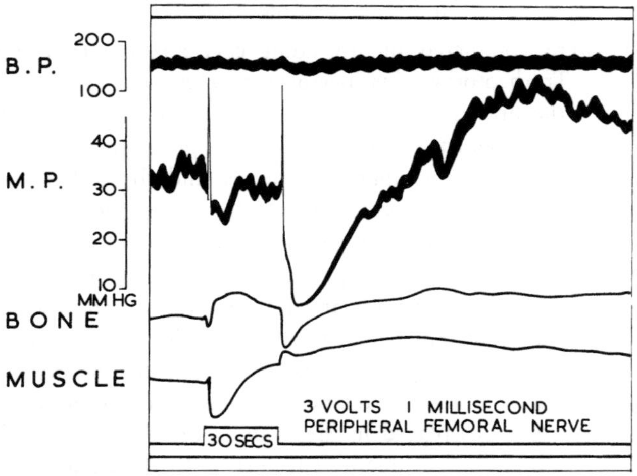

Fig. 1. Upper tracings — Arterial blood-pressure and intramedullary pressure. Lower tracings — Bone blood-flow and muscle blood-flow. The muscle blood-flow falls initially but rises above its resting level during continued stimulation and reactive hyperaemia causes a further increase when nerve stimulation stops. The immediate fall in medullary pressure and bone blood-flow are apparent and the fall and subsequent rise when nerve stimulation is withdrawn is shown

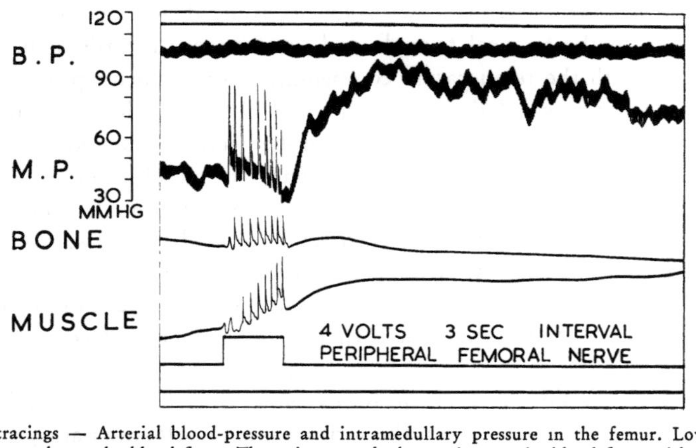

Fig. 2. Upper tracings — Arterial blood-pressure and intramedullary pressure in the femur. Lower tracings —. Bone blood-flow and muscle blood-flow. There is a gradual rise in muscle blood-flow with repeated nerve stimulation; sudden rises in bone blood-flow and intramedullary pressure occur with each muscle contraction, but the intramedullary pressure gradually falls

(2) Repeated nerve stimulation caused intermittent muscle contractions each temporarily reducing the muscle blood-flow, which however, increased progressively during muscle relaxation. This change was associated with a momentary rise in the intramedullary pressure and the blood flow in bone during each muscle contraction, but there was a gradual fall in medullary pressure after each stimulus (Fig. 2).

Stimulation of the peripheral cut end of the femoral nerve after injection of decamethonium caused a fall in muscle blood-flow without affecting the circulation in bone.

Discussion

The simultaneous rise in arterial pressure, intramedullary pressure and blood flow and in muscle blood-flow which occurred when the proximal cut end of the femoral nerve was stimulated could be ascribed to a central effect on arterial pressure similar to stimulating a dorsal nerve root. The surprising feature was the sudden increase in intramedullary pressure and blood flow in bone like that shown by Trueta and Valderrama (1965) in dogs.

The fall and subsequent rise in muscle blood-flow during continuous stimulation of the distal cut end of the femoral nerve suggests that during muscle contraction the pressure on the muscle veins empties them. Sustained or rapidly repeated contraction probably increases muscle blood-flow by arteriolar and capillary dilatation; an effect of the products of local metabolism in spite of raised intramuscular tension. Muscle relaxation further increased blood flow due to vasodilatation with vessels unrestricted by external compression. The gradual fall in medullary pressure and blood flow in bone which was observed may have been a passive effect owing to the diminished resistance in the vascular bed of the overlying muscle.

The present studies suggest the possibility of a passive role of intra-medullary blood-vessels during phases of varying blood flow in muscle; that muscle contraction squeezes blood into bone via venous channels is the more attractive idea, because blood flow and intramedullary pressure tend to follow a similar pattern; that muscle occludes the veins during its contraction and therefore causes a barrier to outflow from bone is hardly acceptable, because blood returning from the femur may escape from veins above the level of the contracting muscle. It may be that under certain conditions the circulation in the medulla may act by a venturi effect in respect of vessels in the surrounding soft tissues.

In some circumstances such as fracture of a long bone the haemodynamic system of the medulla is destroyed and these effects would be abolished. Destruction of the haemodynamic system may account for the oedema of the lower limb which is so well-known after bony injury and prolonged immobilisation, and for the high incidence of venous thrombosis after operations on the hip (Tubiana and Duparc, 1961).

Vascular connections between muscle and bone may be important collateral channels for the spread of tumour cells. They may also be of importance in providing ischaemic muscle or bone with an alternative route for a blood supply (Zucman, 1960).

In the present studies no direct effect of nerve stimulation on the circulation in bones was found. However, there is little doubt that changes in muscle blood-flow have a considerable influence on the circulation in bone through the osseomuscular circulation which Heald (1951) originally described.

Summary

Stimulation of the proximal and peripheral cut ends of the femoral nerve in anaesthetized cats had no direct effect on the circulation in bone. The changes in blood flow in muscle affected the circulation in underlying bone and the physiological implications of this are discussed.

Acknowledgements

I wish to thank Sir Herbert Seddon, Dr. Angus McPherson, the Joint Clinical Research Committee of the Institute of Orthopaedics and the National Fund for Poliomyelitis Research for encouragement and help.

References

Cecchi, E., e A. Fiumicelli: Sull'esistenza di una circolazione umorale tra osso e muscolo. Reumatismo **4**, 371 (1952).

Heald, C. B.: An inquiry into the treatment of fibrositis with observations on vascular communications between bone and muscle. Lancet **II**, 659 (1951).

Shaw, N. E.: Observations on the intramedullary pressure and blood flow in bones. Clin. Sci. **24**, 312 (1963).

— Observations on the physiology of the blood vessels in bone. Ann. roy. Coll. Surg. Engl. **35**, 214 (1964).

Trueta, J., and J. A. F. de Valderrama: Muscle contraction and intraosseous circulation. J. Bone Jt Surg. **47 B**, 186 (1965).

Tubiana, R., and J. Duparc: Prevention of thrombo-embolic complications in orthopaedic and accident surgery. J. Bone Jt Surg. **43 B**, 7 (1961).

Zucman, J.: Studies on the vascular connections between periosteum, bone and muscle. Brit. J. Surg. **48**, 324 (1960).

A Biomolecular Survey of Calcification

F. G. E. Pautard

Astbury Department of Biophysics, Leeds University, Leeds, Yorksh., England

Deposits of inorganic calcium salts are so familiar to biologists that they seldom warrant close attention and are dismissed frequently as waste products. In spite of an increasing awareness that mineralization is a highly organized process, however, it is immediately apparent from the literature that we derive most of our ideas about the ultrastructural basis of calcification from studies of bone. There is little correlative data from other tissues containing calcium phosphate, and the few publications on the molecular structures associated with calcium carbonate in invertebrates are sufficient to emphasize the lack of information about the nature and genesis of the same salt in plants. The present grossly unbalanced state of knowledge is best illustrated by an appeal to mass. The investigations of calcium phosphate in vertebrates far exceed all other studies of calcium salts, yet bone, dentine and enamel are the least abundant mineralized tissues, constituting a fraction of a percent of the calcium oxalate in plants, where the nature of the inorganic substances present seems to have been neglected and where there appear to be no reports of the ultrastructure in the literature.

There is, therefore, only fragmentary evidence for any comparison of the molecular arrangements present in calcified structures throughout nature, and although each type of calcium salt has a common basis in chemistry, it has yet to be demonstrated that there is a common cellular plan of mineralization.

The following survey is designed to compare, at a macromolecular level, analogous structures and analogous calcium deposits in a variety of animals and plants. Certain features have been selected to comment on the three principal problems of distribution, structure and genesis.

Distribution

Comprehensive reports and reviews of the relative amounts of mineral matter in animals (Clarke and Wheeler, 1922) and in plants (Pobeguin, 1954) serve as a useful guide to the distribution of calcium salts in nature, but there are gaps in our knowledge caused by lack of information about clearly defined crystalline salts (as opposed to calculations based on chemical assay of cations and anions) and by the precise geography of "mixed" salts within a single tissue or cell. It is well known, for example, that many crustaceans contain calcium phosphate as well as carbonate in their hard parts, yet until recently (Pautard and Trautz, in press) no species has been found with crystallographic verification of bone salts, although the usual well-defined X-ray diffraction pattern of calcite found in carbonate-rich invertebrates might well conceal a second, less crystalline, phase of phosphate. The absence of precise information about the relationship of anions to calcium has led to the erroneous generalization that calcium phosphate is confined to the vertebrates, calcium carbonate to the invertebrates and calcium oxalate to the plants. In fact, all three salts are to be found in all three situations without any clear demarcation between them, as can be seen by the distributions set out in Table 1.

Table 1. *Distribution of calcium carbonate, oxalate and phosphate in normal biological structures*

Subject	Carbonate	Oxalate	Phosphate
Invertebrata	Shells, tests, exo- and endoskeletons, spines and otoliths.	Insect eggs. Larval cuticles. Associated with carbonate	Protozoa Coelenterata Arthropoda Brachiopoda
Vertebrata	Calcified keratin. Eggs of birds and reptiles. Statoconia. Associated with bone.	Associated with bone. In soft tissue	Bone, dentine enamel. Calcified keratin
Thallophyta Bryophyta Pteridophyta	Cell inclusions	Algae Most mosses and ferns	Bacteria
Gymnosperms Angiosperms	Cell inclusions	Found in all species	Heartwood

The most widely reported calcium salt in plants and animals is the carbonate, ranging from the shells and tests in the Protozoa, through the hard exoskeletons of invertebrates to the eggs of birds and statoconia in man, from intracellular granules in bacteria through spherulites in algae to a wide variety of inclusions in cystoliths, tracheids and leaf parenchyma in angiosperms. The occurrence of calcium phosphate has been less well recorded, partly because bone has dominated the phosphate scene and partly because much of the salt present in tissues other than vertebrate is less crystalline than the more abundant carbonate and may hence be undetected. Deposits of crystalline bone salt have been recorded in invertebrates, in the Protozoa (PAUTARD, 1959), in the Arthropoda (PAUTARD and TRAUTZ, in press) and in the Brachiopoda (KLEMENT, 1938). In the vertebrates, the familiar "phosphatic" structures of bone, dentine and enamel have been supplemented by the calcified keratins, many of which contain appreciable quantities of salt (PAUTARD, 1963). In plants, reports of deposits of bone salts have been confined to the bacteria (ENNEVER, 1963) although there are records of other forms of calcium phosphate in various types of heartwood. Calcium oxalate in the form of intracellular crystals of diverse shapes and sizes is widely distributed in plants, often, as in the case of some xerophytes, constituting over half the dry weight of the plant. Reports of oxalate in animals are numerous, although scattered. Crystals of this salt are often found in the invertebrates, particularly in the Arthropoda, where deposits are found in insect egg shells and are resorbed during embryonic development (for example, MOSCONA, 1948). In the vertebrates, calcium oxalate in pathological stones and calculi is a familiar substance; in normal conditions there is evidence that oxalate is found as a constituent of hard tissues (in fish scales, for instance — NISHIHARA, 1954) and it is likely that small quantities are present in soft tissues as well (JOHNSON and PANI, 1962).

The present evidence, then, suggests that calcium in the form of carbonate, phosphate and oxalate is very widely distributed, can be found in one form to the exclusion of others in animals and plants and often in individual species. Nowhere, however, can we find evidence which confines any one salt to any one group. Instead, we see a wide panorama of calcium salts with almost every variation and combination in different subjects.

Structure

At a molecular level, the structure of calcified tissues is resolved as a partnership between inorganic deposits and organic substances. This partnership varies widely in the amount and ordering of the mineral and organic phases, and we can find examples of different proportions of different salts in the same organic milieu and similar proportions of similar salts in different organic milieu. There are wide variations, too, in the order and crystallinity of the two phases. The three principal calcium salts can be found in crystalline and non-crystalline states in organic environments varying from frankly fibrous proteins and polysaccharides to diffuse indeterminate stroma with no apparent structure.

Mineral phase

While chemical assay of cations and anions can give us figures from which we can calculate plausible structures, the best criterion of a salt is its characteristic X-ray diffraction pattern, which results from an exact arrangement of atoms in a lattice and thus relates the components in a positive geometric way. Unfortunately, X-ray diffraction methods have limitations, particularly in biological subjects, and these are often overlooked in studies of mineral deposits. In the first place, the usual procedures associated with powder analysis, especially where organic enclosure may prevent equilibrium between different types of salt, are not quantitative and it is not profitable to relate the crystallographic evidence to the chemistry. Again, a crystal ceases to give an X-ray diffraction pattern below a certain limiting size (about 50 Å in the case of apatite, for instance) and in many mineralized tissues the inorganic particles are at, or below, the threshold of detection; the term "amorphous" applied to such a state is misleading. Finally, a small proportion of crystals of detectable size will give a clear characteristic X-ray diffraction diagram in the presence of relatively large amounts of "amorphous" material of the same, similar or different chemical composition (PAUTARD, 1964). There is thus no reliable means of estimating the structure of all the inorganic particles in a given tissue and no way of deciding if the crystalline species that is present represents the total inorganic content. The situation is further complicated by comparisons between X-ray diffraction data and observation in the electron microscope. While measurement of the size of crystallites from electron micrographs can confirm the upper, or average, sizes calculated from the width of selected reflexions in the X-ray diffraction patterns, it cannot be assumed that all dense, crystal-like structures are, in fact, crystalline, particularly as the instances of demonstrable *single* crystals by electron diffraction are very few.

With these reservations in mind, however, it is still possible to detect a wide range of crystallinity of calcium salts, varying from colloidal suspensions (for example calcium phosphates in cestodes — BRAND *et al.*, 1960) to crystals of optical size (oxalates in plants — POBEGUIN, 1943) and even larger crystals visible to the unaided eye (calcite in sea urchin spines). An important aspect of the structure of the inorganic phase, in spite of the wide diversity of forms, is the remarkable *constancy* of the deposits in each calcified tissue. While it is true that there are numerous chemical variations in minor cations (Mg, Sr, Na, K, etc.) and minor anions (F, SiO_3, SO_4) and mixtures of calcium salts often occur, each mineralized structure seems to be characterized by a careful control of crystallite shape and size. Even in shells hardened by calcium salts at some distance, apparently, from any cells, the crystallite size remains constant in the mature structure, as shown in the valve of *Lingula unguis* by KELLY *et al.* (1965). In pathological conditions, a certain semblance of constancy is sometimes retained in regions of the inorganic deposit (GONZALES and SOGNNAES, 1960, report a laminated, regular structure in dental calculus) but more usually the crystallite size, shape and distribution tends to be random.

In normal tissues, the crystal characteristics of the three principal calcium salts appear to remain relatively constant also. Calcium carbonate is found most frequently in the form of calcite, occasionally as aragonite; both forms are sometimes found together. Calcium phosphate occurs almost universally as an apatite, or in a closely related crystallographic state. Calcium oxalate appears as several hydrates, the optical characteristics of which have been long established (for example, FREY, 1929). The X-ray crystallography of the oxalate, however, has been confined mostly to comparative powder measurements (in a recent survey, WALTER-LEVY et STRAUSS [1962], list the monohydrate, the dihydrate, a 2.25 hydrate, but question the existence of a trihydrate) although there are some limited data for the lattice of the tetragonal polyhydrates (HONEGGER, 1952). Recently, measurements of the lattice parameters of single crystals of monoclinic monohydrate raphides isolated from *Yucca* have enabled us (ARNOTT *et al.*, in press) to establish the dimensions of the unit cell together with some information about the spatial arrangement of the calcium atoms.

Organic phase

It is unfortunate that the extensive investigation of bone collagen over the past few years has tended to obstruct serious survey of the nature of other organic substances associated with calcium salts in biological tissues. An almost universal preoccupation with collagen structure and chemistry has obscured the fact that there are numerous subjects which contain bone salts associated with other proteins and with polysaccharides. Even in enamel, where it has been suggested on chemical (EASTOE, 1960) and crystallographic (PAUTARD, 1961) grounds that collagen might be absent, the heterogeneous nature of the sparse organic phase has left us with the possibility that collagen-like proteins, or macromolecules with some features in common with collagen, might play a direct part in calcification. From considerations of bones and teeth alone it is not easy to divorce collagen entirely from some specific association with calcium phosphate, but if we look at the wider panorama of calcification we find that there is no evidence for a close association of any one calcium salt with any

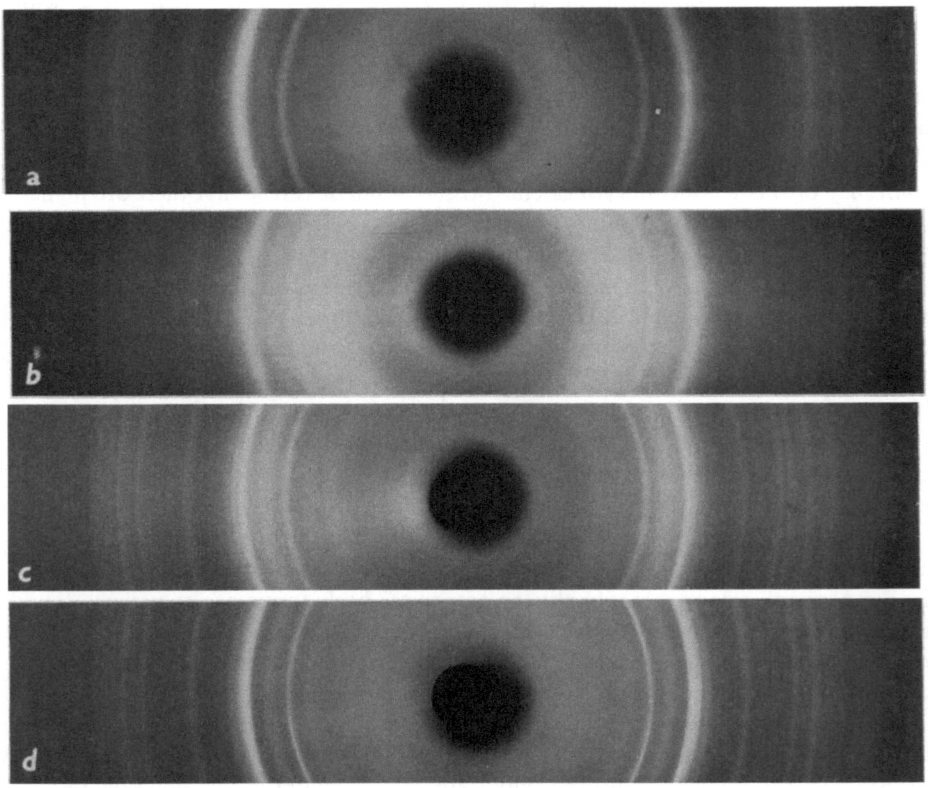

Fig. 1. X-ray powder diffraction diagrams (CuK α radiation) from four subjects each containing calcium phosphate. a. Tip of dorsal spine of *Ictalurus punctatus*. b. Fringe fibre tip of baleen from *Balaenopterus borealis*. c. Tip of chela of *Squilla* species. d. Shell of *Lingula unguis*

one organic substrate and no real grounds for assuming that the "choice" of a particular calcium salt for a particular structure is connected with the nature of the fibrous macromolecules which are present.

This feature of *interchange* of mineral with respect to the organic composition of the tissue is best illustrated by first comparing a range of structures based on one type of calcium salt and then examining analogous structures with two different types of mineral deposit. In Fig. 1 the X-ray powder diffraction photographs have been arranged to compare four subjects, each of which contains crystalline inorganic deposits closely resembling bone salt; the four examples are chosen from different phyla (two invertebrate, two vertebrate) and each is associated with a different molecule. Fig. 1 a is the diagram from the tip of the dorsal spine of the Channel Catfish, *Ictalurus punctatus*. This subject, though of lower vertebrate origin, is typical of bone and contains collagen as the principal organic component. On the other hand, the specimen in Fig. 1 b from Sei whale *(Balaenopterus borealis)* baleen contains crystallites of bone salt essentially similar to those found in Fig. 1 a, but in this case the organic component is keratin and collagen is absent (PAUTARD, 1965). In Fig. 1 c and 1 d, the inorganic salt closely resembles that in Fig. 1 a and 1 b, but the main organic component in both cases is the polysaccharide chitin, in the α-form in the case of the chela of the Mantis Shrimp *Squilla* in Fig. 1 c and probably in the β-form in the case of the shell of the brachiopod *Lingula unguis* in Fig. 1 d.

Analogues structures often contain mixtures of calcium salts, but in some cases one or another crystalline species predominates, occasionally in adjacent tissues. This is particularly true in the keratins, where bone salts have been demonstrated crystallographically, but where "amorphous" calcium deposits, probably of carbonate as well as phosphate, have been suggested (PAUTARD, 1963). Fig. 2 a shows a quadrant X-ray diffraction pattern of Sei whale baleen. The fibre axis is vertical and the c-axis of the hydroxyapatite crystallites (judging from the meridional disposition of the 002 reflexion) is generally parallel to the axis of the α-helices (shown by the orientation of the reflexion at about 5.1 Å on the meridian). On the other hand the diffraction diagram of the tip of the anterior dorsal papillae of the tongue of a bull (Fig. 2 b) shows "spotty" reflexions of calcite, suggesting crystals of large (about 1 micron) size not oriented with respect to α-helices. Close inspection of the original diffraction pattern shows a second series of unoriented reflexions corresponding to the apatite spacings in Fig. 2 a. In Fig. 2 c, the crystallographic pattern from the chela of *Squilla* closely resembles that from the Sei whale baleen fibre in Fig. 2 a, but there is no evidence for any orientation of the crystallites with respect to the axis of the appendage, which is vertical. In Fig. 2 d, a similar structure — the chela of the small crab *Callinectes* found in the same area as the shrimp in Fig. 2 c gives an unoriented diffraction pattern of calcite of smaller crystal size than the comparable salt in Fig. 2 b. Thus, in one set of comparisons, we have large and small crystals of calcite and apatite, oriented and unoriented and as discernable mixtures in two analogous subjects, both of epidermal origin, containing keratin in one case and α-chitin in the other.

From the above, and from other, comparisons it is apparent that the mineral phase and the organic phase are not linked by the specific nature of the calcium salt and the protein or the polysaccharide framework. At least, this cannot be true in the gross sense, for where there are oriented fibrous macromolecules there can usually be found also oriented crystallites of one salt and another. The term "matrix", which is customarily assigned to collagen in bone, tends to be misleading when applied to the organic moiety of other forms of calcification. Collagen is a relatively homogeneous fibrous protein which is the bulk of the organic substance oriented with bone salts, but in the calcified keratins, which are also fibrous and also oriented, the horny material of the "matrix" is not one protein, but a family of proteins, each of which

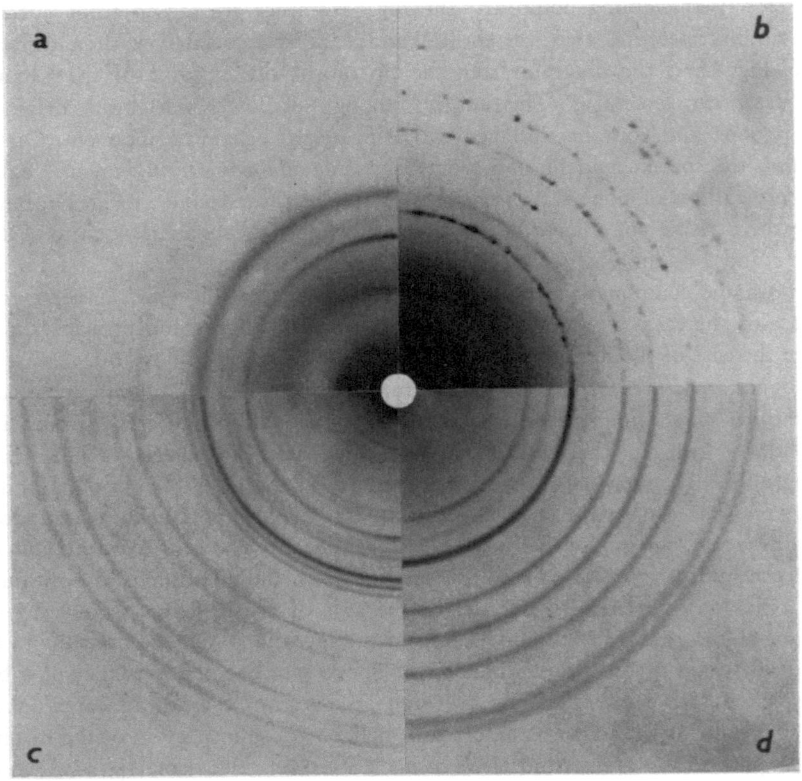

Fig. 2. Comparison of X-ray Laue diffraction diagrams (CuK radiation, fibre axis vertical) from two pairs of structures of epidermal origin. a. Fringe fibre tip of baleen from *Balaenopterus borealis*. b. Tips of anterior dorsal papillae from bovine tongue. c. Tip of chela of *Squilla* species. d. Tip of chela of *Callinectes*

is comparable to collagen in a mechanical sense. Again, in the calcified chitins (for instance KELLY *et al.*, 1965) the principal *oriented* organic component is the polysaccharide, but protein in some unknown configuration is present also and in this case the "matrix" consists of a complex partnership in which the protein tends to diminish as calcification increases.

The diversity of organic molecules and macromolecules associated with calcium salts prompts me to suggest the term *topographical matrix* to describe the skeletal, usually fibrous, framework laid down in partnership with the mineral phase. This term conveys the idea of an architectural arrangement of stable, frequently insoluble structures which are often oriented with the inorganic crystals and which can be distinguished from the more labile and sparse "ground substances" which fill the interstices of the fibrous network. The topographical matrix is related to the calcium deposits in some way, but we are not committed to thinking of one macromolecule or of any specific relationship between macromolecule and mineral. We can regard the topographical matrix as a fabric which may, or may not, be mineralized, and which may, or may not, play a direct role in the calcification process.

Genesis

Our present ideas about calcification are based largely on studies of bone, and it is understandable that there are numerous theories as to the initiation, growth and control of calcium phosphate crystals with respect to collagen. In many ways, however, the position has changed little from that proposed in the comprehensive survey by NEUMAN and NEUMAN in 1953, which examined the problems of calcium deposition in bone in terms of ion exchange and crystal structure, solubility and growth and which laid down certain guiding principles. Not the least of the persistent errors examined in the survey were those of the many calculations of solubility products, which were not considered as applicable to solids of variable composition. The failure to arrive at a satisfactory equation to account for the necessary ions in a lattice of basic calcium phosphate led to the idea of crystallization, as opposed to precipitation, and in the words of NEUMAN and NEUMAN (1953) the situation was apocryphal even for acid salt because "It has been shown that the K_{sp} of $CaHPO_4$ must be exceeded for *precipitation* to occur, yet *calcification* occurs in individuals whose blood levels of calcium and phosphate are well below this product".

This conclusion, that apatite could form only by crystallization, principally because of "*the blood levels of calcium and phosphate*" led to the suggestion that calcification takes place on sites within the matrix which form specific nucleation centres. As a result, there have arisen several general theories to explain the process of nucleation in terms of bound phosphate and bound calcium, either to collagen or to some closely allied part of the matrix. Mineralization has been thus explained in terms of physical chemical factors causing an epitactic growth of crystals from ions migrating freely through the extracellular organic phase, in contrast to the earlier views of ROBISON (1932) which supposed that there was some local enzyme mechanism which precipitated the calcium salt at the calcification front. When the bulk of the studies on bone salt and bone collagen changed to explore the new ideas proposed by NEUMAN and NEUMAN (1953), the emphasis shifted towards the chemistry of the cell-free substances and little attention was paid to the role of the cell in laying down the bone salt. Indeed, there is an inherent fallacy in this neglect, for if the calcium and phosphorus destined to make bone salt goes *through* the cell en route to the mineralization zone, then the "*blood levels of calcium and phosphate*" can have no meaning in relation to the inorganic phase in bone other than to decide the *rate* of transfer. We can find, for instance, the present calculations for serum calcium and phosphorus repeated in a recent review by HARTLES (1964) yet we find quoted also the evidence of WHITEHEAD and WEIDMANN (1959) that some, at least, of the phosphate might go through the cell, since inhibition of the ATP production causes lessening of bone salt formation. It would seem that unless it can be clearly established that *all* the ions in bone salt accumulate directly from the serum, any attempt to relate salt formation to the serum ion product is meaningless.

The curious lack of information as to the role of the osteoblast in the transference of ions to the inorganic phase in bone is not reflected in studies elsewhere; a brief survey of other forms of calcification shows at once that in many cases the cell is entirely responsible for salt formation and leads us to alternative suggestions as to how mineralization might take place.

Before reviewing some recent experiments on bone, however, the results of some of our present studies on the formation of calcium oxalate and calcium carbonate are of interest.

Calcium oxalate

A common form of calcium oxalate in plants — the monohydrate — is found within specialized cells in bundles (often as many as 2500) of lath- or needle-shaped crystals up to 200 microns long and about 1 micron square in section. The bundles of raphides are remarkably regular and each crystal is roughly parallel to its neighbour. It is usually supposed that these deposits are "waste products" and it is believed generally that the crystal arrangements arise within vacuoles, each crystal being enclosed within some sort of sheath (see Scott, 1941). Since the crystal cells develop rapidly, often in the root tip soon after it emerges from the seed, development of the mineral can be traced. The present ultrastructural and biophysical studies of raphides in plants (Arnott and Pautard, in press; Arnott, in press) suggest that the crystals do not arise in a haphazard manner but are laid down by a complex cell organization which involves the formation of *chambers* in which the inorganic material develops.

In *Yucca,* for example, these chambers are irregular when they are first formed and they soon become filled with electron-dense material which does not give an electron diffraction pattern. Later, as the chambers assume the characteristic tapering profile of the oxalate crystals, the contents become crystalline and there is evidence that the vacuole in which the chambers develop contains a detailed fine structure of tubes and membranes. In *Lemna,* the chambers occur in sequence at regular intervals between two membranes; here again the system becomes loaded with an electron-dense, non-crystalline substance during the earlier phases of growth.

The large intracellular crystals of calcium oxalate, then, might not arise by continuous growth from a single site nucleated by some fibrous orienting surface, but by the rearrangement of a mobile inorganic mixture within compartments which have been prefabricated in the vacuolar substance.

Calcium carbonate

Most of our information about the molecular basis of calcium carbonate formation comes from the studies of shell development in molluscs, crustaceans, and echinoderms. The evidence (for example, in the sand dollar *Echinarachnius* [Bevelander and Nakahara, 1960), in Crassostraea (Jodrey, 1953) and in the crustacean exoskeleton (Travis, 1963) suggests that the epidermal cells play a major role in laying down the organic phase. In *Mytilis,* the whole of the mantle calcium has been reported (Rao and Goldberg, 1954) to turn over in 24 hours. The method by which the mineral is transported to the developing shell is, however, a matter of dispute. Some authors (for instance Wilbur, 1964) assume that the ions are extruded by the cell into the extrapallial fluid; in some cases, the presence of crystals within the mantle cells has been reported (Bevelander, 1953).

Our present studies of the ultrastructure of the cells in apposition to the developing shell in *Pinna* and *Pedalium* (Arnott *et al.*, in press) show that the mantle edge extends during the active phase into long filaments which have a detailed fine structure and characteristic bulbous termini, which may become associated with the inner surface of the shell to be incorporated into the familiar lacelike mosaic of conchiolin reported by GREGOIRE (1957).

Calcium phosphate

Raphide formation in plants is essentially an intracellular process and shell formation in molluscs in possibly so, but in bone, dentine and enamel, calcification is generally considered to be an extracellular process in which the role of the cell is to provide the matrix. Precisely how the mineral gets into the "matrix" is not clear, but it is assumed that the ions migrate somehow from the serum fluids. In other structures containing bone salts, however, the relationship between the cell and the mineralization front is quite clear. In *Lingula,* where the crystallites develop in laminae within the shell, the mantle cells are firmly attached to the inner wall. In baleen, the deposits of salt are *within* the cell and there is no evidence for discontinuity between mineral and keratin (PAUTARD, 1965). The close connection between the intracellular deposits of apatite in baleen and the extracellular deposits in bone leaves us with an ultrastructural anomaly which now seems to be resolved. In baleen, the crystallites are usually surrounded by less dense, leaf-like structures (arrowed D in Fig. 3 a inset) whereas in the past no comparable structures have been observed in bone, although opinion as to the fine structure of the calcifying front has varied. Earlier reports (ROBINSON and CAMERON, 1956) suggest that crystals are laid down "within a fraction of a micron of the bone cells"; later, SHELDON and ROBINSON (1957) reported that the osteoblast could carry out metabolic transfer between the extracellular space and the calcified regions. Recently, it has been stated that there is a clear zone between osteoblast and mineral (ASCENZI *et al.*, 1963; FRANK, 1963) while CAMERON (1961) comments that mineral appears in cartilage beyond invading capillaries and at a distance from any cell. On the other hand, DUDLEY and SPIRO (1961) observed structural modifications of the cell surface at the site of contiguity, and HANCOX and BOOTHROYD (1964) have described short processes extending from the cell to the bone edge.

Our present experiments on newborn mouse bone (ARNOTT *et al.*, in press) using modifications of the fixation techniques recommended by SABATINI *et al.* (1964) suggest that there is a considerable amount of ultrastructure within the osteoblast and within numerous filamentous processes which spread from the cell to the mineralized front. Moreover, where a section has been cut by good fortune in the plane of the filament, the filopodia can be traced directly into the body of the crystallites as a delta of electron-dense material (arrowed D in Fig. 3 b) which closely resembles the leaf-like structures (c. f. Fig. 3 a) so often observed in baleen. In these areas, a faint electron diffraction pattern of apatite can be observed; nowhere can we find any periodic deposition of "nuclei", either on the collagen fibres which are always present, or as rows of electron-dense dots. The calcifying delta simply appears to spread out, like a stain, into the organic substances adjacent to the filopodia.

In enamel, present opinion favours the view that the ameloblast is separated from the mineral front by a continuous membrane. Some authors (FRANK *et al.*, 1960; TRAVIS and GLIMCHER, 1964) state that the organic phase forms a framework which faithfully copies the outlines of the crystallites; there is no suggestion as to whether this framework is created by the crystals or by the cell. RÖNNHOLM (1963), on the other hand, in a detailed study of amelogenesis, makes it clear that the pattern of the organic stroma *before* mineralization so closely resembles the crystal arrangement that detailed analysis is essential to distinguish the one from the other.

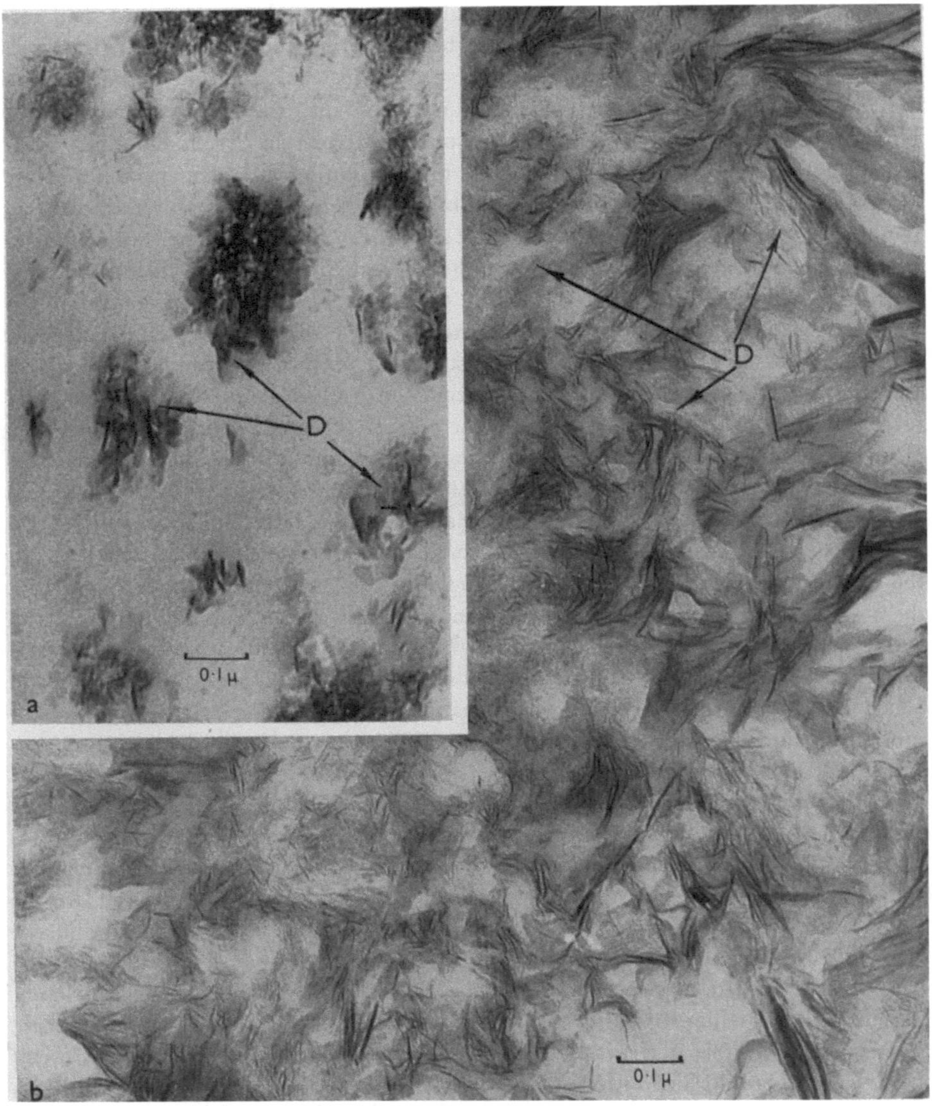

Fig. 3. Electron micrographs of analogous mineralized tissues. a. T.S. Fringe fibre tip of baleen from *Balaenopterus borealis*. Unfixed ×130,000. b. Edge of mineralizing zone in the epiphysis of newborn mouse femur. Fixed glutaraldehyde/cadmium chloride ×130,000. Areas of electron-dense peripheral material are arrowed D

Our own studies of amelogenesis in the rat agree closely with those of RÖNNHOLM (1963) except that improved fixation techniques suggest that the edge of the ameloblast might be continued into fine ribbon-like processes which are first loaded with electron-dense substances that later become crystalline as the elongated chambers reach their final size.

Our opinion is that the cell plays a more direct part in the formation of the mineral deposits in bone and enamel than has been accepted hitherto, but we are still left with a need to explain how the salt actually crystallizes in the organic phase. It is possible, even in such widely differing subjects as bone, baleen and *Lingula* shell that there is some common factor in the organic phase responsible for specific nucleation of the mineral. In baleen, however, we have so far been unable to find any significant evidence for bound phosphorus or serine phosphate in any fraction of cells containing small (2%) or large (25%) amounts of salt. We have detected a small amount of calcium in the EDTA-soluble, nondialysable portion of cell extracts which increases with increasing mineralization and although this would tend to support the present view of URIST (1964) that calcification is attended by increase in bound calcium, we cannot say that calcification in baleen is closely associated with those features claimed as significant in bone.

Some conclusions

A general theory of calcification is not possible without further study of tissues other than bones and teeth. Indeed, there may be no general theory of calcification and each type of deposit may have to be considered separately. It seems likely, though, that there is some biological principal underlying all processes of mineralization. A biomolecular survey of calcification produces the surprising conclusion that bone and enamel seem to be the exception to the general rule that mineralization is basically an *intracellular* event which is under the closest control until the mineral substances are occluded, or "pinched off", by the cell. Even in the highly complex silica skeletons of the diatoms, it has been shown recently by REIMANN *et al.* (1965) that every part of the mineral is encapsulated in an organic sheath.

A tentative general hypothesis for mineralization is illustrated diagrammatically in Fig. 4, the basis of which is to assume that the cell creates the image of the mineral. Improving techniques of studying ultrastructure seem to increase the certainty that the cell is an enormously complicated structure right down to each macromolecule; to suggest that *all* normal mineralization is the filling of chambers specially created to receive a chosen salt is to ask no more than what we would expect of a cell. Such a prospect solves many problems at once; it explains the regularity of crystal deposits, their sequence of formation and their precise location; it removes the necessity to look for specific arrangements in the topographical matrix — any structure will do, providing it has a hole in it; it spares us the impossible physical chemistry of calculating ion products and it leaves us with new possibilities as to the function of many mineralized tissues.

If the cell participates directly in the laying down of salt, however, we are left with new problems as to how this is accomplished. The possibility that the cell may "pump" inorganic structures has been enhanced by recent observations (GREENWALT *et al.*, 1964) on mitochondria which accumulate "amorphous" calcium phosphate. Even in pathological conditions, the involvement of mitochondria (see BOYCE and KING, 1963, for a review of the position) has been repeatedly emphasized, and the transition from "amorphous" to crystalline states in such structure may be a matter of metastable particles (for instance, EANES *et al.*, in press) rather than metastable solutions.

And if mitochondria are involved in the metabolic transfer of mineral to a site, then it is likely that there will be genetic information separate from the nucleus to do so, and we can look forward to the exciting possibility that the evolution of mineralization may be separate from the cell which makes use of it.

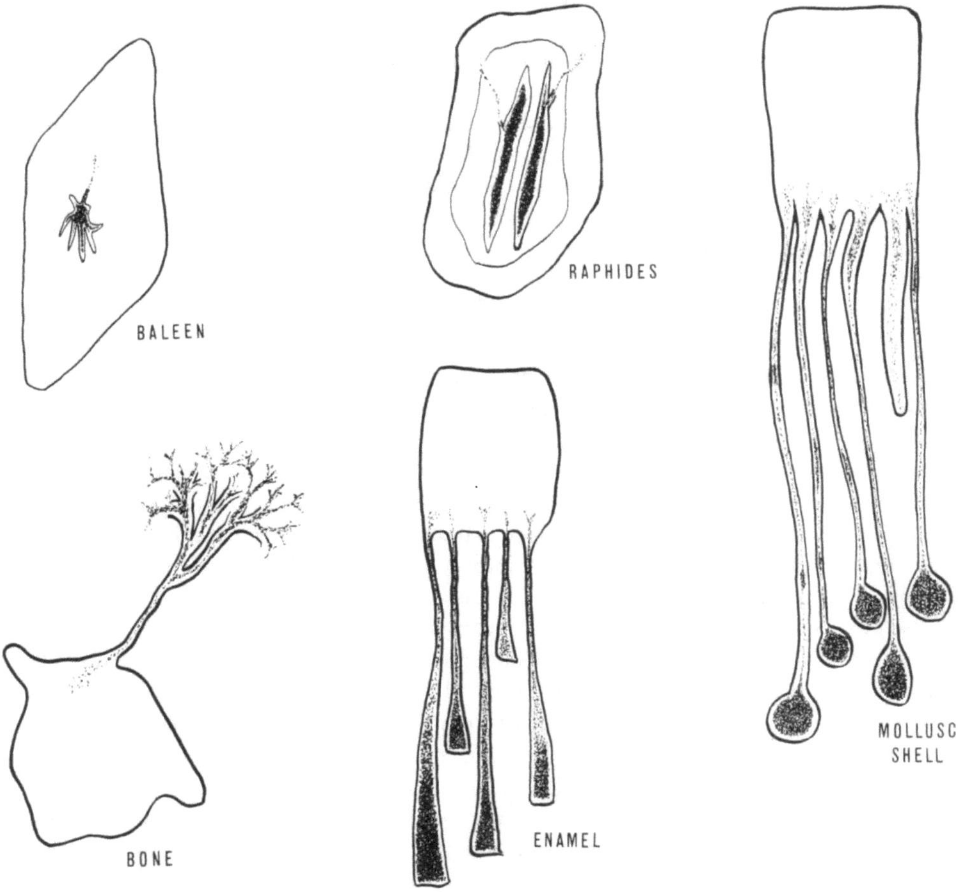

Fig. 4. Diagram of intracellular mineralization of comparable tissues. The pathway of the calcium salts within each cell is shaded tentatively

References

ARNOTT, H. J.: Studies of calcification in plants. 3rd European Symposium on Calcified Tissues (in press).

—, G. BEVELANDER, and F. G. E. PAUTARD: (in press).

—, and F. G. E. PAUTARD: (in press).

— —, and H. STEINFINK: Nature (Lond.) (in press).

ASCENZI, A., C. FRANÇOIS, and D. S. BOCCIARELLI: On the bone induced by oestrogens in birds. J. Ultrastruct. Res. 8, 491 (1963).

BEVELANDER, G.: Interactions between protein elaboration and calcification in molluscs. Anat. Rec. **117**, 568 (1953).

—, and H. NAKAHARA: Development of the skeleton of the sand dollar *(Echinarachnius parma)*. In Calcification in Biological Systems. SOGNNAES, R. F. (ed.). Washington: Amer. Ass. Advanc. Sci. 1960, p. 41.

BOYCE, W. H., and J. S. KING: Present concepts concerning the origin of matrix and stones. Ann. N. Y. Acad. Sci. **104**, 563 (1963).

BRAND, T. VON, T. I. MERCADO, M. V. NYLEN, and D. B. SCOTT: Observations on function, composition and structure of cestode calcareous corpuscles. Exp. Parasit. **9**, 205 (1960).

CAMERON, P. A.: The fine structure of osteoblasts in the metaphyses of the tibia of the young rat. J. biophys. biochem. Cytol. **9**, 583 (1961).

CLARKE, F. W., and W. C. WHEELER: The inorganic constituents of marine invertebrates. U.S. Geol. Survey **124**, (1922).

DUDLEY, H. R., and D. SPIRO: Fine structure of bone cells. J. biophys. biochem. Cytol. **11**, 624 (1961).

EANES, E. C., I. H. GILLESSEN, and A. S. POSNER: Intermediate states in the precipitation of hydroxyapatite. Nature (Lond.) (in press).

EASTOE, J. G.: Organic matrix of tooth enamel. Nature (Lond.) **184**, 411 (1960).

ENNEVER, J.: Microbiologic calcification. Ann. N. Y. Acad. Sci. **109**, 4 (1963).

FRANK, R. M.: Etude au microscope électronique de l'ossification en milieu conjonctif. Ann. Histochim. **8**, 25 (1963).

—, R. F. SOGNNAES, and R. KERN: Calcification of dental tissues with special reference to enamel ultrastructure. In Calcification in Biological Systems. SOGNNAES, R. F. (ed.). Washington: Amer. Ass. Advanc. Sci. 1960, p. 162.

FREY, A.: Calciumoxalat-Monohydrat und Trihydrat. In Linsbauer's Handbuch der Pflanzenanatomie. Berlin: Gebrüder Borntraeger **1929**, p. 81.

GONZALES, F., and R. F. SOGNNAES: Electron microscopy of dental calculus. Science **131**, 156 (1960).

GREENAWALT, T. W., C. S. ROSSI, and A. L. LEHNINGER: Effect of active accumulation of calcium and phosphate on the structure of the rat liver mitochondria. J. Cell Biol. **23**, 21 (1964).

GREGOIRE, C.: Topography of the organic components in mother of pearl. J. biophys. biochem. Cytol. **3**, 797 (1957).

HANCOX, N. M., and B. BOOTHROYD: Ultrastructure of bone formation and resorption. In Modern Trends in Orthopaedics. CLARK, J. M. P. (ed.). London: Butterworths 1964, p. 26.

HARTLES, R. L.: Calcification. In Modern Trends in Orthopaedics. CLARK, J. M. P. (ed.). London: Butterworths 1964, p. 53.

HONEGGER, R.: The polyhydrates of calcium oxalate. Vjschr. Naturforsch. Ges. **97** (1952).

JODREY, L. H.: Studies on shell formation. III. Measurement of calcium deposition in shell and calcium turnover in mantle tissue using the mantle-shell preparation and Ca^{45}. Biol. Bull. **104**, 398 (1953).

JOHNSON, F. A., and K. PANI: Histochemical identification of calcium oxalate. Arch. Path. **74**, 347 (1962).

KELLY, P. G., P. T. P. OLIVER, and F. G. E. PAUTARD: The shell of *Lingula unguis*. In Calcified Tissues. RICHELLE, L. J., and M. J. DALLEMAGNE (eds.). Liège: Université de Liège 1965, p. 334.

KLEMENT, R. VON: Die anorganische Skelettsubstanz, ihre Zusammensetzung, natürliche und künstliche Bildung. Naturwissenschaften **26**, 145 (1938).

MOSCONA, A.: Utilization of mineral constituents of the egg shell by the developing embryo of the stick insect. Nature (Lond.) **162**, 62 (1948).

NEUMAN, W. F., and M. W. NEUMAN: The nature of the mineral phase of bone. Chem. Rev. **53**, 1 (1953).

NISHIHARA, H.: Calcium oxalate content of fish scales. Sci. Rep. Saitama Univ. Sec. **B 1**, 1939 (1954).

PAUTARD, F. G. E.: Hydroxyapatite as a developmental feature of *Spirostomum ambiguum*. Biochim. biophys. Acta **35**, 32 (1959).

PAUTARD, F. G. E.: An X-ray diffraction pattern from human enamel. Arch. oral Biol. **3**, 217 (1961).
— Mineralization of keratin and its comparison with the enamel matrix. Nature (Lond.) **199**, 531 (1963).
— The molecular organization of bone. In Modern Trends in Orthopaedics. CLARK, J. M. P. (ed.). London: Butterworths 1964, p. 1.
— Calcification of baleen. In Calcified Tissues. RICHELLE, L. J., and M. J. DALLEMAGNE (eds.). Liège: Université de Liège 1965, p. 347.
—, and O. R. TRAUTZ: (in press).
POBEGUIN, T.: Les oxalates de calcium chez quelques Angiospermes. Etude physico-chimique. Ann. Sci. nat. Bot. **11/4**, 1 (1943).
— Contribution à l'étude des carbonates de calcium. Ann. Sci. nat. Bot. **15**, 29 (1954).
RAO, K. P., and E. D. GOLDBERG: Utilization of dissolved calcium by a pelecypod. J. cell. comp. Physiol. **43**, 283 (1954).
REIMANN, B. E. F., J. C. LEWIN, and B. E. VOLCANI: Studies on the biochemistry and fine structure of silica shell formation in diatoms. I. The structure of the cell wall of *Cylindrotheca fusiformis*. J. Cell Biol. **24**, 39 (1965).
ROBINSON, L. A., and D. A. CAMERON: Electron microscopy of cartilage and bone matrix at the distal epiphyseal line of the femur in the newborn infant. J. biophys. biochem. Cytol. **2**, 253 (1956).
ROBISON, R.: The Significance of Phosphoric Esters in Metabolism. New York: University Press 1932.
RÖNNHOLM, E.: The structure of the organic stroma of human enamel during amelogenesis. J. Ultrastruct. Res. **3**, 368 (1963).
SABATINI, D. D., F. MILLER, and R. S. BARNETT: Aldehyde fixation for morphological and enzyme histochemical studies with the electron microscope. J. Histochem. Cytochem. **12**, 57 (1964).
SCOTT, F. M.: Distribution of calcium oxalate crystals in *Ricinus communis* in relation to tissue differentiation and presence of other ergastic substances. Bot. Gazette **103**, 225 (1941).
SHELDON, H., and R. A. ROBINSON: Electron microscope studies of crystal-collagen relationship in bone. J. biophys. biochem. Cytol. **3**, 1011 (1957).
TRAVIS, D. F.: Structural features of mineralization from tissue to macromolecular levels of organization in the decapod crustacea. Ann. N. Y. Acad. Sci. **109**, 177 (1963).
—, and M. J. GLIMCHER: The structure and organization and relationship between the organic matrix and the inorganic apices of embryonic bovine enamel. J. Cell Biol. **23**, 447 (1964).
URIST, M. R.: Recent advances in physiology of calcification. J. bone Jt Surg. **46**, 889 (1964).
WALTER-LEVY, L., et R. STRAUSS: Sur la répartition des hydrates de l'oxalate de calcium chez les végétaux. C. R. Acad. Sci. **254**, 1671 (1962).
WHITEHEAD, R. G., and S. M. WEIDMANN: The effect of parathormone on the uptake of ^{32}P into adenosine triphosphate and bone salt of kittens. Biochem. J. **71**, 312 (1959).
WILBUR, K. M.: Shell formation and regeneration. In Physiology of Mollusca. WILBUR, K. M., and L. M. YONGE (eds.). New York: Academic Press 1964, p. 343.

Bone Mineral Metabolism in the Rat*

L. J. Richelle**, C. Onkelinx, J.-P. Aubert

Institut de Thérapeutique Expérimentale, Université de Liège, Liège, Belgique;
Institut Pasteur, Paris, France

Introduction

Numerous attempts have been made to describe the evolution of bone tissue with time. The model which has been applied to such descriptions is quite simple: bone is considered as a mass of a homogeneous material which is being formed and destroyed at finite rates.

Such models do not allow to take into account existing variations in the proportions of organic to mineral material in the microscopic structures of bone, i. e. the existence of a range of specific gravities. *A fortiori,* possible variations in the chemical composition of the mineral phase in these same structures are ignored.

Actually, the finding of a range of specific gravities implies that the turnover rate of the organic matrix and the turnover rate of the mineral phase are not identical functions of time. Variations in the Ca/P ratios of the microscopic structures of bone would have the same implications regarding calcium and phosphorus turnover rates.

It has been shown by Deakins (1942) for teeth, and later by Robinson (1960) for bone, that in a constant volume of calcified tissues, the amount of organic material does not change with time; the specific gravity of this volume increases because water is progressively replaced by mineral.

One theoretical representation which can be based upon the data of Robinson leads one to consider bone as being made up of a population of elementary volumes. The evolution with time of the number of these elementary volumes is the result of two processes: one corresponds to the appearance of new elementary volumes and the other to the destruction of existing ones. From Rowland *et al.* (1959), it is known that the amount of mineral present, expressed in g hydroxyapatite per cm^3 varies between 1.11 and 1.50, respectively for the least and the most calcified structures (diaphyseal cow bone). One can calculate therefrom the range of expected specific gravities which extends from 1.65 up to 2.25 mg/mm^3 (Richelle, 1964).

In our theoretical representation, we will assume that elementary volumes of bone appear with a specific gravity 1.65 mg/mm^3. This implies that bone does not exist as such below that value.

The evolution with time of the specific gravity of a given elementary volume is determined by its progressive mineralization raising its value from 1.65 up to a maximum equal to 2.25 mg/mm^3, provided it is not destroyed before reaching the maximal value.

It is indeed considered that resorption can affect elementary volumes irrespective of their degree of mineralization. Moreover, it can be assumed, as opposed to the processes involved in bone formation, that bone destruction bears synchronously on all the constituents. The elementary volume is destroyed as a whole, at the specific

* This work has received the support of the U.S. Public Health Service, National Institute of Dental Research, Grant nr. DE-01931-01-02.

** Chargé de Recherches du FNRS.

gravity and chemical composition it had reached. Such a representation permits a formal analysis of the system.

Thanks to experimental data, obtained from combined kinetic analysis of calcium metabolism and a technique of microsampling of bone tissue, the formal analysis leads to the definition of mathematical expressions for the various functions.

It is the purpose of this paper to establish and discuss a particular aspect of the analysis, namely the kinetics of the process of mineralization in the rat.

Experimental

Material and methods

All experiments were done with female Wistar R rats. The animals were fed a powder diet containing 0.65% Ca, 0.69% P, 1 i. u. vitamin D per gram and distilled water *ad libitum*.

Every experimental animal was studied by the method of Aubert and Milhaud (1960) to measure the parameters of calcium metabolism. This requires the determination of a chemical and radiochemical balance and the analysis of the serum disappearance curve of a single dose of Ca^{45} injected intravenously.

Diaphyseal bone samples from these animals were separated into fractions of progressively increasing specific gravities by successive centrifugations in mixtures of toluene and bromoforme (Herman and Richelle, 1961; Richelle, 1964). All the chemical and radiochemical determinations were carried out, with the aid of automatic machines. The experimental data as obtained from the records of the machines, were transferred to punched cards and processed through an IBM 7040 digital computer. The programme computed the individual data, analysed them statistically and proceeded to the evaluation of the complete set of data, in terms of a logical analysis based upon the selected model. All the methods and techniques are detailled elsewhere (Onkelinx *et al.*, 1965).

Abbreviations

The following abbreviations will be used:

t, time corresponding to the age of the animal;

ω, time corresponding to the age of an elementary volume of bone;

δ, the specific gravity;

[Ca], mass of calcium per unit volume;

M, mass; M_{Ca} refers to mass of calcium, M_P refers to mass of phosphorus, M_b refers to mass of bone;

N, number of elementary volumes which are present;

N_f, number of elementary volumes which have been formed;

N_d, number of elementary volumes which have been destroyed;

f_M, frequency distribution of the mass;

f_N, frequency distribution of the number of elementary volumes.

All these parameters can be written as functions of one another; in this case, the independent variable is written between parentheses. For example, the evolution of the mass with time will be written $M(t)$ and the value of the function at a given time t_i will be referred to as $M(t_i)$.

Results

1. *Functions M(t)*

It is possible to establish experimentally for given samples of bone (in this case, the long bones of the rat), a series of functions $M(t)$, namely $M_b(t)$, $M_{Ca}(t)$, $M_P(t)$, for the diaphysis, the epiphysis or both.

Between age 30 days and 120 days, these functions can be expressed by an equation of the following type:

$$M(t) = \frac{M_{max.}}{1 + \alpha\, e^{-kM_{max.}\, t}} \tag{1}$$

where, $M_{max.}$ is the limit value of the function when time becomes large,

$\alpha = \frac{M_{max.}}{M_0} - 1$, M_0 being the value of the function at time 0,

k is a constant (units: $M^{-1}\, t^{-1}$).

The numerical values of the parameters of Eq. 1, are derived from the linear transformation of Eq. 1, that becomes:

$$\ln\left[\frac{M_{max.}}{M(t)} - 1\right] = \ln \alpha - k\, M_{max.}\, t \tag{2}$$

Since the value of $M_{max.}$ is unknown, fitting the points to the best straight line was realized by an iterative procedure, in which $M_{max.}$ was assigned values ranging between $\pm 20\%$ of the experimental value at time 150 days. The best fitted line was selected by an analysis of variances, based on the F test of Snedecor.

Table 1 gives in the different cases, the numerical values of the parameters of Eq. 1. Fig. 1 shows $M_{Ca}(t)$.

In order to correlate kinetic data calculated from measurements done *in vivo*, with data derived from specific gravity separations of diaphyseal samples, it is important to know whether or not the diaphysis gives a good picture of bone metabolism, as a whole.

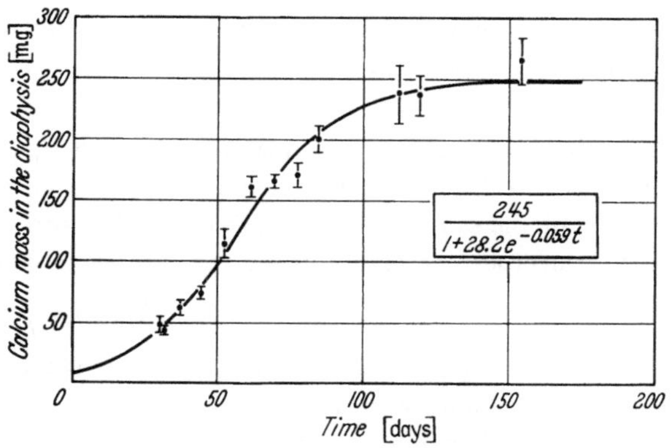

Fig. 1. Mass of calcium (M_{Ca}) in the diaphysis of the long bones of rats as a function of their age (t). The points represent mean values for groups of six animals. The deviations shown correspond to two standard deviations. The mass is measured in mg and the age in days

One comparison which can be done is to relate the evolution with time of the mass of calcium deposited in the diaphysis on one hand, and in the whole skeleton on the other. These latter data exist in the literature (Sherman and MacLeod, 1925) and can be expressed by an equation similar to Eq. 1:

$$M_{Ca}(t) = \frac{2100}{1 + 29.8\, e^{-0.055\, t}} \tag{3}$$

where M_{Ca}, the total mass of calcium in the body, is expressed in mg, and t, the age of the rat, in days. This equation is valid for female rats between 30 and 120 days.

Though we did not measure the total mass of calcium in our experimental animals, it is possible to evaluate it, by calculating a cumulative calcium balance, between 30 and 120 days. This gives a function of time, which is expressed in Eq. 4:

$$M_{\mathrm{Ca}}(t) = \frac{2292}{1+22.1\,\mathrm{e}^{-0.051\,t}} \qquad (4)$$

where M_{Ca}, the cumulative calcium balance, is expressed in mg, and t, the age of the rat in days. This expression has been derived by the iterative procedure used for the other $M(t)$ functions, but in the absence of variances of the mean cumulated values, selection was made on the basis of minimal deviation of the experimental points from the regression line, and of the t test of Student.

Table 1. *Numerical values for the parameters of Eq. 1*

$$M\,(t) = \frac{M_{\mathrm{max.}}}{1+\alpha\,\mathrm{e}^{-kM_{\mathrm{max.}}\,t}}$$

Sample [1]		$M_{\mathrm{max.}}$ (mg)	α	$k\,M_{\mathrm{max}}$ (day^{-1})	F [2]
Diaphysis	Mass	1047	17.4	0.053	1.87
	Phosphorus	127	19.5	0.053	1.42
	Calcium	245	28.2	0.059	0.92
Epiphysis	Mass	883	17.8	0.056	1.38
	Phosphorus	92	21.9	0.054	0.81
	Calcium	185	27.3	0.057	2.81

[1] The sample "diaphysis" and "epiphysis" refers respectively to the diaphysis and epiphysis of the long bones (upper and lower legs).

[2] In our experimental conditions ($\nu_1 = 8$; $\nu_2 \cong 50$), the value of F for $p < 0.05$ is 2.13.

The comparison of the values for α and $k\,M_{\mathrm{max.}}$ in Eq. 3 and Eq. 4 with those reported in Table 1 for the calcium in the diaphysis shows that in the three cases, they are of the same order of magnitude. Therefore, it is permissible to consider that, for our purposes, the diaphysis is a representative sample of the skeleton.

2. Function $N(t)$

In order to obtain the function $N(t)$, that is the evolution of the total number of elementary volumes with the age of the animal, one has to transform the functions $M(t)$, expressed in units of mass into functions expressed in number of elementary volumes.

This transformation is possible if at a given time, one knows the mean specific gravity and the mean calcium content per unit of bone mass. From the series of $N(t_i)$ values thus obtained, Eq. 5 has been derived in a way similar to that used for Eq. 1:

$$N(t) = \frac{5202}{1+14.6\,\mathrm{e}^{-0.048\,t}} \qquad (5)$$

where, $N(t)$, the total number of elementary volumes present is expressed in number of mm^3, and t in days.

By derivation, one obtains the rate of growth of the population, given by

$$\frac{\mathrm{d}N}{\mathrm{d}t} = 0.926 \times 10^{-5}\,N\,(5202 - N) \qquad (6)$$

3. *Function* $f_N(\omega)$

In a population, the elements of which are continuously renewed by processes of appearance and disappearance, it is possible, at a given time, to define an age for every element of the population and to draw the curve expressing the frequency distribution of the population as a function of the age of the elements.

In the kinetic analysis of bone metabolism, it is necessary, therefore, to distinguish two types of time functions: in the first case, the time is measured by the age of the animal and is refered to as t; in the second case, the time is measured by the age of the elementary volumes and is refered to as ω. Hence, for an animal of age t_i, the range of ages for the elementary volumes will extend from 0 up to t_i.

For any given age of the animal, i. e. for every particular value of $N(t)$, there exists a corresponding function of frequency distribution $f_N(\omega)$, so that

$$\int_0^{t_1} f_N(\omega)\, d\omega = N(t_1) \tag{7}$$

As $N(t)$ is known (Eq. 5), in order to calculate $f_N(\omega)$, it is necessary to know either the function of formation or the function of destruction of the elementary volumes. Because, as mentionned earlier, the process of bone destruction appears to bear synchronously on all the constituents of bone, the experimental values of the intensity of calcium removal from bone obtained by the kinetic analysis of calcium metabolism *in vivo* can be used to establish the mathematical expression of the function of destruction. This transformation is done by the same procedure as used to obtain Eq. 5. One gets Eq. 8:

$$N_d(t) = \frac{4452}{1 + 14.8\, e^{-0.051\, t}} \tag{8}$$

Eq. 8 expresses the evolution with the age of the animal (t), of the total number of elementary volumes which have been destroyed, expressed in number of mm^3. Hence the rate of destruction can be written:

$$\frac{dN_d}{dt} = 1.199 \times 10^{-5}\, N\, (4452 - N) \tag{9}$$

Comparison of Eqs. 6 and 9 shows that the rate of growth and the rate of destruction are given by functions which, for all practical purposes, can be considered identical. Identity of Eqs. 6 and 9 simplifies the mathematical treatment. A more general solution when these equations are not identical is possible, but will not be presented here.

The behaviour of the population of so-called elementary volumes can, therefore, be described in a general manner by the following equations:

a) the rate of growth is given by

$$\frac{dN}{dt} = k\, N\, (N_{max.} - N) \tag{10}$$

b) the rate of destruction is given by

$$\frac{dN_d}{dt} = k\, N\, (N_{max.} - N) \tag{11}$$

c) it follows that the rate of appearance is given by

$$\frac{dN_f}{dt} = k_f\, N\, (N_{max.} - N) \tag{12}$$

with $k_f = 2\,k$.

The mathematical analysis of the system defined by Eqs. 10, 11 and 12 shows that there exists a series of functions $f_N(\omega)$, such as, at any time t_i,

$$f_N(\omega) = 2\,\alpha\,k\,N^2_{\max.}\,[1+\alpha\,e^{-kN_{\max.}\,t_i}]\,\frac{e^{-kN_{\max.}\,(t_i-\omega)}}{[1+\alpha\,e^{-kN_{\max.}\,(t_i-\omega)}]^3} \tag{13}$$

with $0<\omega<t_i$.

Eq. 13 can also be written in a simpler form:

$$f_N(\omega) = \frac{2\,N(t_i-\omega)\,N'\,(t_i-\omega)}{N(t_i)} \tag{14}$$

where $N'(t)$ is the derivative function of $N(t)$.

Eqs. 13 and 14 are formally correct only if the total number of elementary volumes present at time t_i, does not include elementary volumes, already existing at $t=0$ and not yet destroyed at $t=t_i$, meaning that the age of these volumes would be greater than t_i. Practically, it is difficult to take this number into account, which is actually small and becomes rapidly negligible when the age of the animal increases. Fig. 2 shows three such functions for $t_i = 31$, 61 and 119 days.

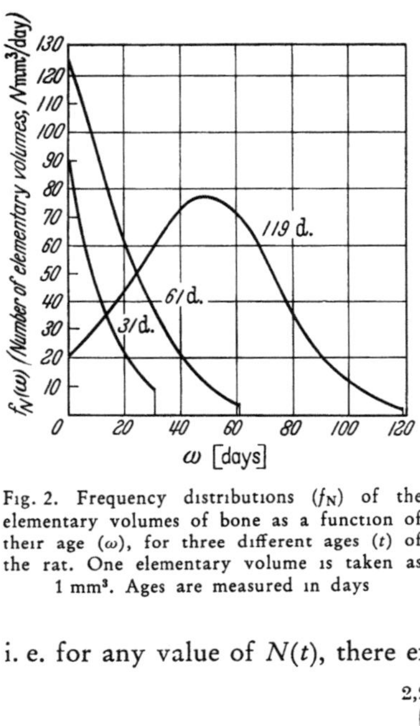

Fig. 2. Frequency distributions (f_N) of the elementary volumes of bone as a function of their age (ω), for three different ages (t) of the rat. One elementary volume is taken as 1 mm³. Ages are measured in days

4. *Function* $f_N(\delta)$

Separation of bone samples into fractions of increasing specific gravities yield values, which have been expressed in terms of percentage of the total sample calcium or phosphorus content, found for a given interval of specific gravities (RICHELLE, 1964). In the theoretical representation developed here, such values express the frequency distribution of the population of elementary volumes for finite intervals of specific gravities. For any given age of the animal, i. e. for any value of $N(t)$, there exists a theoretical function $f_N(\delta)$, such as

$$\int_{1,65}^{2,25} f_N(\delta)\,d\delta = N(t_i) \tag{15}$$

where δ is the specific gravity of the elementary volumes expressed in mg/mm³.

Fig. 3 shows three histograms for $t_i = 31$, 61 and 119 days. These histograms could be used to draw the curve expressing $f_N(\delta)$, if the class interval of specific gravity was sufficiently small, which is experimentally impractical.

5. *Function* [Ca] (ω)

It is the purpose of this paper to establish an expression describing the kinetics of the mineralization process.

There are several possibilities; one of them is to determine the function of calcification [Ca] (ω), i. e. the kinetics of calcium deposition in any elementary volume. As we know particular values of $f_N(\delta)$ and the mean calcium content of a volume of bone, corresponding to a given specific gravity interval, it is possible to calculate the corresponding values of the function $f_N([Ca])$, expressing the frequency distribution of the population as a function of the calcium content of the elementary volumes.

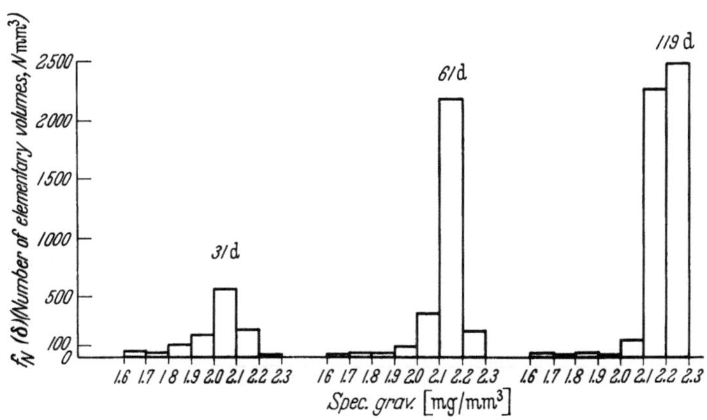

Fig. 3. Frequency distribution (f_N) of the elementary volumes of bone as a function of their specific gravity (δ), for three different ages (t) of the rat. One elementary volume is taken as 1 mm³. The specific gravity is measured in mg/mm³ and the age in days

If we had a mathematical expression for $f_N([Ca])$ as it is the case for $f_N(\omega)$ (Eq. 13), it would be possible to determine the function of calcification $[Ca](\omega)$ in the following way:

$$\text{As } f_N(\omega) = \frac{dN(t_i)}{d\omega} \text{ (see Eq. 7) and } f_N([Ca]) = \frac{dN(t_i)}{d[Ca]} \text{ (see Eq. 15)}$$

it follows that

$$\frac{d[Ca]}{d\omega} = \frac{f_N(\omega)}{f_N([Ca])} \tag{16}$$

By integration, Eq. 16 would give the unknown function $[Ca](\omega)$.

Practically, however, if drawing histograms for $f_N([Ca])$ is possible, there is no obvious linear transformation which would permit to obtain a simple and secure mathematical expression for the corresponding function. Therefore, the function $[Ca](\omega)$ has been established by calculating particular values of the function. This was done as follows.

By integrating the particular function $f_N(\omega)$ corresponding to any given time t_i, one obtains a new function, $N(\omega)$. The known values of $f_N([Ca])$, at given t_i, can be used to calculate particular values of the integral of this latter function i. e. $N([Ca])$. In this way, it is possible to find for every particular value of [Ca], the corresponding value of ω.

Fig. 4 shows for all the animals, the calculated values of [Ca] plotted as a function of ω. Using the classical linear transformation, one finds that $[Ca](\omega)$ can be described by a single hyperbolic function, which can be written

$$[Ca] = 0.175 + \frac{0.285\,\omega}{\omega + 3.6} \tag{17}$$

where [Ca] is the calcium content, expressed in mg present in the elementary volume (taken as 1 mm³ of bone) and ω is the age of the elementary volume expressed in days. The analysis of the adjustement of the hyperbolic function to the experimental points will be presented together with the refined solution of the model, unbiased by the assumed identity of Eqs. 6 and 9. The line in Fig. 4 represents values of [Ca] calculated from Eq. 17.

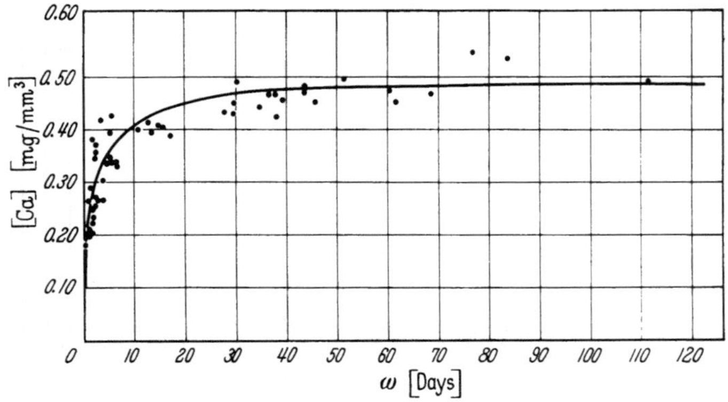

Fig. 4. Function of calcification [Ca] (ω). The calcium content [Ca] of an elementary volume is shown as a function of the age of the elementary volume (ω). The calcium content is expressed in mg/mm³ and the age in days

Discussion

It is possible to proceed further with this type of analysis and distinguish for instance in the $\bar{v}_{0+}$ as defined by kinetic analysis, the part due to the appearance of new elementary volumes as opposed to the mineralization of already existing ones.

We shall limit ourselves in the present paper to the discussion of the function [Ca] (ω).

The equation of the function of calcification is of the type

$$[\mathrm{Ca}] = [\mathrm{Ca}]_0 + \frac{([\mathrm{Ca}]_{\mathrm{max.}} - [\mathrm{Ca}]_0)\omega}{\omega + \tau} \tag{18}$$

where $[\mathrm{Ca}]_0$ is the calcium content of the elementary volume for $\omega = 0$;
$[\mathrm{Ca}]_{\mathrm{max.}}$ is the maximum calcium content of the elementary volume;
τ is a constant, which is the time of half maximum calcium increase.

Such a function had been predicted and sketched with a good approximation by Robinson in 1958 on the basis of autoradiographic and microradiographic observations.

The rate of calcification, that is the derivative of Eq. 18 is given by

$$\frac{d[\mathrm{Ca}]}{d\omega} = \frac{\tau([\mathrm{Ca}]_{\mathrm{max.}} - [\mathrm{Ca}]_0)}{(\omega + \tau)^2} \tag{19}$$

which is identical with

$$\frac{d[\mathrm{Ca}]}{d\omega} = \frac{1}{\tau([\mathrm{Ca}]_{\mathrm{max.}} - [\mathrm{Ca}]_0)}([\mathrm{Ca}]_{\mathrm{max.}} - [\mathrm{Ca}])^2 \tag{20}$$

Eq. 19 and 20 show that the rate of calcification decreases rapidly as time and calcification increase. This does not agree with the proposed diagramatic representation of Neuman and Neuman (1958), which assumed a constant rate of mineral acquisition up to 70% of maximum calcification. Eq. 20 characterizes the kinetics of a reaction of the second order, the significance of which remains to be established.

Because of the complexity of the system and, moreover, of the existence of isoionic exchange, it is evident that no simple description of the radioactive calcium incorporation to the elementary volumes can be proposed. It is possible however to test the validity of the function of calcification by another experimental approach. Eq. 18 can be used to calculate the age of an elementary volume as a function of its calcium content, which is given by

$$\omega = \tau \frac{[\mathrm{Ca}] - [\mathrm{Ca}]_0}{[\mathrm{Ca}]_{\mathrm{max.}} - [\mathrm{Ca}]} \tag{21}$$

On the other hand, the age of the elementary volumes can be determined experimentally by labelling collagen with radioactive proline. In such an experiment, at the time of the injection, only the collagen of the forming elementary volumes is labelled. Later, the maximum specific activity of the collagen hydroxyproline indicates the calcium content of the elementary volumes formed at the time of the injection. This measurement, done at different times after the injection, permits to establish on other experimental data, the function $\omega\,[\mathrm{Ca}]$. The actual data (Lapiere, 1965) are in agreement with the values calculated from Eq. 21.

Conclusions

This report represents an attempt to develop a formal analysis taking into account the heterogeneity of bone tissue In this analysis, bone is considered as a heterogeneous population of elementary units. The evolution of the system and of its elements has been described by a series of time functions.

A set of these functions (Eqs. 10, 11 and 12) describe the evolution of the population as a whole. They are obviously simplified expressions of the underlying phenomena, which involve the complex processes of cellular activity. Such expressions would be of little help if one attempted to study specifically these processes in growth or aging.

However, general expressions of this type, which describe the evolution of the whole system are nevertheless useful as operational definitions. They make it possible to give numerical values for the rate of growth, the rate of appearance and the rate of destruction of the elements of the population. Indeed, these values are necessary in order to analyse the kinetic events which take place in individual elements of the population.

Among the various events taking place, we have limited ourselves in this paper to the study of the calcification. A hyperbolic function has been found to describe adequately the kinetics of this process. It remains to be shown what are the actual phenomena responsible for this type of kinetic behaviour.

References

Aubert, J.-P., et G. Milhaud: Méthode de mesures des principales voies du métabolisme calcique chez l'homme. Biochim. biophys. Acta **39**, 122 (1960).

Deakins, M.: Changes in ash, water, and organic content of pig enamel during calcification. J. dent. Res. **21**, 429 (1942).

Herman, H., et L. Richelle: Le calcium échangeable de la substance minérale de l'os étudiée à l'aide du Ca-45. VII. Activité comparée de fractions d'os total de densité differente. Bull. Soc. Chim. biol. **43**, 273 (1961).

Lapiere, Ch. M.: The remodelling of the bone matrix. This book, p. 20.

NEUMAN, W. F., and M. W. NEUMAN: The Chemical Dynamics of Bone Mineral. Chicago: The University of Chicago Press 1958, p. 107.
ONKELINX, C., L. J. RICHELLE, and J. DEBRAS: Automatic samples and data processing in studies of calcium metabolism in rats. Symposium on Radioisotope Sample Measurement Techniques in Medicine and Biology. Vienna 1965.
RICHELLE, L. J.: One possible solution to the problem of the biochemistry of bone mineral. Clin. Orthop. **33**, 211 (1964).
ROBINSON, R. A.: Chemical analysis and electron microscopy of bone. In Bone as a Tissue. RODAHL, K., J. T. NICHOLSON, and E. M. BROWN (eds.). New York: McGraw-Hill Book 1960, p. 186.
ROWLAND, R. E., J. JOWSEY, and J. H. MARSHALL: Microscopic metabolism of calcium in bone. III. Microradiographic measurements of mineral density. Radiat. Res. **10**, 234 (1959).
SHERMAN, H. C., and F. L. MACLEOD: Calcium content of the body in relation to age, growth and food. J. biol. Chem. **64**, 429 (1925).

Physico-chemical Methods for the Identification of Microcrystalline Basic Calcium Phosphates Prepared in Vitro

P. LERCH, C. VUILLEUMIER

Institut für anorganische und physikalische Chemie der Universität, Bern, Schweiz;
Institut de Radiophysique Appliquée, Université de Lausanne, Lausanne, Suisse

I. Introduction

The method of synthesis of hydroxyapatite proposed by HAYEK (1960), which consists of the reaction of $Ca(NO_3)_2$ in the presence of NH_3 with Na_2HPO_4, permitted us by changing the conditions of the proceedings to obtain two specific kinds of phosphates:
hydroxyapatite (HA) $Ca_{10}(PO_4)_6(OH)_2$
hydrated tricalcium phosphate (TCPH) $Ca_9(PO_4)_6 \cdot 1/2\, H_2O$.
For a better understanding of the synthesis mechanism of these components, and to obtain a criterion which would permit the verification of the nature of the hydroxyapatite during synthesis, we thought that it would be interesting to measure the variations of pH during this procedure; commonly, it seems that this operation takes place as a simple neutralization.

The conclusions of this method should make it possible to discuss the composition and structure of other calciumorthophosphates analogous to those mentioned above, which might play a part in the processes of calcification, such as octocalcium-orthophosphate (OCP) $Ca_8H_2(PO_4)_6 \cdot H_2O$.

For this purpose, we will use results already obtained (LERCH and VUILLEUMIER, 1964 a, b; VUILLEUMIER, 1965) in X-ray and electron diffractions, specific area measurements and especially thermogravimetric (TG) and differential thermal analysis (DTA).

II. Experimental part and results

The proportions of Ca^{++} and PO_4^{---} were varied, thus giving excesses up to 200% of each ion. The reactives were permanently stirred at 25 °C under N_2 during

48 hr, to prevent reactions with atmospheric-CO_2. pH was continuously measured by a combined glass electrode and registered.

Two kinds of curves were obtained: one by an excess of Ca^{++} or stoichiometric mixture, the other by excess of PO_4^{---}.

The first type of curve (Fig. 1) shows an initial and fast neutralization, which appears after PO_4^{---} is added to the $Ca(NO_3)_2+NH_3$ mixture. In one minute the pH falls from 10.7—10.5 down to 8.8—8.5 and stabilises during a period of 4—8 hr at an approximate value of 8. After this a new fall of pH occurs which lowers the pH to 6.5 to 5.3.

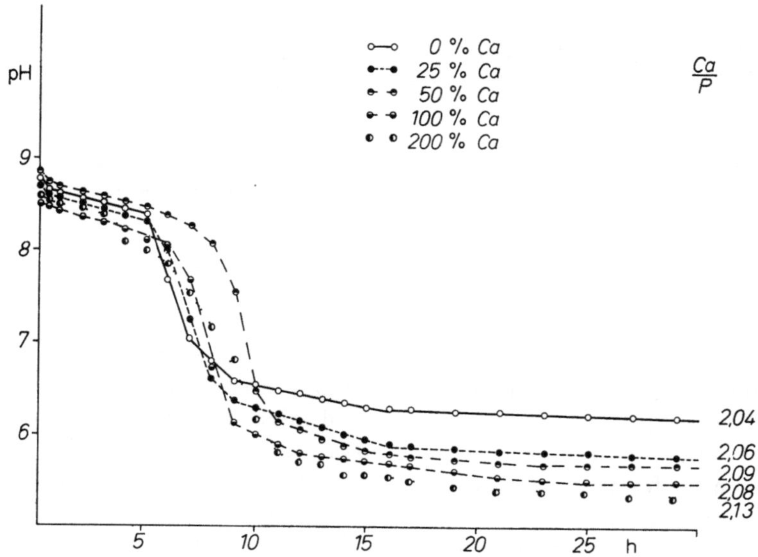

Fig. 1. pH-curve of HA

The higher the excess of Ca^{++} is, the larger becomes the fall, and the sooner it appears. After this second step the pH reaches its final value in about ten hours. This end-pH depends directly upon the Ca/P-ratio; i. e. for an end-pH of 5.30 (200% Ca^{++} excess) a Ca/P of 2.13 is obtained.

X-ray diffraction patterns show the diagram of the hydroxyapatite of small dimensions. Norelco X-ray diffraction gives a dimension along the c-axis of about 300 Å. The specific area measured by the method of B.E.T. is 110 ± 5 m²/g. Electron micrograph show needles, which are mostly agglomerated to bigger and needlelike aggregates with dimensions of 1200×120 Å. Such aggregates show a calculated specific area of about 100 m²/g, which is in good agreement with the measured B.E.T. area. Single needles can sometimes be seen with similar dimensions as those given by Norelco. The Ca/P (2.04—2.13) indicates that the preparations obtained in the described way, can be attributed to HA. Indeed, the TG and the DTA confirm this. The TG curve is really the one of the HA, with the characteristic points at 100 °C, 300 °C and 500 °C, giving waterlosses of 1.5 moles, 1.0 moles, 0.5 moles and a total waterloss of 2.0 moles at 1000 °C if we subtract 1.5 moles waterloss up to 100 °C, which can be attributed to adsorbed water. The DTA curve corresponds with the TG curve showing an endothermic peak at 100 °C and an exothermic one at 330 °C, followed by a slow exothermic rise corresponding to a slow dehydration of the thermogravimetric curve. X-ray analyses at the mentioned temperatures show that the structure of the product does not change except the reflexes becoming sharper.

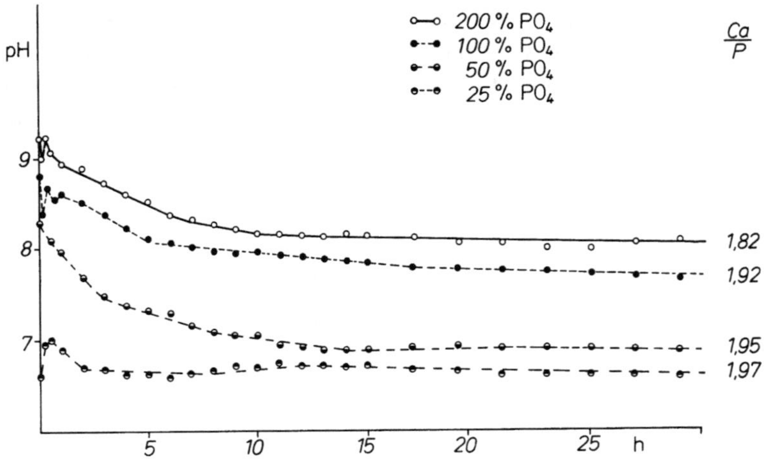

Fig. 2. pH-curve of TCPH

The pH curves obtained by a mixture containing an excess of PO_4^{---} show a totally different behaviour. One observes a steady decrease of the pH towards its end-value (Fig. 2). The curves show a fast and initial neutralization, which is followed by a slow decrease, ending more quickly as the excess of PO_4^{---} becomes larger. As in the former curves there is a direct relation between the end-pH and the Ca/P. The preparations obtained in this way show similar X-ray diffraction patterns as the former products, similar dimensions and similar electron micrographic appearance. The Ca/P indicates that the preparations are TCPH. So do the TG and DTA diagrams. We have again characteristic points at 100 °C, 300 °C and 500 °C corresponding to waterlosses of about 1.5, 1.0, 0.5 moles and an entire new step between 700 °C and 740 °C, corresponding to a waterloss of 0.5 moles. The total waterloss is 2.0 moles up to 1000 °C. The DTA-curve also gives a new endothermic peak at 700 °C, which corresponds with the 0.5 moles waterloss and which can easily be attributed to the transformation of the calcium phosphate to β-TCP. This transformation can be shown by X-ray analysis at the mentioned temperatures.

Formation of HA or TCPH depends essentially on the end-pH which is given by the concentration of the reactives. The following equation was found between Ca/P and end-pH:

$$\mathrm{Ca/P} = 2.65 - \frac{\mathrm{pH}}{10} \qquad (1)$$

This equation shows that in physiological media we can expect a TCPH with a Ca/P of 1.92 according to several authors.

We have identified the product wich appears during the intermediary step of the synthesis of HA. The isolated product shows an amorphous X-ray diffraction pattern and an amorphous electron micrographic appearance which are similar to the amorphous parts of the OCP obtained by the method of WATSON and ROBINSON (1953). The specific area of the intermediary product is $130 \pm 10\ m^2/g$ according to the electron micrograph. The suspension of the amorphous product in water leads to crystalline material of hydroxyapatite X-ray diffraction patterns with the same pH-curve as the HA. The Ca/P ratio of the amorphous product is the same as the one for its water suspension at any time and pH, and also the same as that for the end product of the uninterrupted Hayek synthesis. TG- and DTA-curves of the amorphous product are very different to those of HA (Fig. 3). The characteristic temperatures are now 100 °C, 170 °C and 300 °C, representing waterlosses of about 8 moles (adsorbed water), 1.8 and 0.2—0.3 moles. The total waterloss up to 1000 °C is 3.2 to 3.3 moles. The DTA-curve corresponds with the TG-curve except for one exothermic peak at 680 °C.

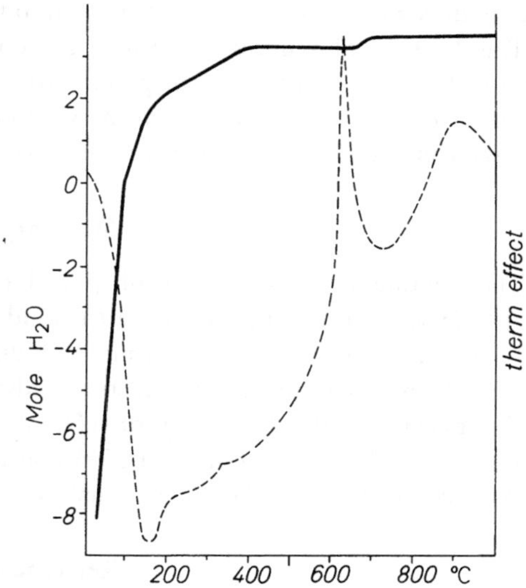

Fig. 3. thermic curves of amorphous product

These curves resemble those of a mixture of TCPH and OCP, which are shown in Fig. 4. X-ray analysis shows that the product remains amorphous up to 600 °C. At 650 °C the reflexes of the α-TCP appear thus corresponding to the exothermic peak of the DTA. At 650 °C we can observe the X-ray pattern of β-TCP. Therefore, we can state that the amorphous product is a mixture of TCPH and OCP. If we consider the pH of the intermediary step as the end-pH, we find according to equation (1) a Ca/P ratio about 1.84. The discrepancy in the experimental value can be explained by surface adsorption of Ca^{2+}. This shows us that global chemical analyses are unsufficient to determine the real nature of hydroxyapatites. In aqueous suspension the amorphous product is hydrolized and the pH decreased.

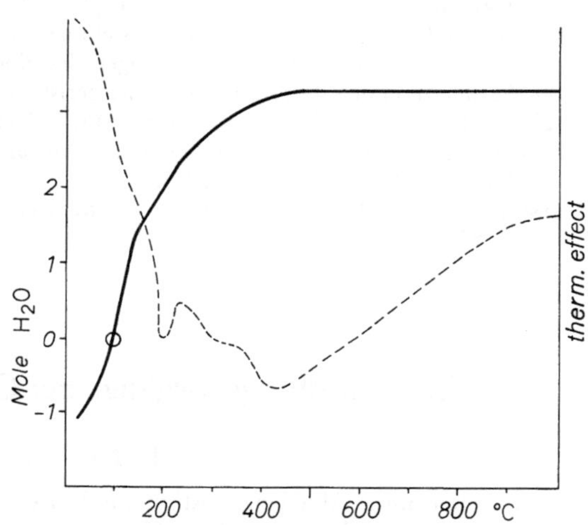

Fig. 4. thermic curves of OCP

III. Conclusions

HA is formed in two distinct steps: formation of the amorphous product then hydrolization to the final HA. TCPH is formed directly as shown by X-ray diffraction patterns which are crystalline from the very beginning. The synthesis can be steered either to HA or to TCPH by influencing the end-pH. It would even be possible to obtain OCP by this method if an end-pH of at least 9 could be obtained. Such required end-pHs can be obtained by excesses of Ca^{2+} or PO_4^{---}. It is quite logical to use excesses of Ca^{++} and PO_4^{---} to obtain the final-pHs required and no other buffers which could bring impurities into the reactives.

The different pH-curves found during the formation of HA and TCPH and the fact to obtain intermediary amorphous products in the case of HA, and the formation of crystalline products from the very beginning in the case of TCPH, brings us to the conclusion that the TCPH is a real and distinct phase.

Summary

The continuous measurement of pH during the hydroxyapatite synthesis of Hayek (1960) distinguishes two different kinds of reaction mechanism depending on Ca^{++}- or PO_4^{---}-excesses. By thermic and diffraction methods it was possible to establish the nature of the final products and also one intermediate amorphous product, which appears at the beginning of HA-synthesis (Ca^{2+}-excess or stoicheiometric mixture). With PO_4^{---}-excess, the TCPH appears from the beginning of the reaction.

We wish to thank the Fonds National Suisse, for support of this research.

References

Hayek, E., H. Newesely, W. Hassenteufel, und B. Krismer: Zur Bildungsweise und Morphologie der schwerlöslichen Calciumphosphate. Mh. Chem. **91**, 249 (1960).

Lerch, P., und C. Vuilleumier: Die Herstellung und Identifizierung von Hydroxylapatiten mit ähnlichen Dimensionen wie diejenigen des Knochens. Chimia **18**, 20 (1964 a).

— — Etude thermique de préparations microcristallines d'hydroxylapatites et d'autres phosphates de l'os préparés in vitro. Chimia **18**, 392 (1964 b).

Vuilleumier, C.: Die Herstellung, Identifizierung und das thermische Verhalten von Hydroxylapatiten. Diss. Univ. Bern 1965.

Watson, M. L., and R. A. Robinson: Collagen-crystal relationships in bone. II. Amer. J. Anat. **93**, 1583 (1953).

Umwandlungsvorgänge bei Calciumphosphaten

H. Newesely

Kristallchemische Abteilung, Institut für Kariesforschung und Forschungsgruppe für Mikromorphologie im Fritz-Haber-Institut, Berlin-Dahlem, Deutschland

Bei mikromorphologischen Untersuchungen an der Remineralisationsschicht der Zahnoberfläche bzw. in Zahnbelägen wurden Calciumphosphatkristallite mit verschiedenen Ausbildungsformen festgestellt (Johannsson, 1965; Mühlemann *et al.*, 1964; Lenz und Newesely, 1964; Lenz *et al.*, 1964; Schroeder, 1964; Höhling *et al.*, 1962). Die Zuordnung zu bestimmten Strukturtypen war jedoch nicht immer mit Sicherheit möglich.

Mit Unterstützung der Deutschen Forschungsgemeinschaft, Bad Godesberg.

Die Untersuchungen werden in „Monatshefte für Chemie" (Wien: Springer) ausführlich veröffentlicht.

In diesem Zusammenhang erschien es wichtig, in vitro genauere Angaben über die Existenz- und Umwandlungsbedingungen der Calciumphosphate unter den dort zutreffenden chemischen Reaktionsumständen — also auch im schwach sauren pH-Bereich und bei erhöhter Temperatur — zu erhalten; dies um so mehr, als in den verfügbaren älteren Arbeiten noch nicht das Auftreten des Oktacalciumphosphates bei der Hydrolyse des Brushits bekannt war (D'Ans und Knütter, 1953) bzw. diese sich auf Aussagen bei Raumtemperatur beschränkten (Moreno *et al.*, 1960).

Wir untersuchten die Zusammensetzung und Struktur der kristallisierten Calciumphosphate, die bei homogener Reaktion im pH-Bereich von 4,0—7,0, im Temperaturbereich von 20—80 °C und im Konzentrationsbereich von 0,01 m—0,1 m auftreten.

Material und Methode

Homogene Kristallisation wurde in der Weise erreicht, daß genau eingestellte Calcium- und Phosphatlösungen vorsichtig zu einem vorgelegten großen Volumen Pufferlösung (0,2 m Natriumacetat, pH und Temperatur vorgegeben) zugefügt wurden. Als schwacher Komplexbildner sollten die Acetat-Ionen außerdem die Lösungsumgebung in vitro dem Mundmilieu angleichen.

Die Übersättigung ist so gering gehalten, daß sich Kristallkeime erst nach Stunden oder Tagen aus dem homogenen Medium bildeten. Die hierbei entstehenden Kristallisationsprodukte erwiesen sich im mikroskopischen Bild als einheitliches Material; es wurde sodann davon jeweils der analytische Gehalt von Calcium und Phosphat sowie der Strukturtyp festgestellt.

Beim Übergang zu höheren Konzentrationen entstehen Fällungsprodukte. Diese eigneten sich nicht für die angestrebte Identifizierung, da sie — obwohl auch sie zum Teil einen kristallinen Charakter hatten — doch nicht mit Sicherheit einheitlich zusammengesetzt sind (Newesely, 1964).

Ergebnisse

Im homogenen Bereich des Temperatur/pH/Konzentration-Diagramms treten Brushit, Oktacalciumphosphat und Monetit auf; Hydroxylapatit wurde nur im Fällungsgebiet gefunden.

Brushit, das Dicalciumphosphat-Dihydrat (Calciumhydrogenphosphat-Dihydrat), entsteht im gesamten pH-Bereich, wird jedoch oberhalb pH = 6,3 bei physiologischen Bedingungen (Temperatur $\sim$ 40 °C) in Oktacalciumphosphat umgewandelt. Zwischen pH = 5,0 und 6,0 erfolgt diese Umsetzung erst bei höheren Temperaturen (60—70 °C). Die Existenzbedingungen des Oktacalciumphosphats umfassen somit den pH-Bereich von 5,0—7,0 und den Temperaturbereich von 30—70 °C.

Die Bildungsbedingungen des wasserfreien Dicalciumphosphats, Monetit, schließen sich an die des Oktacalciumphosphats gegen niedrigere pH-Werte (pH $<$ 4,5), an die des Brushits gegen höhere Temperatur ($>$ 60 °C) an.

Die Ergebnisse dieser Messungen bezogen sich auf das reine System CaO–P_2O_5–H_2O (inclusive Natriumacetat).

Angaben über die Umwandlungsvorgänge in Gegenwart von Begleitionen liegen bereits an anderer Stelle vor. In Gegenwart von 1—2% Magnesiumionen bildet sich β-Tricalciumphosphat, Whitlockit (Trautz *et al.*, 1954; Hayek und Newesely, 1958), bei Zusatz von $>$ 50 μg Fluorid/Liter der Lösung wird die Oktacalciumphosphat-Struktur instabil und geht in die Apatit-Struktur über (Newesely, 1961).

Diskussion und Zusammenfassung

Nach den vorliegenden Ergebnissen kristallchemischer Untersuchungen an Calciumphosphaten, die bei homogener Reaktion in schwach saurem Medium entstanden, ist bei der Ausbildung von Remineralisationsschichten und Zahnbelägen die Existenz von Dicalciumphosphat-Dihydrat (Brushit), β-Tricalciumphosphat (Whitlockit), Oktacalciumphosphat und Apatit — insbesondere letztere auch in Form von Fällungsprodukten — möglich. Die Existenzbedingungen des wasserfreien Dicalciumphosphats (Monetit) werden hingegen in der Umgebung der Zähne kaum erreicht werden.

Literatur

D'Ans, J., und R. Knütter: Zur Abgrenzung der Existenzgebiete der Dicalciumphosphate und des Apatits. Angew. Chem. **65**, 578 (1953).

Hayek, E., und H. Newesely: Über die Existenz von Tricalciumphosphat in wässeriger Lösung. Mh. Chem. **89**, 88 (1958).

Höhling, H.-J., W. Wannenmacher, und F. Güllenstern: Über den Zahnstein. Dtsch. Zahnärztebl. **16**, 144, 704 (1962).

Johannsson, B.: Remineralisation of slightly etched enamel. J. dent. Res. **44**, 64 (1965).

Lenz, H., and H. Newesely: Maturation and remineralisation of enamel. Proc. ORCA **11**, 95 (1964).

—, K. Rossinsky, und H. R. Mühlemann: Elektronenoptische Studien der Oberfläche und der Tiefen des initialen künstlichen White Spot. Schweiz. Mschr. Zahnheilk. **74**, 654 (1964).

Moreno, E. C., W. E. Brown, and G. Osborn: Stability of dicalcium phosphate dihydrate in aqueous solutions and solubility of octocalcium phosphate. Soil Science **24**, 99 (1960).

Mühlemann, H., H. Lenz, and K. Rossinsky: Electron optical appearence of rehardened enamel. Helv. odont. Acta **8**, 108 (1964).

Newesely, H.: Changes in crystal types of low solubility calcium phosphates in the presence of accompanying ions. Proc. ORCA **8**, 174 (1961).

— The behavior of the poorly crystallized calcium phosphates. Gordon Res. Conf. on dissolution and crystallisation of calcium phosphates. Meriden N. H. 1964.

Schroeder, H. E.: Two different types of mineralisation in early dental calculus. Helv. odont. Acta **8**, 117 (1964).

Trautz, O. R., E. Fessenden, and M. C. Newton: Magnesian whitlockite in ashed dental tissue. J. dent. Res. **33**, 687 (1954).

Some Observations on the Nature of Bone Mineral

J. MacGregor

Bioengineering Unit, University of Strathclyde, Glasgow, Scotland

Few will deny that there is a very rapid ionic exchange between the mineral component of the skeleton and the calcium (Ca^{++}) and inorganic phosphate (P^{---}) ions of the circulating body fluids. The mechanism which governs this exchange and the question of whether a true physicochemical equilibrium exists is much more controversial.

Nordin (1957) was the first to demonstrate that whole bone powder would produce and maintain consistent products of the concentrations of calcium and phosphate ions in buffers in equilibrium with it. In subsequent contributions

MacGregor and Nordin (1960, 1962) and MacGregor (1964 a, b) developed the suggestion that bone mineral could be said to have a "solubility product" in terms of $\{Ca^{++}\}^3 \{PO_4^{---}\}^2$ * at physiological pH, temperature and ion strength. We have never suggested that bone was "tri-calcium phosphate", only that the behaviour of powdered bone going into solution *in vitro* could best be described in terms of that ion product.

The studies were extended to rat bone and also to child bone (MacGregor, 1962) and data such as those shown in Fig. 1 were obtained. It can be seen that at equilibrium (see MacGregor and Nordin, 1960 for experimental details), the calcium concentrations in all three series of experiments were similar and dependent only on the pH of the buffer employed. On the other hand, the concentrations of inorganic phosphate are relatively independent of pH but rise from about 0.2 mM for human adult bone to about 0.4 mM for powdered child bone and 1.0 mM for bone from growing rats. Consequently, when the empirical ion products were calculated they were consistent for equilibrations with each material, but very different for bone from different sources. Nevertheless, it was clear that the equilibrium concentrations were related to the blood levels of $\{Ca^{++}\}$ and $\{P^{---}\}$ in each case and it was concluded that if bone mineral had an "equilibrium constant" then either there were specific ion effects unallowed for in both child and rat plasma and appropriate equilibrating fluids (rather unlikely), or there was a pH gradient between bone and plasma from rat to child to human adult (possible), or thirdly that the bone salt of rats and children was qualitatively different from that of adults (MacGregor, 1964 b). This last alternative was thought to be unlikely but very recently MacGregor and Brown (1965) presented evidence to support the view that bone mineral is first laid down as octocalcium phosphate (OCP) which then slowly hydrolyses to hydroxyapatite (HA). The anatomical skeleton, therefore, would be composed of "reactive" and "unreactive" bone having predominantly OCP and HA in the lattice respectively — young actively growing bone having proportionally more of the former. It is interesting that Ibsen and Urist (1964) have independently shown that homogenised bone fragments labelled with tetracycline yield more pyrophosphate than equivalent amounts of unlabelled moities from the same mix (see also McLean, 1965, p. 6) when heated to 325 °C for one hour.

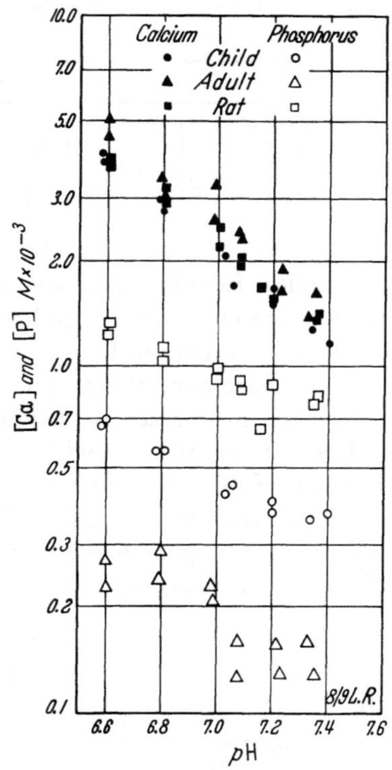

Fig. 1. The concentrations of calcium and phosphate at equilibrium in equilibration experiments with human adult, child and rat bone

The presence of OCP stoichiometry in child bone and calf bone mineral was demonstrated by calculation of the chemical potential relationships from equilibration

* The brackets { } are used to imply "the concentration of".

data. However, if it is true that OCP is present then, being more reactive than hydroxyapatite, the ion product representing its stoichiometry should be more constant than any other possible products at equilibrium. I have calculated the various ion products for the child bone data along with their distributions, standard errors and coefficients of variation. These data are shown in the following Table:

	Mean	SE	Coeff. Varn.
pK $\{Ca^{++}\}\{HPO_4^{=}\}$	6.246	0.15910	0.02545
pK $\{Ca^{++}\}^8\{HPO_4^{=}\}^2\{PO_4^{\equiv}\}^4$	64.714	0.20547	0.00318
pK $\{Ca^{++}\}^3\{PO_4^{\equiv}\}^2$	26.112	0.15884	0.00608
pK $\{Ca^{++}\}^{10}\{PO^{\equiv}\}^6\{OH^-\}^2$	95.011	0.84535	0.00890

It is clear from the coefficients of variation that the OCP product is undoubtedly the most constant of the "equilibrium constants", and the presence of OCP in the bone powder is confirmed.

If new bone mineral is laid down as OCP then even in the adult a proportion of the skeleton must react as OCP with consequent elevation of the equilibrium ion product in terms of Ca^{++} and P^{---}. As the parathyroid glands specifically ensure the constancy of $\{Ca^{++}\}$, it follows that variations in the rate of new bone formation (and hence the proportion of OCP) might be expected to result in variations in plasma inorganic phosphate levels. Certainly a raised plasma inorganic phosphate is a feature of acromegaly and low values are found in hypopituitarism (Astwood, 1955). Studies with human growth hormone (Gershberg, 1960) have also shown that the administration of the hormone is accompanied by a prompt rise in plasma inorganic phosphate concentration.

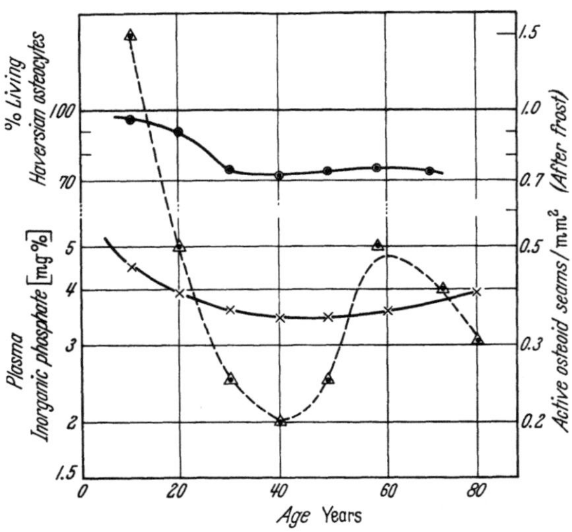

Fig. 2. The relationship of % lining osteocytes (○), and active osteoid seam count (△) with regression curve of plasma inorganic phosphate concentration and age (×)

There have recently been many developments in quantitative histology. Frost has vigorously led the field and has associated active bone formation with many parameters, such as the number of foci of formation per mm^3 (Frost, 1964), the number of "active seams" per mm^2 (Frost, 1963), the percentage of live osteocytes (Frost, 1963). The last two of these parameters have redrawn from Frost's data and are shown in Fig. 2. Also shown is the mean regression line of inorganic phosphate, concentrations (y) on age (x) in normal women (Greenberg *et al.*, 1960):

$$\log_{10} y = 0.73072 - 0.009610\, x - 0.000102\, x^2 + 0.016700 \log_{10} x$$

In each case there are high values in the young which fall to a minimum around the age of 40 before a further rise in later years. The general trend is highly suggestive.

It is interesting to speculate that in osteomalacia where the mineralisation of osteoid is retarded, the observed low phosphate concentrations may be the result rather than the cause of the condition, although in several cases secondary hyperparathyroidism with increased renal clearance of phosphate may also be a factor.

In carefully controlled experimental conditions, however, it may be that a critical evaluation of plasma phosphate levels will indicate the trend in the rate of new bone formation.

In conclusion, I would like to commend caution to those workers who assess "calcification" and "calcifiability" *in vitro*. Dr. H. FLEISCH has kindly made available his data on the "formation products" of calcium phosphate precipitation on to collagen in vitro. The appropriate calculations for determining the stoichiometry of the equilibrium at the point of precipitation have been made using the chemical potential method as described in MACGREGOR and BROWN (1965). The results are shown in Fig. 3. A good fit was obtained and the regression coefficient was such that the Ca : P ratio of the equilibrium was not significantly different from 1 (in fact Ca : P = 6.6 : 6). In this case, therefore, $CaHPO_4$ must have been the dominant phase, and not the OCP or HA found when *bone* is present. It may be of interest here to mention in parenthesis that an unselected group of renal calculi equilibrated at pH 7 in vitro have also shown the presence of OCP (MACGREGOR *et al.*, in press).

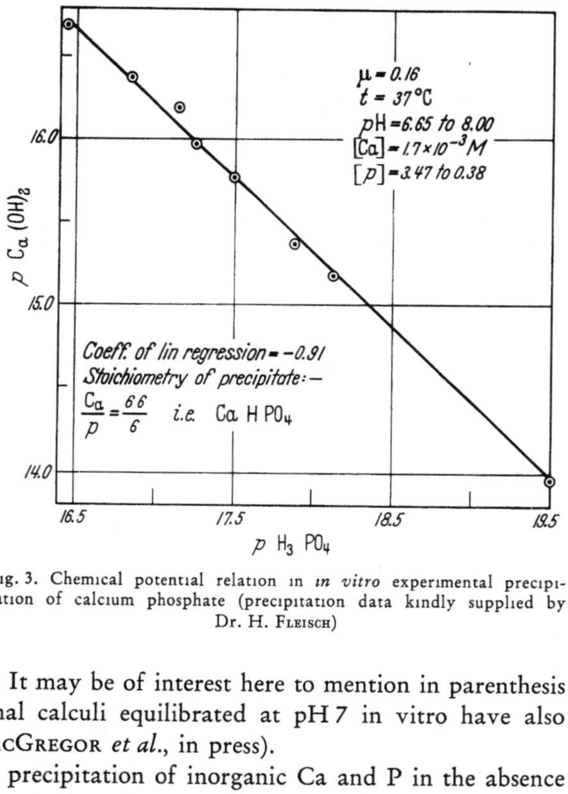

Fig. 3. Chemical potential relation in *in vitro* experimental precipitation of calcium phosphate (precipitation data kindly supplied by Dr. H. FLEISCH)

It appears probable that the precipitation of inorganic Ca and P in the absence of formed bone or an "active" template does not represent either the process of *in vivo* calcification nor even the physical-chemical equilibrium conditions for bone mineral and, therefore, appropriate limitations should be set on the interpretation of such data.

References

ASTWOOD, E. B.: Growth hormone and corticotropin. In The Hormones. PINCUS and THIMMAN (eds.). New York: Academic Press 1955, p. 235.

FROST, H. M.: Bone Remodelling Dynamics. Springfield: Charles C. Thomas 1963.

— Bone Biodynamics. Springfield: Charles C. Thomas 1964, p. 315.

Gershberg, H.: Metabolic and renotropic effects of human growth hormone in disease. J. clin. Endocr. 20, 1107 (1960).
Greenberg, B. G., R. W. Winters, and J. B. Graham: The normal range of serum inorganic phosphorus and its utility as a discriminant in the diagnosis of congenital hypophosphataemia. J. clin. Endocr. 20, 364 (1960).
Ibsen, K. H., and M. R. Urist: Relationship between pyrophosphate content and oxytetracycline labelling of bone salt. Nature (Lond.) 203, 761 (1964).
MacGregor, J.: The relationship between bone powder and its ions in solution in tissue fluids. Thesis. University of Glasgow 1962.
— The relationship between calcium and phosphate ions in bone mineral and tissue fluids. In Bone and Tooth. Blackwood, H. J. J. (ed.). Oxford: Pergamon Press 1964 a, p. 351.
— Blood-bone equilibrium. In Bone Biodynamics. Frost, H. M. (ed.). Springfield: Charles C. Thomas 1964 b, p. 409.
—, and W. E. Brown: Blood-bone equilibrium in calcium homeostasis. Nature (Lond.) 205, 359 (1965).
—, and B. E. C. Nordin: Equilibration studies with human bone powder. J. biol. Chem. 235, 1215 (1960).
— — Equilibration studies with human bone powder. II. The role of the carbonate ion. J. biol. Chem. 237, 2704 (1962).
—, W. Robertson, and B. E. C. Nordin: Equilibration studies with renal calculi. Brit. J. Urol. (in press).
McLean, F. C.: Internal remodelling of compact bone. In Calcified Tissues. Richelle, L. J., and M. J. Dallemagne (eds.). Liège: Université de Liège 1965, p. 1.
Nordin, B. E. C.: The solubility of powdered bone. J. biol. Chem. 227, 551 (1957).

The Osteon Calcification as Revealed by the Electron Microscope

A. Ascenzi, E. Bonucci

Istituto di Anatomia Patologica dell'Università di Pisa, Pisa, Italia

The aim of the present study is to investigate for the first time the dynamics of osteon calcification using the electron microscope. For this purpose a special technique was devised to examine osteons in which the calcium content as well as the orientation of the anisothropic components had been previously established.

Materials and method

Longitudinally sectioned specimens from femoral ox-shafts were fixed in neutral formol and ground on a glass plate to a thickness of about 30—40 micra. A careful examination was made in order to select osteons at the initial stage of calcification (i.e. having the lowest amount of calcium as determined microradiographically) and osteons which had reached their highest degree of calcification. The units were chosen in such a way that under the polarizing microscope they appeared evenly bright according to the marked longitudinal spiral course of the fibres in successive lamellae.

At this stage wedge-shaped bone fragments with a portion of the chosen osteon on top were dissected from the section, according to the technique described by Ascenzi and Fabry (1959). Once the technique was mastered, it was easy to prepare from each osteon two specimens shaped as in Fig. 1. They were dehydrated in alcohol and embedded in Araldite. In the resin blocks the specimens were orientated in such a way as to obtain respectively ultrathin sections, (a) tangentially orientated as regards the lamellae, (b) running radially and (c) cross-orientated in respect to the osteon.

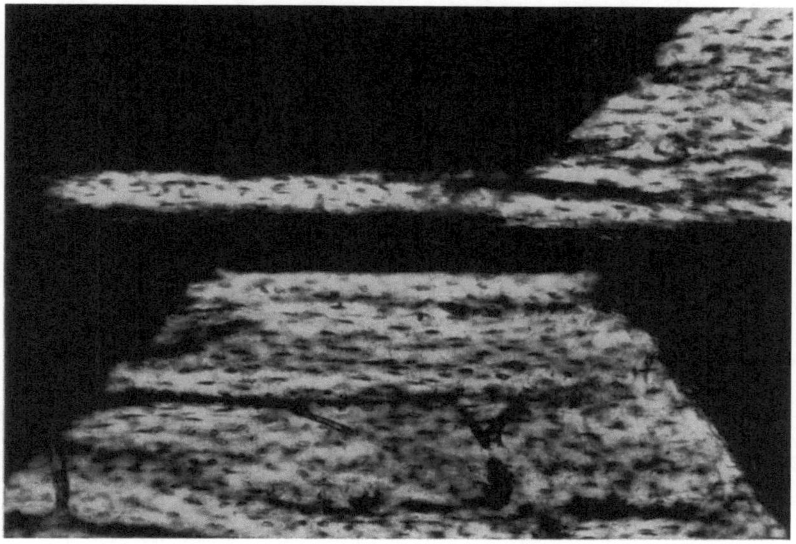

Fig. 1. Two dissected specimens showing on top a longitudinal portion of the same osteon. Polarizing microscope. × 75

The osteons were sectioned with a Porter-Blum microtome fitted with a diamond knife. A Siemens Elmiskop I electron microscope was used to examine the sections.

For particular purposes the specimens were decalcified by EDTA before embedding. Decalcification was also carried out on ultra-thin sections, using phosphotungstic acid, which also gives good staining of the collagen fibrils.

Results

In osteons at the initial stage of calcification, the calcium salts show two different features at the level of the lamellae (Fig. 2). The first is a series of parallel bands which are separated by clear interbands and run almost perpendicular to the osteon axis. The bands have an average width of 400 Å and the interbands reach 250 Å. These values indicate that the parallel banding identifies the broad bands at the major collagen periods. Here small spots appear measuring no more than 10 Å across. These spots which apparently represent foci of crystal inception or centers of nucleation (see Glimcher, 1959) fuse in linear or needleshaped crystallites which span the band regions, reaching a maximum width of 40—45 Å.

The second feature met in the lamellae of the osteons during the initial stage of calcification are bundles of needle-shaped crystallites considerably longer than those at the level of the broad band. Generally they have a longitudinal orientation as regards the osteon axis. Owing to their length the crystallites can cover two or many major collagen periods. The thickness averages 40—45 Å.

Transitional figures are found between the needle-shaped crystallites lying at the level of the cross-bands and the bundles of elongated needle-shaped crystallites.

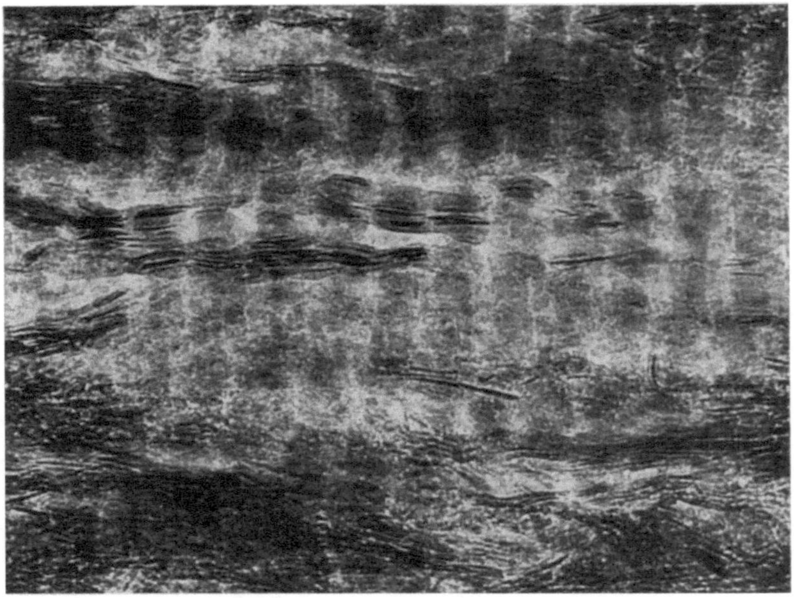

Fig. 2. Ultrathin longitudinal section of an osteon at the initial stage of calcification. Explanation in text. × 125.000

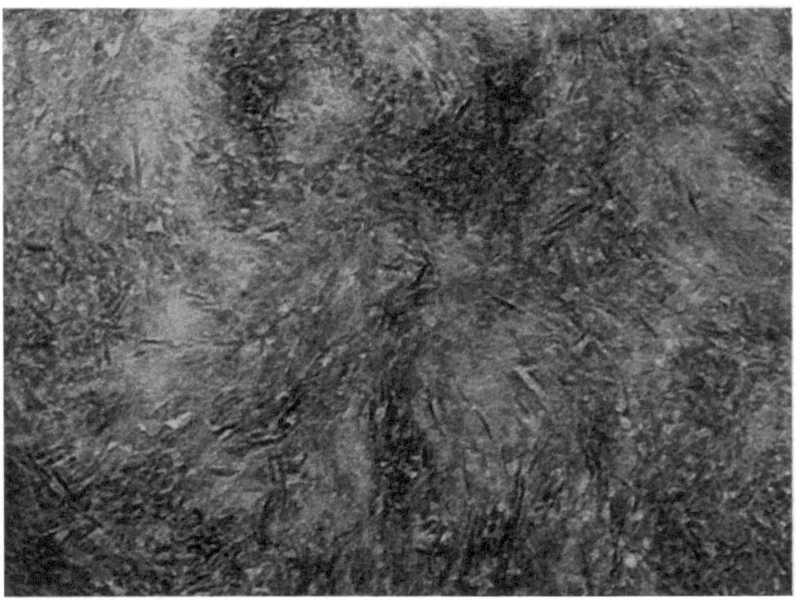

Fig. 3. Ultrathin cross-section of an osteon at the initial stage of calcification. Explanation in text. × 60.000

In ultra-thin cross-sections crystallites are evenly distributed according to their penetration into the collagen fibrils (Fig. 3).

In contrast with the lamellae, the interlamellar cementing zones show only one feature, the calcified bands are missing or very rare. The crystallites have the same shape and about the same size, but they are irregularly distributed and orientated in all directions forming at some points whorled figures.

In fully calcified osteons the lamellae show no appreciable qualitative differences from those of osteons in the initial stages of calcification (Fig. 4). However, compari-

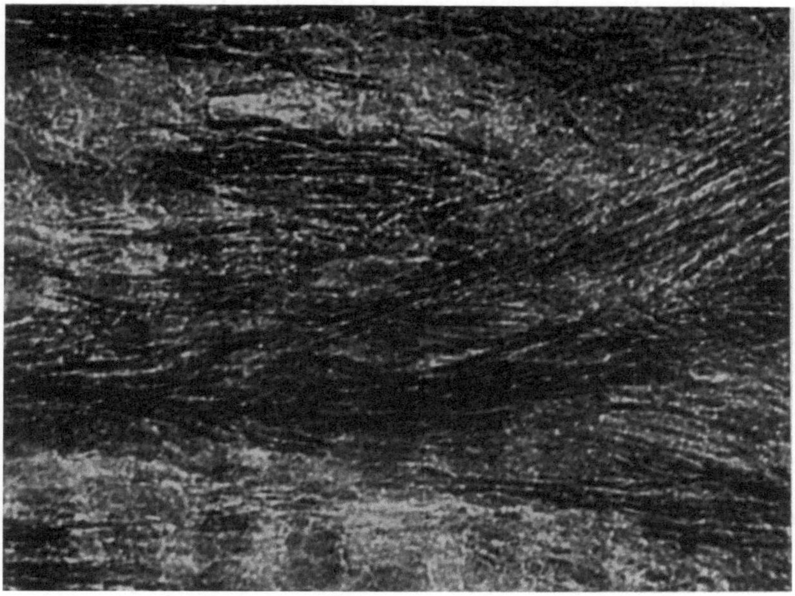

Fig. 4. Ultrathin longitudinal section of a fully calcified osteon. Explanation in text. × 185.000

son of micrographs from osteons both at the initial stage of calcification and from fully calcified ones suggests that the number of needle-shaped crystallites increases in the latter. The surfaces covered by elongated crystallites as well as those covered by calcified bands were measured in 56 micrographs. The results show that the areas covered by needle-shaped crystallites are predominant in the osteon in the initial stage of ossification and correspond to about 69 per cent. The same areas increase by 14 per cent, when osteons complete their ossification going up to 83 per cent. The statistical analysis shows that the differences between the two mean values are highly significant, t being 6.334 for $P = 0.05$. This value is only indicative. In order to obtain more reliable data on the actual increase of calcium it would be necessary to consider the spatial distribution, density and dimensions of the calcified material in the two types of apatite deposition as the cross-banding has a lower opacity to the electron beam than the other calcified areas. At the moment this problem presents difficulties which still have to be solved.

In the fully calcified osteons the interlamellar cementing zones are formed almost entirely of needle-shaped crystallites, which makes it difficult to establish whether the calcium salts are actually increased. However, the absence or scarcity of areas covered by calcified bands, in which calcium is obviously low, supports the view that the interlamellar zones are more highly calcified than the lamellae.

Ultra-thin sections obtained from previously decalcified osteons at the final stage of ossification did not show, after treatment by phosphotungstic acid, any qualitative difference from those of osteons at the initial stage of ossification. In the lamellae the fibrils are closely packed in bundles and are preferentially orientated according to the osteon axis, although the bundles interweave frequently at small angles. Conversely, in decalcified osteons the interlamellar cementing zone is composed of thin fibrils irregularly orientated in all directions. The thick banded fibrils are few or completely lacking. Where present, they show a cross-, or strongly oblique orientation and pass through one lamella to the next.

Conclusions

The investigation under the electron microscope of the dynamics of the osteon calcification reveals that after a sudden initial penetration of a large percentage of the matrix by elongated needle-shaped crystallites, the apatite is laid down more slowly and the areas covered by needle-shaped crystallites get larger at the expense of the areas in which calcium is laid down only at the level of the main cross-banding of the collagen fibrils.

A detailed paper on this subject is in press for the "J. of Ultrastructure Res.".

References

Ascenzi, A., and C. Fabry: Technique for dissection and measurement of refractive index of osteons. J. biophys. biochem. Cytol. **6**, 139 (1959).

Glimcher, M. J.: Molecular biology of mineralized tissues with particular reference to bone. Rev. mod. Phys. **31**, 359 (1959).

Collagen and Apatite in Hard Tissues and Pathological Formations from a Crystal Chemical Point of View

H. J. Höhling, H. Themann, J. Vahl

Institut für Medizinische Physik, Münster, Deutschland

During recent years electron microscopical investigations have been carried out by us on ultrathin sections of dentine, cementum and bone (Höhling, 1960, 1961, 1963 a, b, c, 1964; Höhling and Pfefferkorn, 1964; Vahl and Höhling, 1964/65). In these four examples of apatite mineralization on collagen we found the same morphological phenomena on electron microscopical examination.

On one hand we observed light-looking, elongated formations all of the same length, arranged parallel and in rows (Fig. 1, arrow 1) which were identified as apatite-crystallites by means of a combination of electron "small-area" diffraction with dark-field observation. On the other hand, we observed strands of thinner (ϕ 60—80 Å), dark-looking, longer formations frequently of unequal length which in general ran parallel to the rows of light-looking crystallites (Fig. 1, arrow 2). We observed these formations only in the peritubular zone of the dentine and concluded by means of the above mentioned methods that they, too, were apatitic, although we had first assumed them to be collagen subfibers without apatite.

Concerning the thin, dark-looking, apatitic formations (Fig. 1, arrow 2) we concluded that: 1. they are formed earlier than the above mentioned light-looking crystallites, 2. they are in a more disordered stage of crystallinity. We reached the first conclusion from the fact that in the initial stages of collagen mineralization in myositis ossificans, cementum, dentine or turkey leg tendon (NYLEN *et al.*, 1960) only the thin, dark-looking formations could be seen. In the case of myositis ossificans we observed (THEMANN and HÖHLING, 1964—1965), as GLIMCHER (1961) did in the case of bone and collagen mineralization in vitro, first the so-called "dots" out of which the very thin, dark, rodlike formations develop.

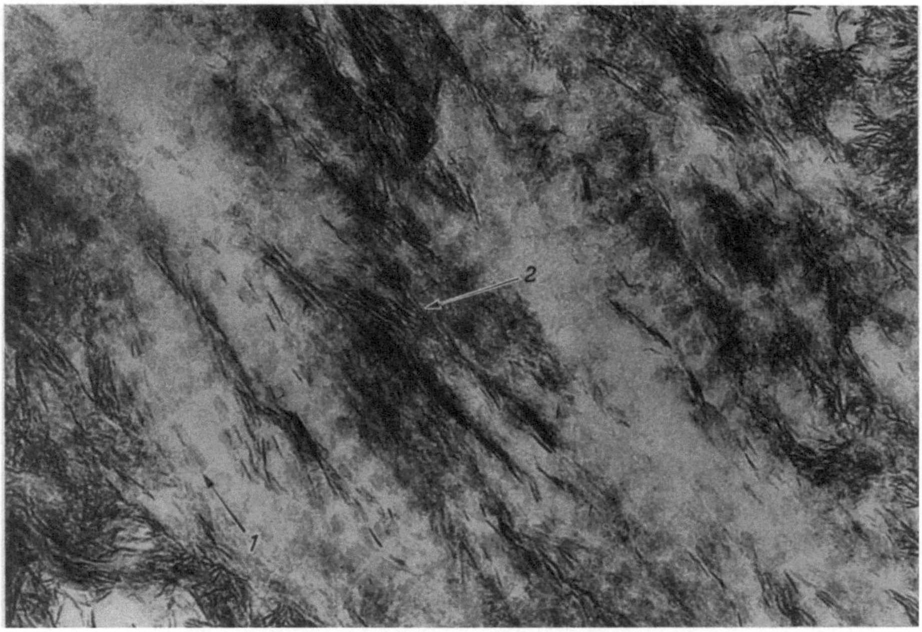

Fig. 1. Ultrathin section of myositis ossificans Arrow 1 shows the light-looking apatite crystallites, parallel arranged in rows with a distance from one row to the next in the range of 650±50 Å. Arrow 2 shows the thin (ϕ 60—80 Å) dark looking apatitic formations described in the paper. Magnification: 82 000 : 1

We reached our second conclusion i.e. that they are not apatite crystallites with a fully developed crystal-lattice, from several independant observations. REIMER (1962, Fig. 1) found on electron microscopic examination of thin metal foils that they looked darker in a more amorphous state and that they became lighter in appearance when converted into a more crystalline state. The dark appearance of the thin apatitic formations might therefore, result from poor crystallinity. Furthermore, the fact that they show relatively few electron diffraction lines, that they are often bent, that they are of unequal thickness throughout their whole length and that they are very thin, might support the conclusion that they are still in an initial state of crystallinity.

The interaction of ions which leads to the "binding" of phosphate with the side groups of the collagen fibres as matrix presumably accounts for the fact that the lattice of these nuclei is still in a less organized state. Moreover, we concluded that by this reciprocal action collagen subfibers ("spiral lattices" according to Sasisekharan and Ramachandran, 1957) are "cemented", for the diameter of these dark apatitic elements (60—80 Å) is within the range of the diameter which might be assumed for collagen subfibers from equatorial low angle diffraction spots got by Ramachandran and Sasisekharan (1960). By this apatitic "cementation" of collagen subfibers the macromolecular arrangement and thus the cross-striation of the collagen fibers is lost.

We concluded that the light-looking apatite crystallites (Fig. 1, arrow 1) are generally formed from the thin, dark-looking apatitic formations when there is a sufficient delivery of ions for apatite formation and sufficient micro-space for expansion of the crystallites in width because in the areas of the dark-looking apatitic formations the thicker, lighter-looking apatite formations mentioned above gradually develop. The fact that these elements gradually become lighter may result from an increasing organization of the atoms in the lattice.

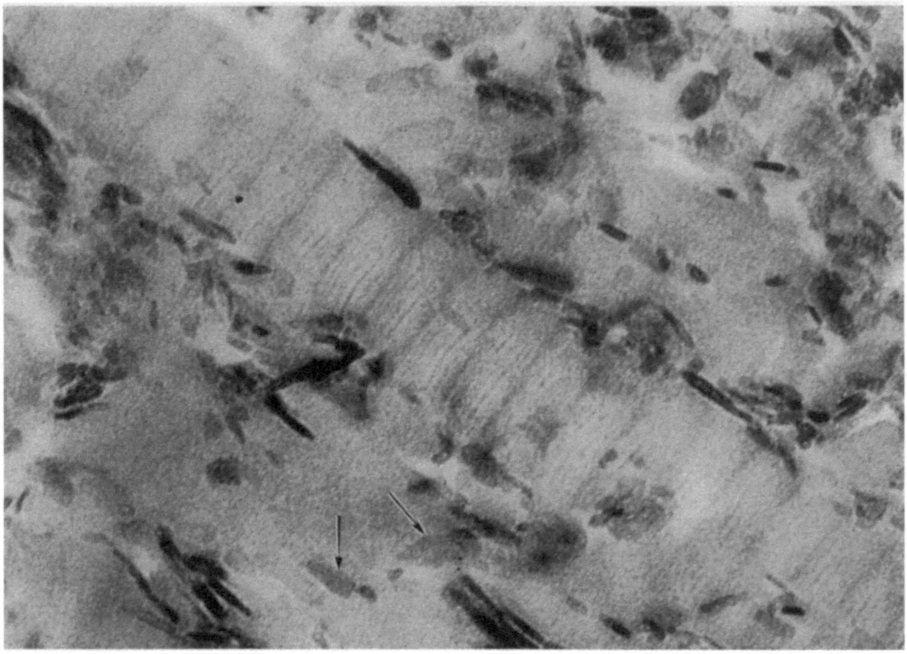

Fig. 2. Ultrathin section of carious dentine. By the decomposition of the thin, dark looking apatitic formations "cemented" collagen-subfibres were set free again and could combine to thicker collagen fibres with cross-striation. (The arrows indicate light-looking apatite crystallites which lie at random in carious dentine.) Magnification: 198 000 : 1

It was observed that the distance from one row of the light-looking parallel apatite crystallites to the next lies within the range of the collagen macro-period (640 Å-period) (Carlström and Glas, 1959; Glas, 1962; Quigley and Hjørting-

Hansen, 1962; Höhling, 1963 a, b, 1964; Höhling and Pfefferkorn, 1964). Thus we concluded that the macromolecular arrangement of collagen influences the length of the apatite crystallites.

Following the results of Hodge and Petruska (1963, Fig. 9) we assume that the nuclei develop on certain "dark bands" of the collagen cross-striation within the so-called "hole zone". In the area of the "hole zone" the nuclei grow in length (and also in thickness), until they reach the "overlap zone" of the macroperiod in which there seems to be a blocking force which prevents further growth in length (Höhling, 1964; Höhling *et al.*, in press, Fig. 5).

In the case of dentine caries as an example of hard tissue decay we made the following observations. In carious dentine it is mainly the thin, dark-looking apatitic formations which are decomposed. But the light-looking crystallites are also affected and disorganized in their arrangement. By the decomposition of the thin, dark-looking apatitic formations the "cemented" collagen subfibers are set free but then combine again to form thicker collagen fibers with the characteristic cross-striation and macromolecular arrangement. (Of course this is not a new formation of collagen fibers but only a lateral aggregation of subfibers to thicker fibers which already existed before mineralization, in embryonic dentine.) These carious changes are shown in Fig. 2.

During further carious attack the macromolecular arrangement of collagen is destroyed and the thicker collagen fibers are decomposed into their subelements. By

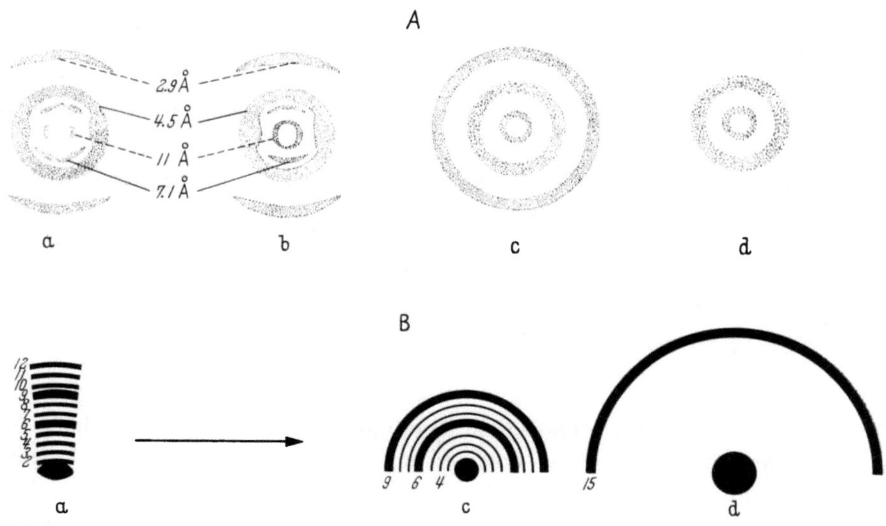

Fig. 3. Diagrammatical representation of x-ray wide angle — and low angle — patterns for sound and diseased tendon. The loss of reflexions from the sound to the diseased state (in the figure from left to right) is the same as from sound demineralized to carious additionally demineralized dentine. But for carious dentine there was seldom reached the stage *d*, in which only the 4.5 Å- and 11 Å reflexion had remained

combined x-ray diffraction and infrared-absorption analysis we found that the collagen decay caused by dentine caries occurs in the same way as the collagen decay described by us for human tendon and meniscus (Dahmen and Höhling, 1962; Höhling and Dahmen, 1963; Höhling, 1963 c; Höhling *et al.*, 1965; Höhling and Pfefferkorn, in press).

In Fig. 3 the x-ray patterns of sound and diseased human tendon are represented diagrammatically with the effect of increasing disease shown from left to right in the figure. In the upper row wide angle patterns are seen in the lower row low-angle patterns. Above all there is a loss of the 7.1 Å- and 2.9 Å-reflexions together with a loss of the reflexions of the 640 Å period. This loss indicates *changes* in the *polypeptide* chain. Such changes in the wide angle range have also been observed by us in carious dentine.

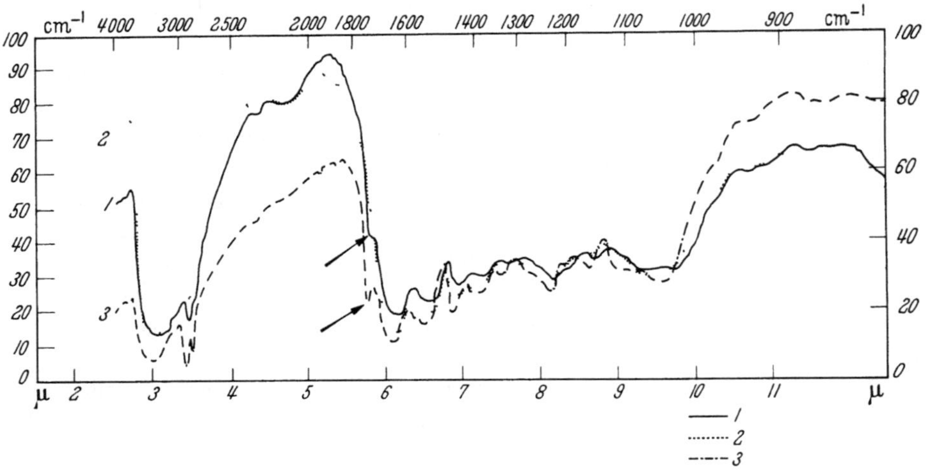

Fig. 4. Infrared diagrams of sound dentine collagen (Nr. 2). Carious dentine collagen (weakening of the intensity of the 2.9 Å- and 7.1 Å x-ray reflexions) (Nr. 1) and diseased human tendon (loss of the 2.9 Å- and 7.1 Å x-ray reflexions) (Nr. 3). In the case of carious dentine, diagram Nr. 1 (with collagen not so much decomposed), there is a beginning of a peak, and in the case of diseased tendon, diagram 3 (with more decomposed collagen), a full peak in the range of 5.8 μ. We conclude that it indicates a C=O valence oscillation resulting from broken peptide bonds in the polypeptide chains

In the infrared diagrams (Fig. 4) of samples of carious dentine and diseased tendon, showing decrease or loss of the 7.1 Å- and 2.9 Å-reflexion, we found the same new peak near 1730 cm^{-1}. It lies in the range of a C=O valence oscillation. Since the 2.9 Å- and 7.1 Å-x-ray reflexions had disappeared in the case of these samples we concluded that peptide-bonds were affected or broken. This attack seems to occur when the collagen fibers are split longitudinally to a sufficient degree.

Summary

In the case of collagen mineralization by apatite in dentine, cementum, bone and tissues with myositis ossificans we observed on ultrathin sections: 1. light-looking, elongated apatite crystallites (⌀ ∼ 200 Å) of the same length (∼ 650 ± 50 Å) arranged parallel and in rows. 2. strands of thinner (⌀ 60—80 Å), dark looking and in general longer formations which were found also to be apatitic.

From a variety of observations we concluded that the thin, dark looking apatitic formations were formed earlier than the light-looking, thicker apatite crystallites; that they were still in a more disordered stage of crystallinity and that the light-looking apatite crystallites gradually developed out of them by a change to a better state of atom arrangement in the crystal lattice.

In carious dentine the thin, dark looking apatitic formations which cement the collagen subfibres were first decomposed. The collagen subfibers were then set free and could combine again to form thicker collagen fibrils with typical cross-striations. In the event of further carious attacks the thicker fibres were also affected and split up into subelements. We found by x-ray diffraction and infrared absorption analysis that peptide bonds in the polypeptide chain had been broken.

References

CARLSTRÖM, D., and J. E. GLAS: The size and shape of the apatite crystallites in bone as determined from line-broadening measurements on oriented specimens. Biochim. biophys. Acta **35**, 46 (1959).

DAHMEN, G., und H. J. HÖHLING: Submikroskopische Untersuchungen an gesunden und degenerierten Menisci. Z. Orthop. **96**, 7 (1962).

GLAS, J. E.: Studies on the ultrastructure of calcified tissues. Thesis. Stockholm 1962.

GLIMCHER, M. J.: The role of macromolecular aggregations state and reactivity of collagen in calcification. In Macromolecular Complexes. 6th Annual Symposium Publication. The Ronald Press 1961.

HODGE, H. J., and J. A. PETRUSKA: Recent studies with the electronmicroscope on aggregates of the tropocollagen macromolecules. Aspects of Protein Structure. Proc. Madras Symposium. RAMACHADRAN, G. N. (ed.). 1963.

HÖHLING, H. J.: Untersuchungen elektronenmikroskopischer Schnittbilder an gesundem und kariösem Dentin. Z. Naturforsch. **15**, 753 (1960).

— Elektronenmikroskopische Untersuchungen an gesundem und kariösem Dentin mit Hilfe der Abdruckmethode und der Schnittmethode an kompakter, nicht entmineralisierter Substanz. Z. Zellforsch. **53**, 192 (1961).

— Zur Frage der organischen Matrix in bezug auf Dentin, Zement und Knochen. Arch. oral. Biol. Suppl. p. 265 (1963 a).

— Kollagen und Apatit im menschlichen Hartgewebe. Collagen Symposium Den Haag 1963 b

— Gesundes und degeneriertes Kollagen aus strukturchemischer Sicht. Med.-Naturwiss. Gesellschaft. Münster 1963 c.

— Die Bauelemente von Zahnschmelz und Dentin aus morphologischer, chemischer und struktureller Sicht. Habilitationsschrift University of Münster 1964.

—, und G. DAHMEN: Sublichtmikroskopische Untersuchungen an gesunden und degenerierten Sehnen. Z. Orthop. **97**, 339 (1963).

—, R. KATTERBACH, und H. VOGEL: Elektronenmikroskopische Untersuchungen zur Aufklärung der strukturchemischen Veränderungen bei der Dentinkaries. Dtsch. Zahnärztebl. (in press).

—, und G. PFEFFERKORN: Bestimmung und Verteilung der Kristallite im Hartgewebe. Third Eur. Reg. Conf. electr. Micr. Prague 1964.

— — Biokristallographische Untersuchungen zur strukturellen Veränderung an degenerierten menschlichen Sehnen. Z. Orthop. (in press).

NYLEN, M. U., D. B. SCOTT, and V. M. MOSLEY: Mineralization of turkey leg tendon. II. Collagenmineral relation revealed by electron and x-ray microscopy. In Calcification in Biological Systems. SOGNNAES, R. F. (ed.). Washington: Amer. Ass. Advanc. Sci. 1960, p. 129.

QUIGLEY, M. B., and E. HJØRTING-HANSEN: Crystal arrangement in anorganic bone. Act. odont. scand. **20**, 359 (1962).

RAMACHANDRAN, G. N., and V. SASISEKHARAN: Study of molecular structure of fibres. J. sci. industr. Res. **19 A**, 357 (1960).

REIMER, L.: Änderung des elektronenmikroskopischen Bildkontrastes beim Übergang amorph-kristallin und flüssig-kristallin. Naturwissenschaften **49**, 1 (1962).

SASISEKHARAN, V., and G. N. RAMACHANDRAN: Studies on collagen. II. Cylindrical lattice structure of collagen. Proc. Ind. Acad. Sci. **45**, 363 (1957).

THEMANN, H., and H. J. HÖHLING: Several discussions on the structural connection between collagen and apatite in tissues with myositis ossificans. Inst. med. Phys. Münster 1964/65.

VAHL, J., and H. J. HÖHLING: General aspects of the nature of thin, electron microscopically dark-looking apatitic formations in hard tissues, calculi, salivary stones and pathological collagen mineralizations. Continental European Section I. A. D. R., Straßburg 1964/65.

Studies of Calcification in Plants

H. J. ARNOTT

Cell Research Institute, University of Texas, Austin, Texas, U. S. A.

It has long been known that insoluble calcium salts in the forms of the carbonate, sulfate, and oxalate occur as optically visible crystals in a wide variety of plants (SOLEREDER, 1908). The deposits are commonly considered to be waste products and occur in a variety of shapes, often seeming to fill a cell. Calcium oxalate crystals are by far the most common, and a single cell may contain from one to many hundreds. Crystal cells have been studied by light and polarization microscopy (see reviews in GUILLIERMOND, 1933; KÜSTER, 1956) and the crystals have been studied by various techniques including X-ray and infra-red analysis (POBEGUIN, 1943; WALTER-LEVY, 1962).

The salient features of a variety of crystal cells investigated by ARNOTT and PAUTARD (1965) are: 1. Crystals are produced within active cells as a part of their program of differentiation, usually in meristematic tissues. 2. Crystal formation is not a random event but takes place in a series of biologically organized steps. 3. Crystal development occurs within chambers which first become loaded with an electron dense material and subsequently appear to function as boules in which crystalization occurs, often, but perhaps not always, shaping the crystals.

A previous study of the growing root tip of *Yucca* (ARNOTT, 1962) revealed that raphide cells develop in linear rows with as many as 27 cells in a single file. The present research has shown partly differentiated crystal cells within the zone of active mitosis, in juxtaposition to cells in division and only a few hundred microns from the root tip. In the root zone, where the major growth parameter is cell enlargement, raphide cells are very well differentiated (Fig. 1) and exhibit two characteristics not found in their immediate neighbors. First, they contain a series of electron dense compartments within a crystal vacuole, *i. e.*, the vacuole in which the crystals develop. Secondly, they possess numerous highly differentiated crystaloplastids, *i. e.*, the modified plastids which occur in crystal cells.

The crystal chambers are elongate, and when cut in transverse section have rectangular or rounded profiles. At an intermediate stage in crystal ontogeny, the chambers exhibit an electron-dense material which does not give an electron diffraction pattern; however, after prolonged heating in the electron beam a pattern suggesting calcium oxide is produced, and at the same time obvious changes occur in the electron-dense material. This dense material is rapidly leached by water in sectioning or by the staining of thin sections with uranyl acetate and/or lead citrate. Therefore, it must be studied in unstained preparations rapidly picked up from the trough. Such data indicates that the chambers are not crystals or crystalline at the electron diffraction level, but are merely loaded with an electron-dense material of an unknown nature. The exact manner in which crystallization occurs is also not understood; however, X-ray data (STEINFINK *et al.*, 1965) shows calcium oxalate monohydrate to be present in the mature crystals. The fact that the mature crystals in *Yucca* and other plants often have rounded contours rather than sharp facets, means one cannot overlook the possibility that the crystal compartments act as boules, and are in part responsible for the rounded contours found in many plant crystals.

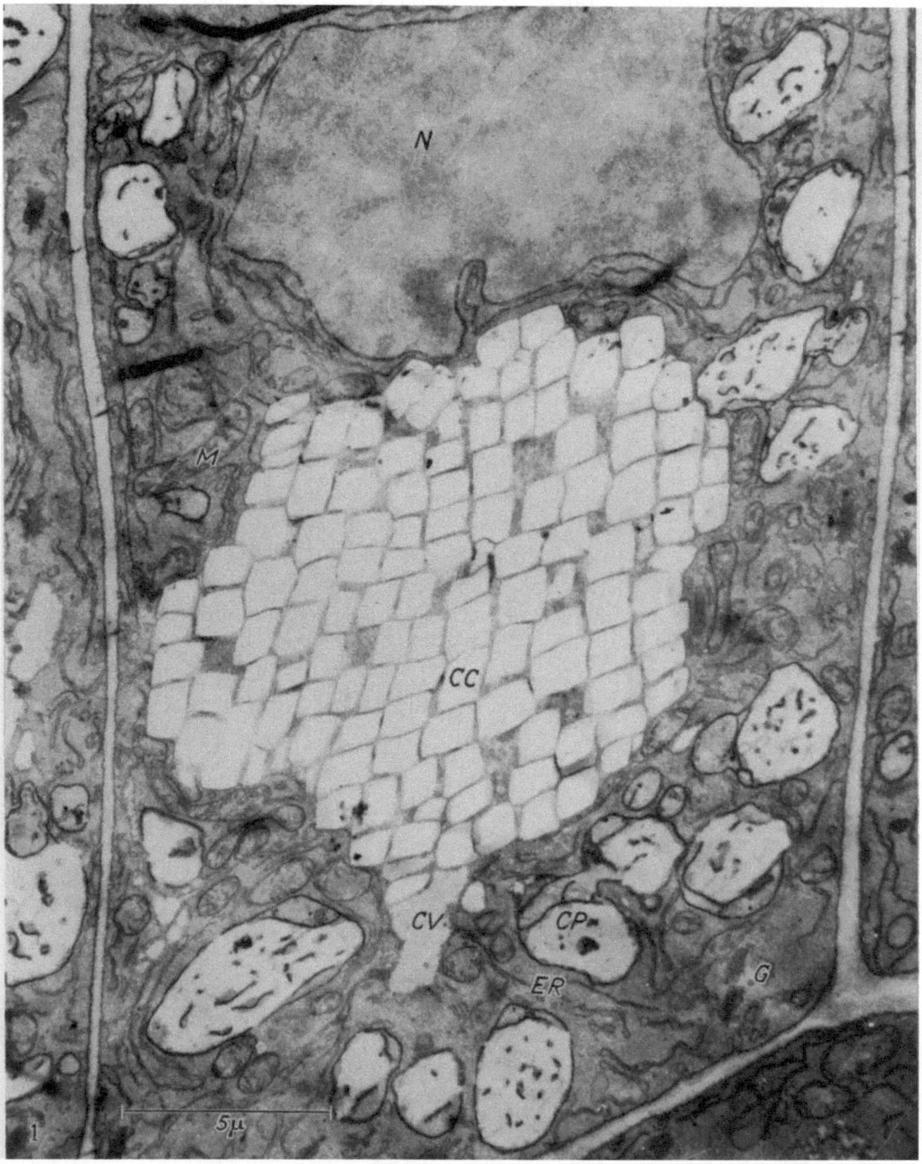

Fig. 1. Crystal cell from the root of *Yucca schidigera*. Crystal chambers cut in transverse section. $KMnO_4$ fixation; post stained lead hydroxide
cc = crystal chambers; cp = crystalloplastids; cv = crystal vacuole; er = endoplasmic reticulum; g = Golgi bodies; lcc = loaded crystal chambers; m = mitochondria; n = nucleus; pp = proplastid; v = vacuole

By enlargement and internal membrane proliferation, proplastids in the raphides of *Yucca* develop into crystalloplastids, characteristic only of crystal cells. These plastids are bounded by a double membrane, the inner of which invaginates at several points to produce the series of internal membranes. Three zones can be observed in these plastids, *viz.*, a relatively dense zone, a transparent zone, and a lamellar zone.

The crystalloplastids are often constricted into segments connected by a narrow isthmus. These plastids appear to degenerate as the crystal cells mature. The plastids do not give an electron diffraction pattern.

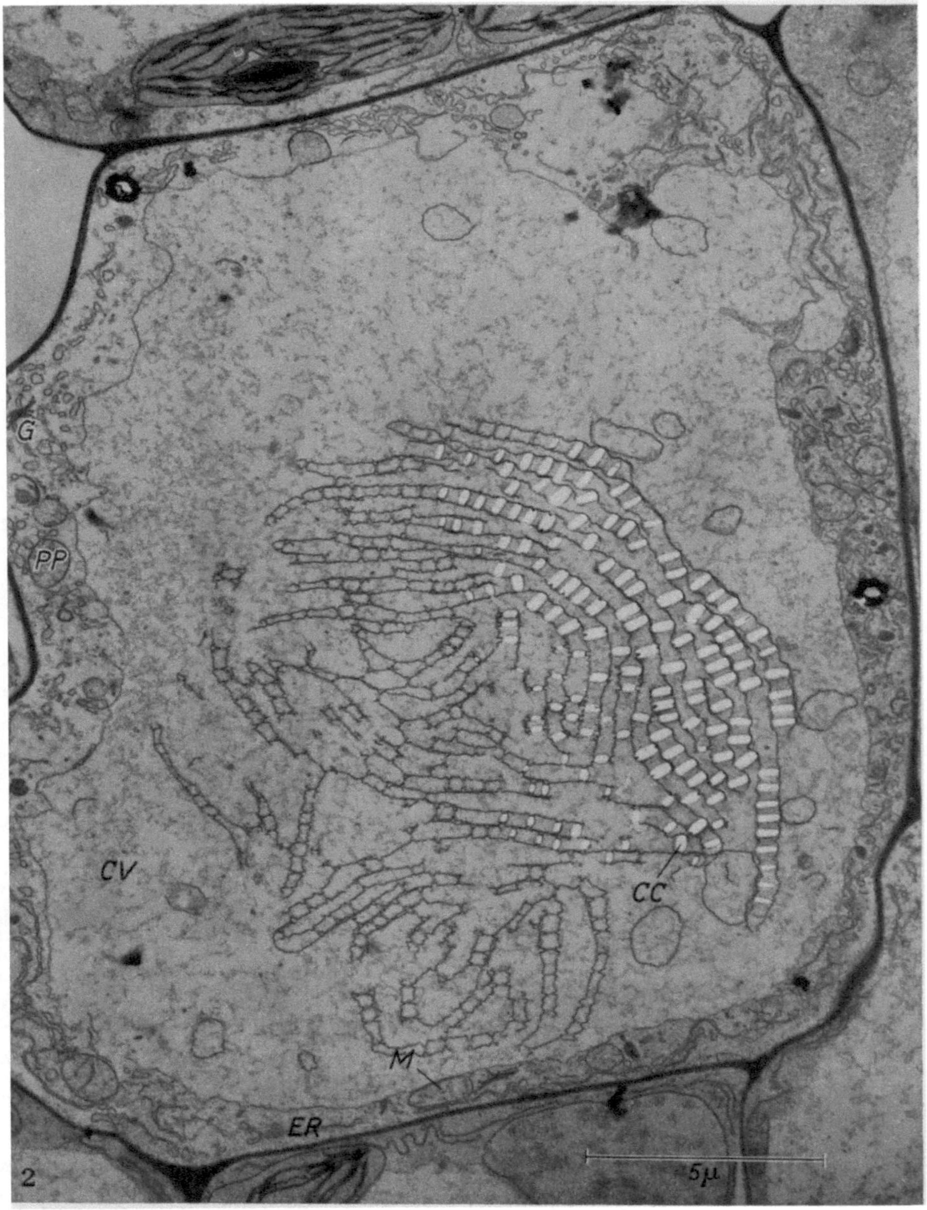

Fig. 2. Transection of a crystal idioblast of *Lemna minor*. A series of paired membranes within the crystal vacuole are in the process of chamber formation. $KMnO_4$ fixation; post stained with uranyl acetate and lead citrate

In isolated crystal cells, raphide idioblasts, of the developing frond of the duckweed, *Lemna minor*, crystal chambers also develop within a crystal vacuole. However, in this case the chambers are formed within a series of "parallel" paired lamellae

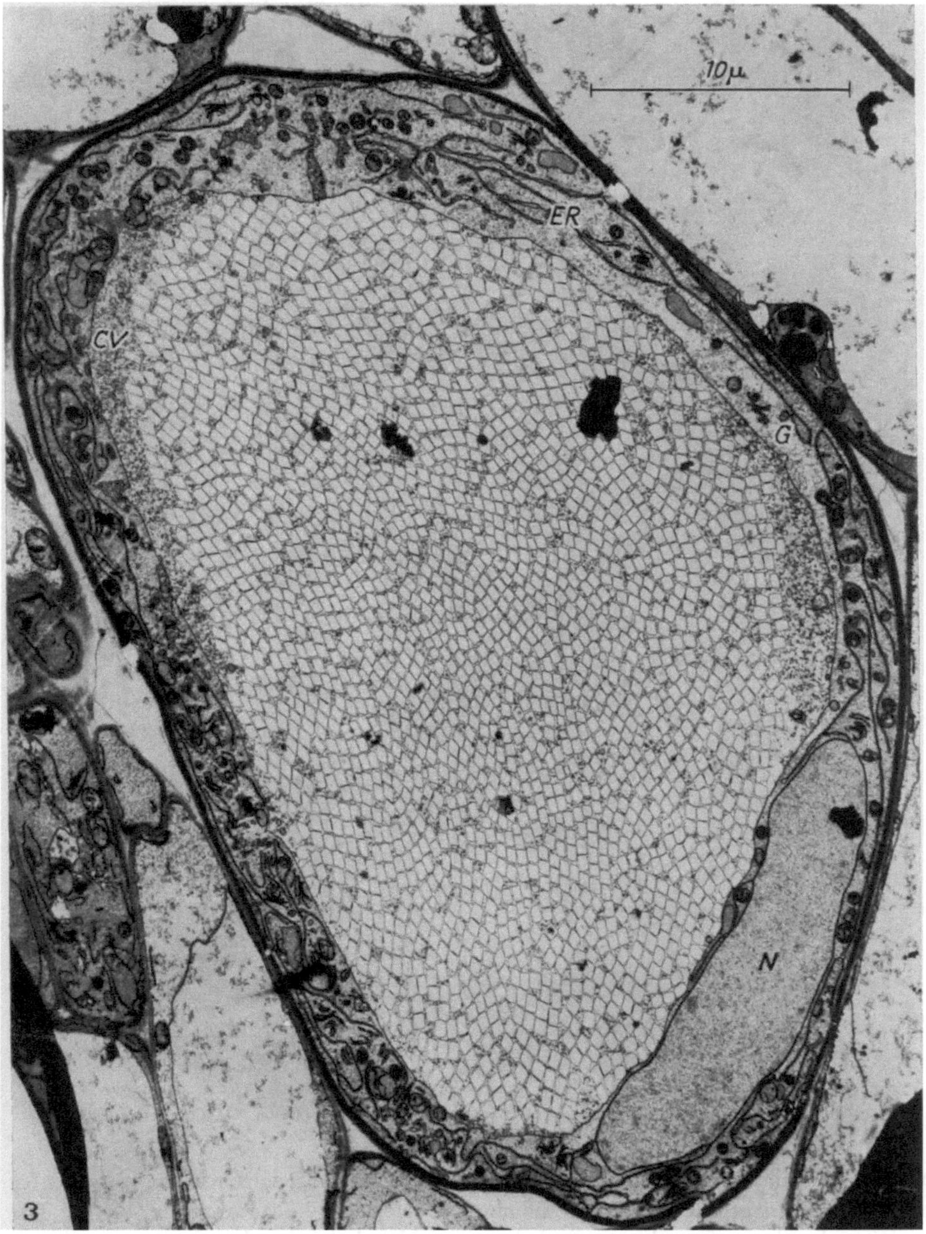

Fig. 3. A developing raphide idioblast of *Eichhornia crassipes* cut transverse to the long axis of the cell. Cell contains ca. 2140 crystal chambers. $KMnO_4$ fixation; post stained with lead citrate

(as many as 15 or more pairs may be present in one cell) extending from the peripheral cytoplasm into the vacuole (Fig. 2). The chambers arise by successive changes in the membranes (Fig. 2). When the paired membranes are cut transverse to the long

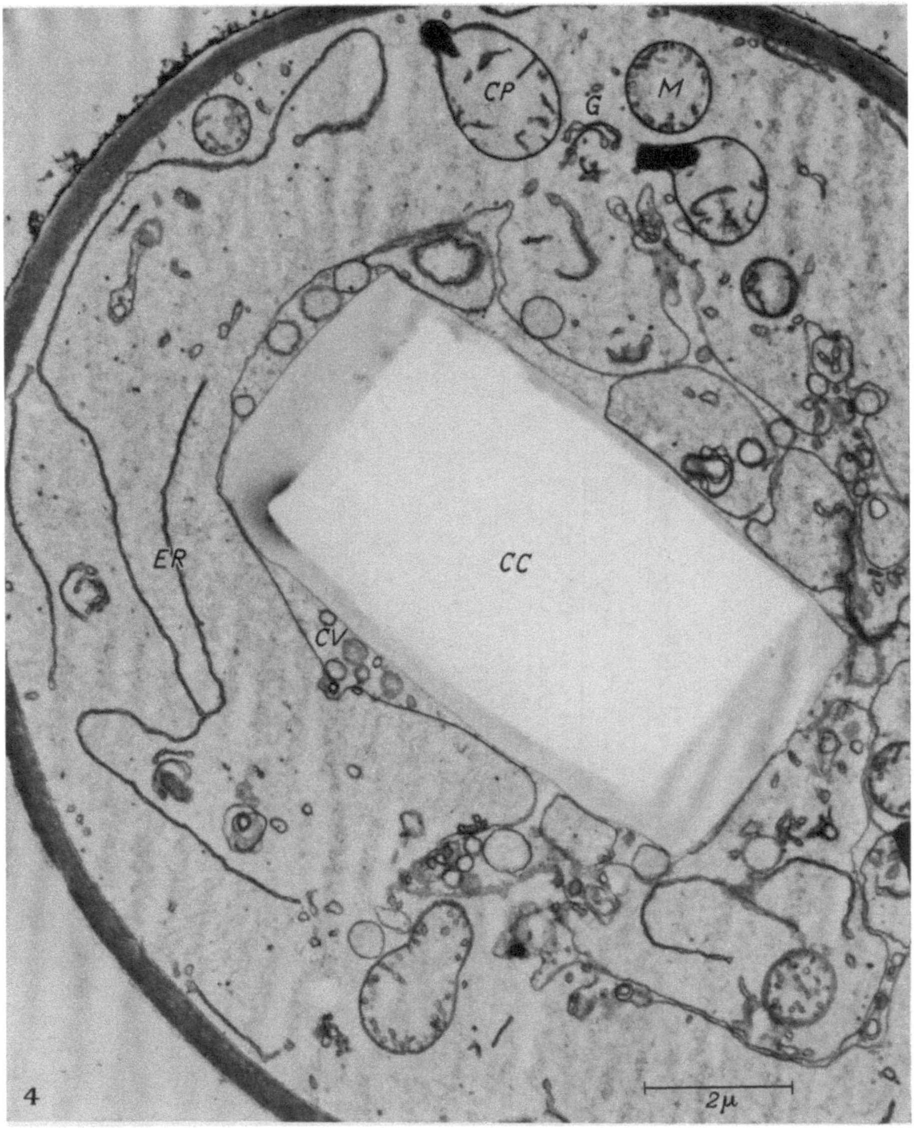

Fig. 4. Transection of styloid idioblast of *Eichhornia crassipes*. Fixation $KMnO_4$ poststained

axis of the cell, a series of hourglass profiles can be seen. By densification at the center of the hourglass profile the crystal chambers develop in a linear sequence (Fig. 2). The growing chambers often show rounded contours but later they become rectangular in transverse section. The electron-dense loaded chambers, at an intermediate stage in development, do not produce an electron diffraction pattern. Mature crystals give an X-ray diffraction pattern characteristic of calcium oxalate monohydrate. No special differentiation of plastids was observed in the *Lemna* idioblasts; however, the cells are exceptionally well provided with Golgi bodies, endoplasmic reticulum and mitochondria.

In the shoot of the water hyacinth *(Eichhornia)*, raphide idioblasts with over 2000 crystals per cell were observed; cells with 2140 (Fig. 3) and 2012 crystals were counted. Paradoxically, in the same tissue cells having only a single crystal per cell are quite common (Fig. 4). In principle, the development of the raphide cell with its many needle shaped crystals and the styloid cells with one (or a few) large tabular shaped crystals is the same. In each case the crystals form within a chamber produced in the crystal vacuole. As in *Lemna*, the crystal chambers of *Eichhornia* are in intimate association with a series of tubules and membranes which extend into the crystal vacuole from the peripheral cytoplasm. In this case it is clear that if a cell is to produce over 2000 crystals in close proximity to each other, it must exercise more or less complete control of the process, *i. e.*, crystal formation in plants may have physical and chemical parameters but it is a biological controlled phenomenon.

Summary

The formation of calcium oxalate crystals in the plants investigated is a biologically controlled process, intimately associated with cellular differentiation. Crystal development occurs by the formation of loaded chambers associated with membranes and tubules; subsequently crystals are formed within these chambers. The possibility that the chamber acts like a boule is suggested.

Acknowledgments

I sincerely thank Prof. W. G. Whaley for his encouragement and for the use of the facilities of the Cell Research Institute. The present research was supported in part by N.S.F. Grant GF-1458 and N.I.H. 5TIGM 789.

References

Arnott, H. J.: The morphology and anatomy of *Yucca*. Univ. Calif. Publ. Bot. 35, 1 (1962).

—, and F. G. E. Pautard: Mineralization in plants. Amer. J. Bot. **52**, 618 (1965).

Guilliermond, A.: Traité de Cytologie Végétale. Paris. E. Le François 1933.

Kuster, E.: Die Pflanzenzelle. Jena: Fischer 1956.

Pobeguin, T.: Les oxalates de calcium chez quelques angiospermes. Ann. Sci. nat. Bot. **4**, 1 (1943).

Solereder, H.: Systematic Anatomy of the Dicotyledons. Oxford: Clarendon Press 1908.

Steinfink, H., F. G. E. Pautard, and H. J. Arnott: Crystallography of calcium oxalates in plants. Amer. J. Bot. **52**, 613 (1965).

Walter-Levy, L., et R. Strauss: Sur la répartition des hydrates de l'oxalate de calcium chez les végétaux. C. R. Acad. Sci. **254**, 1671 (1962).

Crystallographic Identification of Calcium Deposits as Regards their Pathological Nature, with Special Reference to Chondrocalcinosis

R. LAGIER, C. A. BAUD, M. BUCHS

Institut de Pathologie et Institut de Morphologie, Université de Genève, Genève, Suisse

In a paper published in 1962, KOHN *et al.* showed that the "Pseudogout Syndrome" of chondrocalcinosis articularis was accompanied by the presence in synovial fluid of a form of calcium pyrophosphate crystals. By their size, these crystals are comparable with those of sodium urate and therefore are presumably able to induce articular attacks. Moreover, they can produce two types of joint disturbances: a synovial inflammatory reaction that may present a picture similar to that of rheumatoid arthritis; a cartilage deterioration creating the morphological condition of osteoarthrosis, which is found occasionally in several joints. However, these deposits may be observed without clinical signs and found in routine radiographical or post-mortem examination. It is also interesting to note that the histological pictures are in several ways similar to those of gout, in cartilage as well as in reacting synovial membrane, where microtophi can sometimes be observed (LAGIER, to be published).

The purpose of this paper is to study these deposits of chondrocalcinosis and compare them with other tissue calcifications.

Material and techniques

This study is limited to tissue calcifications, excluding mineral deposits in cavities or canals. Tests were performed on 108 samples from 42 cases, collected by means of biopsy or from post-mortem material; each sample was ground and studied by the X-ray diffraction method for crystallographic identification.

Results

Our results are presented in three tables, corresponding to three groups of findings. We have indicated the nature of the different samples and their number, and also given the number of cases (i.e., of subjects) from whom the samples were collected. In some instances specimens of a different nature were obtained from the same case.

Three types of crystals were observed; apatite, whitlockite and calcium pyrophosphate dihydrate.

The first group includes deposits with apatite only and corresponds to a broad spectrum of pathological calcification (Table 1).

The second group is represented by deposits with whitlockite and apatite (Table 2). They were found predominantly in lesions of tuberculous or hydatid disease. In some of these deposits a tuberculous or parasitic origin was only suspected, though the probability was great; here the situations and conditions were different from those of the first group. The relative amount of whitlockite, as compared to that of apatite, was apparently in direct relationship to the degree of inflammatory activity. In some extreme conditions only whitlockite or apatite was observed, the latter occurring in old and stabilized processes.

The third group is that of chondrocalcinosis (Table 3). It includes eight cases of primary chondrocalcinosis, most of these having been found by routine biopsy or post-mortem examination, and only two of these cases were accompanied by clinical

Table 1. *Cases in which the calcareous deposits consisted of apatite (A)*

		No. of cases	No. of samples	A
Calcinosis	circumscripta ("chalk gout")	1	2	+
	universalis	1	3	
	milk-alkali syndrome	1	2	
Atheromatous plaques		2	3	+
Calcified deposits in the shoulder's rotator cuff (so-called peritendinitis calcarea)		1	2	+
Miscellaneous calcifications	pericardium	1	1	+
	meninges	1	2	
	thyroid gland	1	1	
	pancreas	1	1	
	gastrocnemius muscle	1	1	
	leiomyoma uteri	2	4	
	sebaceous cyst	1	1	
	lymph node (gelatinous carcinoma)	1	1	
	osteochondroma	1	2	
	chronic bone infarct	1	1	

Table 2. *Cases in which the calcareous deposits consisted of apatite (A), or whitlockite (W), or a mixture of the two in a single sample (A+W)*

		No. of cases	No. of samples	A	W	A + W
Calcifications in tuberculosis	lung	5	6		+	+
	lymph nodes	3	4	+		+
	vertebral spine	1	1			+
Calcifications in hydatid disease	lung	1	1		+	
	liver	3	3	+	+	+
	spleen	1	2	+		
	parametrium	1	3	+		+
Calcifications presumably of tuberculous origin	brain	1	1			+
Calcifications presumably of parasitic origin	liver	2	3			+
	spleen	1	2			

signs of polyarthrosis. Among the 36 samples of different articular tissues thus examined including fibro-cartilage of synchondroses, 29 instances of calcium pyrophosphate dihydrate were observed. The only case where apatite was mixed with pyrophosphate within the same sample was that of a meniscus from a knee with osteochondrosis dissecans. In six specimens apatite alone was found in calcifications of intervertebral discs; they occurred in two spines containing discal deposits of calcium pyrophosphate in other locations. Nevertheless, in those patients showing

Table 3. *Cases in which the patient presented with chondrocalcinosis articularis. According to their site, the calcareous deposits consisted either of apatite (A), calcium pyrophosphate dihydrate (P), or a mixture of the two in a single sample (A+P). (As in the preceding tables, the type of calcium deposit is indicated by + in the corresponding column)*

		No. of cases	No. of samples	A	P	A+P
Primary chondrocalcinosis articularis	hyaline articular cartilage, synovial membrane, articular ligaments	5	13		+	
	menisci of the knee	3	3		+	
		1	1			+
	intervertebral discs	2	18	+	+	
	symphysis pubis	1	1		+	
	Extra-articular calcifications					
	atheromatous plaques	4	5	+		
	costal cartilage	1	1	+		
	mitral valve	1	1	+		
	fibroma of the ovary	1	1	+		
	meninges	1	2	+		
	phlebolith	1	1	+		
Primary hyper-parathyroidism	hyaline articular cartilage, synovial membrane	1	3		+	
	atheromatous plaques	1	1	+		
Gout (secondary, with osteomalacia)	intervertebral discs	1	2		+	
	intra-osseous calcifications	1	2	+		

signs of primary chondrocalcinosis, different extra-articular calcifications were, as usual, apatite.

The same findings were made in two other forms of chondrocalcinosis. In one of these calcium pyrophosphate was found on the synovial membrane and cartilage of a knee, in a case of primary hyperparathyroidism which had undergone successful surgical removal of a parathyroid adenoma several years before. Unfortunately it was not possible to explore the extra-articular calcification in this case; however, in another case of von Recklinghausen's disease the examination of an atheromatous plaque revealed evidence of apatite.

The other was a case of gout, secondary to polycythemia vera and associated with osteomalacia. This diagnosis was confirmed by X-ray diffraction which showed the presence of sodium urate monohydrate deposits. Radiographs revealed signs of chondrocalcinosis of knee menisci and systematic post-mortem examination permitted the collection of two samples of calcareous deposits found in intervertebral discs.

These calcifications were composed of calcium pyrophosphate, but curious intra-osseous calcareous deposits in the metatarsal bones were identified as apatite.

Discussion and conclusions

We can only interpret the present findings within the limits permitted by the techniques employed. However, this preliminary study has led to certain conclusions.

1. Among the well-known pathological tissue calcifications, a great number are apatite deposits. Of particular interest were those found in the following conditions: calcinosis (circumscripta, universalis, milk-alkali syndrome); atheromatous plaques; constrictive pericarditis or calcification of meninges; intra-osseous calcareous deposits in an osteochondroma or a chronic bone infarct (in the latter this well-known fact corresponded to the "apatite membrane"). In addition to histological data, the presence of apatite in the calcification of the shoulder's rotator cuff (so-called peritendinitis calcarea) is another means of distinguishing it from that of chondrocalcinosis articularis.

2. In calcareous deposits of tuberculous or parasitic origin whitlockite and apatite are present; this substantiates the previous observations of BRANDENBERGER and SCHINZ (1945). The amount of the former is seemingly related to the rate of inflammatory activity of the process. In some rare instances, we find only apatite in old cases.

3. Chondrocalcinosis articularis is characterized by calcium pyrophosphate dihydrate deposits in articular structures, including the fibrocartilage of the menisci, of the intervertebral discs or of the symphysis pubis. In eight cases of primary chondrocalcinosis, asymptomatic or with clinical signs of polyarthrosis, we have confirmed the findings of KOHN *et al.* (1962) and BUNDENS *et al.* (1965) in cases with the clinical picture of "pseudogout". Similar observations were made in two cases of chondrocalcinosis which were accompanied by diagnosed diseases. One of these was primary hyperparathyroidism in which the cartilaginous lesions were histologically similar to those described by BYWATERS *et al.* (1963). The other was accompanied by a uratic gout secondary to polycythemia vera.

All these cases were characterized by the fact that the extra-articular calcifications examined consisted of apatite. If this point were confirmed with visceral calcifications as in nephrocalcinosis, this would imply that calcium pyrophosphate deposits do not correspond to a disease *per se* but are a common denominator in articular tissue, depending on different etiological conditions. In primary chondrocalcinosis these deposits are related to a condition of unknown origin but seemingly associated with a genetic factor (VALSIK *et al.*, 1963); sometimes they are accompanied by a metabolic disturbance like hyperparathyroidism, hemochromatosis (DELBARRE, 1964; DE SEZE *et al.*, 1964) or even gout. The possibility of an association between gout and VON RECKLINGHAUSEN's disease has been suggested (BYWATERS *et al.*, 1963; VIX, 1964). However, in our case of gout there was neither clinical nor pathological evidence of hyperparathyroidism. We did not have the opportunity to examine visceral calcifications of such origin with X-ray diffraction; nevertheless a single examination with the polarizing microscope of nephrocalcinosis in VON RECKLINGHAUSEN's disease showed no crystals of the calcium pyrophosphate type. This observation agrees with those of Caulfield and Schrag (1964) concerning the presence of apatite in experimental nephrocalcinosis with parathyroid extracts, and thus supports the idea advanced above.

As regards the presence of apatite in some articular structures in cases of chondrocalcinosis, it should be noted that it was found in particular locations, i. e. in intervertebral discs and in a knee meniscus. In the intervertebral discs the apatite deposits were macroscopically dissociated from the areas containing calcium pyrophosphate; the presence of the former seemingly corresponded to foci of connective tissue deterioration. The only sample where apatite and pyrophosphate were associated was taken from a remodelled meniscus in a knee suffering from osteochondrosis dissecans. These findings support the idea that chondrocalcinosis reflects a special local disturbance by itself, independent of, even though sometimes adjacent to, other pathological calcifications which occur in a previous tissue deterioration.

References

Brandenberger, E., und H. R. Schinz: Über die Natur der Verkalkungen bei Mensch und Tier und das Verhalten der anorganischen Knochensubstanz im Falle der hauptsächlichen menschlichen Knochenkrankheiten. Helv. med. Acta **12**, suppl. 16, 1 (1945).

Bundens, W. D., Jr., C. T. Brighton, and G. Weitzman: Primary articular-cartilage calcification with arthritis (pseudogout syndrome). J. Bone Jt Surg. **47 A**, 111 (1965).

Bywaters, E. G. L., A. St. J. Dixon, and J. T. Scott: Joint lesions of hyperparathyroidism. Ann. rheum. Dis. **22**, 171 (1963).

Caulfield, J. B., and P. E. Schrag: Electron microscopic study of renal calcification. Amer. J. Path. **44**, 365 (1964).

Delbarre, F.: Les manifestations ostéo-articulaires de l'hémochromatose. Presse méd. **72**, 2973 (1964).

Kohn, N. N., R. E. Hughes, D. J. McCarty, Jr., and J. S. Faires: The significance of calcium phosphate crystals in the synovial fluid of arthritic patients: The "Pseudogout Syndrome". Ann. intern. Med. **56**, 738 (1962).

Lagier, R.: Les manifestations anatomiques de la chondrocalcinose; comparaison avec celles de la goutte. Communication à l'Association libre des pathologistes suisses. Berne 1964 (to be published).

Sèze, S. de, A. Hubault, J. Welfling, M. F. Kahn, et J. Solnica: Les arthropathies des hémochromatoses. Hémochromatose et „chondrocalcinose" articulaire. Leur place dans le cadre des arthropathies métaboliques. Rev. Rhum. **31**, 479 (1964).

Valsik, J., D. Zitnan, and S. Sitaj: Chondrocalcinosis articularis. Section II. Genetic study. Ann. rheum. Dis. **22**, 153 (1963).

Vix, V. A.: Articular and fibrocartilage calcification in hyperparathyroidism: Associated hyperuricemia. Radiology **83**, 468 (1964).

Infrastructural and Crystallographic Study of Experimental Calcifications

A. Policard, C. A. Baud, A. Collet, H. Daniel-Moussard, J. C. Martin

Centre d'Etudes et Recherches des Charbonnages de France, Verneuil-en-Halatte, Oise, France; Institut de Morphologie, Ecole de Médecine, Genève, Suisse

Electron microscopic examinations of experimentally produced calcified deposits led the authors to investigate the nature of the substances deposited both within and outside the cells and to observe the changes induced by different sampling techniques.

Materials and methods

Nephrocalcinosis was produced in rats (Wistar or Long Evans) according to FOURMAN (1959) by daily intraperitoneal injections for 6 to 8 days of 1.5 ml of a 10 per cent solution of calcium gluconate. The animals were killed directly after the last injection or 10 days or so later; the deposits did not appear to be different in either case. Fragments taken from the kidneys were fixed in 1% osmium tetroxide mixture according to SJÖSTRAND and embedded in methacrylate or Epon. At the same time control examinations were made using the light microscope in particular after staining according to VON KOSSA and microincineration.

In another experiment, surgical fibrin sponges impregnated with calcium gluconate were introduced into the peritoneal cavity of Wistar rats. After 5 days fragments were taken as above for light and electron microscopic examination.

Crystallographic examinations were made by electron diffraction (Trüb-Taüber diffractograph and Siemens Elmiskop electron microscope), using thin sections prepared as for the electron microscope. Residues from organs prepared by the method of GABRIEL (1894) were also analysed by X-ray diffraction.

Results

1. Renal deposits

In the kidneys two kinds of deposits are observed. Some, mostly intracellular, of small extent, consist of clusters of needle-shaped crystals 170 Å long and 70 Å wide. They are very similar to the apatite crystals of bone. Others, in large number, appear as very fine granular masses of about 50 Å diameter. They are extracellular and generally found within the basement membrane of the proximal convoluted tubules, which is thickened and modified. The grains are often arranged in concentric layers, like LIESEGANG rings. In exceptional cases small clusters of needle-shaped deposits are found among them. A detailed description was previously reported (POLICARD *et al.*, 1960, 1961).

Occasionally small, dense granulations are seen in mitochondria near the basement membrane. They are similar to those already described in the mature osteocyte (BAUD and DUPONT, 1965).

Electron diffraction studies of selected areas of the intracytoplasmic needle-shaped deposits show patterns consistent with apatite (d = 3.41, 3.09, 2.79, 2.60, 2.26, 1.92, 1.81, 1.71, 1.44, 1.245, 1.160).

The total calcareous residue of the kidney prepared by the method of GABRIEL should correspond to the granular deposits which are by far in the majority. With X-ray diffraction, a pattern similar to that of whitlockite or β tricalcium phosphate is obtained. It may be, however, that the residue was modified by the method of preparation used. Extensive areas in ultrathin sections give an electron diffraction pattern with 10 equidistances (d = 4.05, 3.63, 2.92, 2.43, 2.34, 2.19, 2.04, 1.72, 1.54, 1.49); some of them might correspond to whitlockite.

2. The granulome surrounding the sponges

A direct electron microscopic examination of the granulome shows numerous needle-shaped deposits similar to the intracytoplasmic deposits of the kidneys. The needles, often arranged in small clusters, are found in the residues of the sponge or in cells, often polymorphonuclear leukocytes. The clusters of needle-shaped crystals are separated from the cytoplasm by a vacuole limited by a single cytomembrane.

The ultrathin sections of the material embedded in methacrylate give an electron diffraction pattern which is to be interpreted as a mixture of hydrated acid calcium

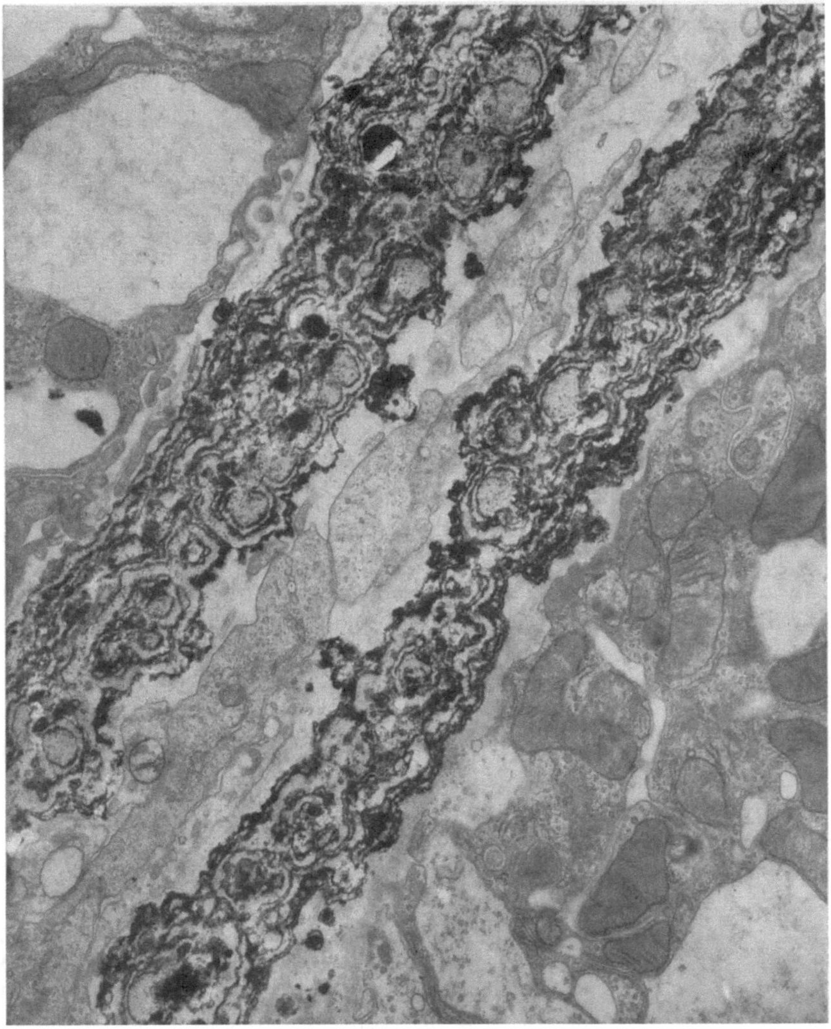

Fig. 1. Periodic extra-cellular deposit in the basal area of two proximal convoluted tubules. After 10 daily calcium gluconate injections and 15 days without injections

orthophosphate or brushite and hydrated calcium metaphosphate (d = 4.26, 4.10, 3.68, 2.96, 2.93, 2.48, 2.45, 2.37, 2.19, 2.08, 1.87).

By extraction with boiling glycerine and potassium hydroxide according to GABRIEL, a mineral fraction is obtained which diffracts X-rays like apatite. There is no disagreement with the result from electron diffraction, since synthetic brushite treated according to GABRIEL is transformed into apatite which can be identified by X-ray diffraction.

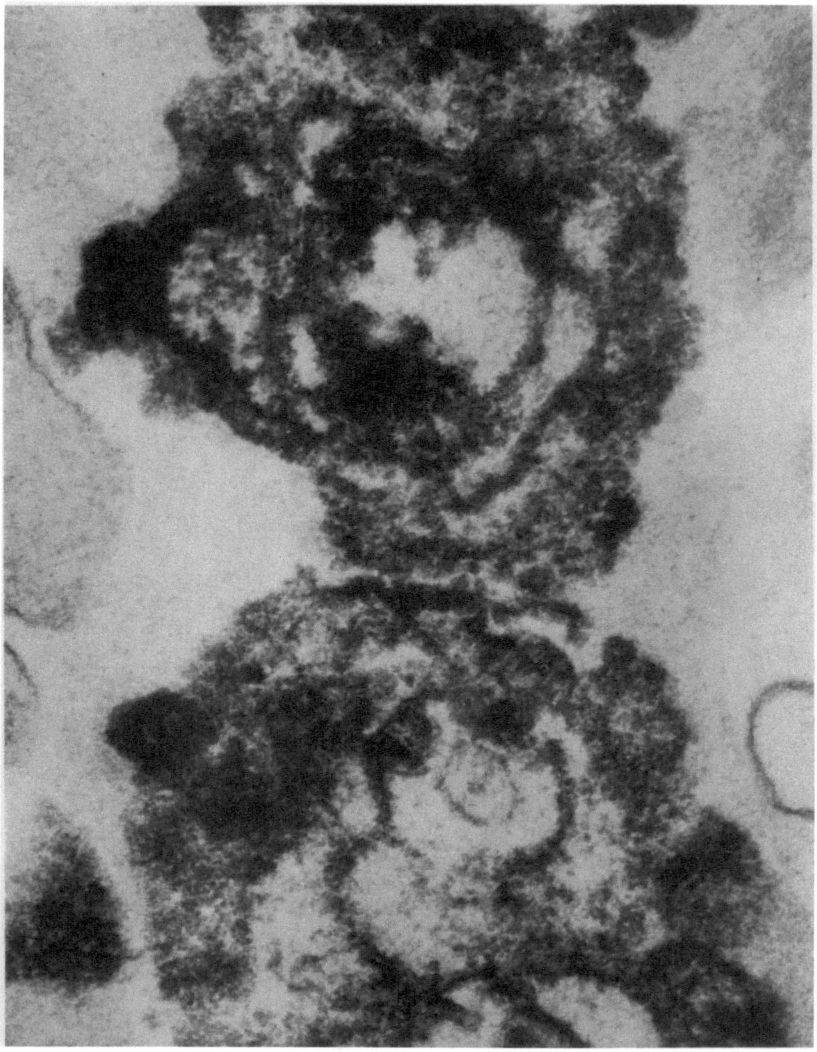

Fig. 2. High magnification of a periodic granular deposit in the basal area of a proximal convoluted tubule. After 9 daily calcium gluconate injections

Discussion

The morphological arrangement of calcium salt depositions varies to a great extent according to their crystallographic form. Various explanations are given concerning the conditions governing the different forms of crystallisation: local pH value, presence of mucopolysaccharides, function of a particular segment of the nephron in the case of the kidney. It will be noted that in the kidney at least, the needle-shaped appearance is clearly observed in the cytoplasm, while the other deposits are extracellular and preferably in the basement membrane which is rich in mucopolysaccharides.

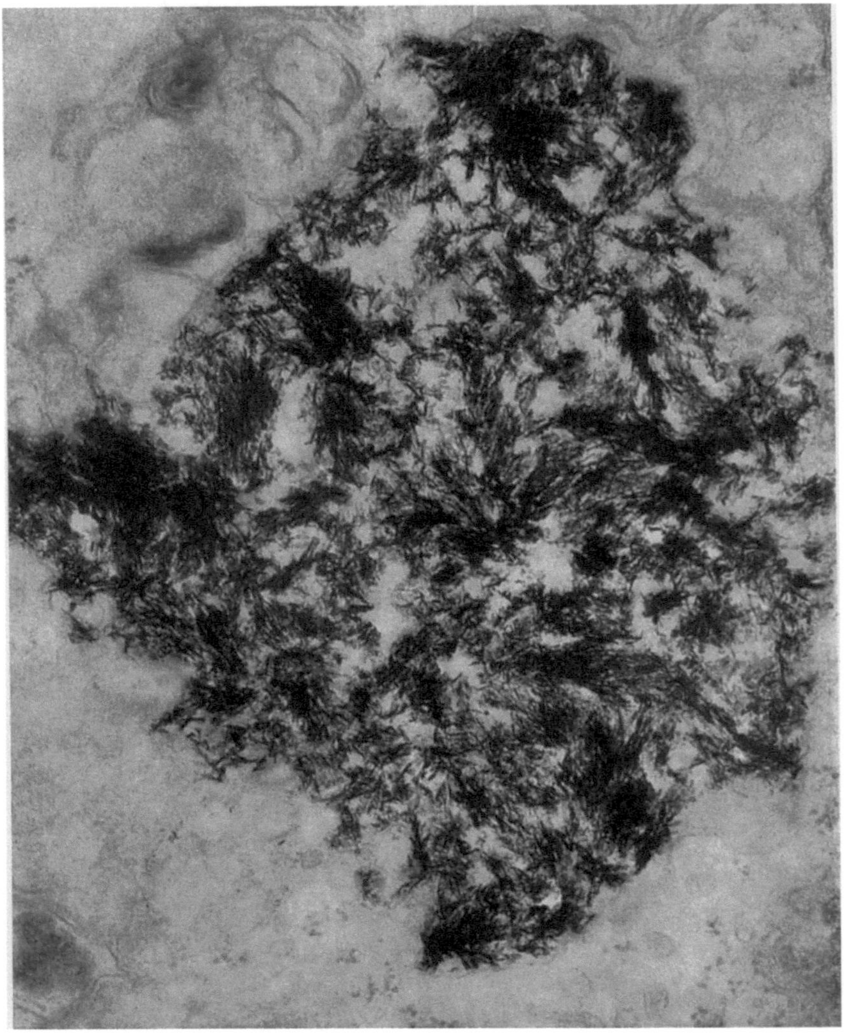

Fig. 3. Needle-shaped intracytoplasmic deposit in a cell of a proximal convoluted tubule. After 9 daily calcium gluconate injections

With the exception of vacuoles around intracellular deposits, which we did not observe, our electron microscopic results are in agreement with those of GIACOMELLI *et al.* (1964) who induced a D hypervitaminosis in rats. In addition, they obtained an electron diffraction pattern of granular deposits which might be interpreted as the pattern of a mixture of apatite and another crystalline phase.

Injecting mice with parathormone CAULFIELD and SCHRAG (1964) obtained numerous needle-shaped intracellular deposits diffracting electrons like apatite.

Granular rosette-like deposits are observed in mitochondria in an early stage. On the other hand, injections of calcium gluconate produce granular deposits arranged in concentric lamellae, located in the basement membrane of the proximal convoluted tubule. They do not diffract the electrons and are ascribed to calcium carbonate and related to the activity of the carbonic anhydrase.

Renal deposits of apatite were observed by GERSHOFF and ANDRUS (1961) in rats fed with a diet rich in calcium and poor in magnesium.

Human extracellular deposits diffracting electrons but giving no interpretable pattern were also observed by GALLE (1962). DEVIK's experiments (1962) provide precise information on the periodic precipitation of calcium phosphates to explain the mechanism of formation of LIESEGANG rings in extracellular deposits.

According to HOWELL *et al.* (1961), the presence of cells, connective tissue fibers and fundamental substance is necessary to induce the deposit of mineral matter around sponges. An enzymatic reaction or other local factors are possibly induced by such elements. Polyvinyl sponges produce a strong reaction which is weakened by a preliminary treatment of the sponges with silicones; sponges of cellulose acetate give a moderate reaction while polyurethane sponges give a negative one.

Acknowledgement

Acknowledgement is made of the assistance given by MISS S. PREGERMAIN, Mrs. NORMAND-REUET, Mr. C. ALEXANIAN for electron diffraction and by Mr. P. HENOC (C.N.E.T. Issy-les-Moulineaux) and Miss S. DURIF for X-ray diffraction.

References

BAUD, C. A., et D. H. DUPONT: La structure submicroscopique des ostéocytes en rapport avec leur fonction. In Calcified Tissues. RICHELLE, L. J., and M. J. DALLEMAGNE (eds.). Liège: Université de Liège 1965, p. 31.

CAULFIELD, J. B., and P. E. SCHRAG: Electron microscopic study and renal calcification. Amer. J. Path. **44**, 365 (1964).

DEVIK, O.: Formation of calcium phosphate studied with Liesegang's Rings. III. Mechanism of ring formation. Kolloid-Z. **181**, 33 (1962).

FOURMAN, J.: Two distinct forms of experimental nephrocalcinosis in the rat. Brit. J. exp. Path. **40**, 464 (1959).

GABRIEL, S.: Chemische Untersuchungen über die Mineralstoffe der Knochen und Zähne. Hoppe-Seylers Z. physiol. Chem. **18**, 257 (1894).

GALLE, P.: Mise en évidence au microscope électronique d'éléments cristallins dans les membranes basales de reins humains pathologiques. Rev. franç. Étud. clin. biol. **7**, 1084 (1962).

GERSHOFF, S. N., and S. B. ANDRUS: Dietary magnesium, calcium and Vitamin B_6 and experimental nephropathies in rats: calcium oxalate calculi, apatite nephrocalcinosis. J. Nutr. **73**, 308 (1961).

GIACOMELLI, F., D. SPIRO, and J. WIENER: A study of metastatic renal calcification at the cellular level. J. Cell Biol. **22**, 189 (1964).

HOWELL, D. S., E. E. DELCHAMPS, and W. RIEMER: Spontaneous mineral deposition in sponge biopsy connective tissue. Proc. Soc. exp. Biol. **106**, 317 (1961).

POLICARD, A., C. A. BAUD, A. COLLET, H. DANIEL-MOUSSARD, et J. C. MARTIN: Etude par microscopie électronique et diffraction des rayons X de divers dépôts calcaires expérimentaux. C. R. Soc. Biol. **155**, 1763 (1961).

—, A. COLLET, H. DANIEL-MOUSSARD, et S. PREGERMAIN: Sur la néphrocalcinome — Recherchez expérimentales au microscope electronique. Presse méd. **68**, 1735 (1960).

Protein Phosphorus and Phosphokinases in Connective Tissue

S. M. KRANE, M. J. GLIMCHER

Departments of Medicine and Orthopedic Surgery, Harvard Medical School,
Massachusetts General Hospital, Boston, Mass., U. S. A.

We have previously discussed the evidence which suggested that interactions betweeen phosphorus and groups on the side chains of the structural proteins of mineralized tissues played a major role in the nucleation of apatite crystals. (GLIMCHER and KRANE, 1962). It was shown that purified, reconstituted collagen fibrils, incubated *in vitro* with inorganic orthophosphate, bound as many as 150—170 moles of phosphorus per mole collagen (GLIMCHER and KRANE, 1964 a). Furthermore the interaction between collagen and phosphate was found to encompass a wide spectrum of bond types from readily dissociable, electrostatic bonds to covalent bonds. Covalently bound phosphorus would be ideally suited for a role in the nucleation process, since such groups would be fixed at specific sites on the molecule as well as have relatively fixed distance, direction and orientation, and still be reactive. Subsequently we were able to demonstrate that ^{32}P-orthophosphate administered to rabbits and guinea pigs *in vivo*, was found associated with both the neutral and acid soluble collagens of skin and healing wounds (GLIMCHER *et al.*, 1964). Furthermore organic phosphorus was detected chemically, in varying amounts in different species, in soft-tissue collagens and gelatins derived from collagens. In addition the single-stranded α chains of several of these gelatins were purified by chromatography on carboxymethyl-cellulose resin columns and shown still to contain the organic phosphorus, with the higher concentration in the α_2 compared to the α_1 chains. C. J. FRANCOIS (personal communication) has recently found organic phosphorus in purified α gelatin chains from chicken bone. VEIS and SCHLUETER (1964) and SCHLUETER and VEIS (1964) have also reported the presence of organic phosphorus in fragments produced by periodate treatment of bovine dentin. We observed that after digestion of the collagens and gelatins with bacterial collagenase and partial acid hydrolysis followed by various chromatographic and electrophoretic procedures, that the organic phosphorus was present in several peptide fractions rich in glycine and serine and containing relatively large amounts of sugar. However, in all but one of these fractions more phosphorus was present than could be accounted for by the content of serine and threonine alone. In addition, the phosphorus linkage was more stable to alkali than is usually found for peptide-bound phosphoserine. It was, therefore, suggested that at least part of the organic phosphorus in collagens was bound to a carbohydrate moiety.

Since tooth enamel is the most highly mineralized of all the calcified tissues in vertebrates, phosphorus analyses were performed on the decalcified, soluble organic matrix proteins of both fetal and adult bovine enamel (GLIMCHER and KRANE, 1964 b). These proteins contained large amounts of organic phosphorus, some fractions as many as 90 residues per 1000 amino acid residues. After partial acid hydrolysis it was possible to identify O-phosphoserine and O-phosphoserine-containing peptides. More recently we have demonstrated the presence of organic phosphorus in the proteins of newly formed enamel from the incisor teeth of adult rabbits and rats.

Although the peptide fractions of dental enamel which we obtained after partial acid hydrolysis, column chromatography and electrophoresis may not have been homogeneous, it is of interest to compare their amino acid compositions to the phosphorus-containing peptides from collagens and phosphopeptides derived from other proteins (Table 1). The similarity of the amino acid composition of these fractions of different proteins is indeed intriguing.

Table 1. *Predominant amino acids of phosphorus-containing peptides of various phosphoproteins*

Source	Amino Acids	Reference
Enamel proteins (calf embryo)	*Ser*, Asp, Glu, Gly, Leu	GLIMCHER and KRANE, 1964 b.
Gelatin (guinea pig skin)	Ser, Asp, Glu, *Gly*, Ala	GLIMCHER *et al.*, 1964
Fibrinogen (human)	Ser, Asp, Glu, *Gly*, Ala, Leu	BLOMBACK *et al.*, 1963
Ovalbumin	Ser, Asp, Glu, Ileu, Ala	FLAVIN, 1954
Ovalbumin	Ser, Asp, Glu, Leu, Ala, Val	PERLMANN, 1952
Casein (human)	Ser, Glu, Thr, Ileu	MELLANDER, 1963

When it was shown that the enamel matrix proteins contained phosphoserine, we considered the possible pathways of synthesis of the protein-phosphorus linkages. BURNETT and KENNEDY (1954) had demonstrated the presence of enzymatic activity in liver mitochondria which catalyzed the transfer of the terminal phosphoryl from ATP to protein-bound serine of casein. RABINOWITZ and LIPMANN (1960) purified protein phosphokinases from yeast and calf brain and further characterized the reaction. These protein phosphokinases catalyze the phosphorylation of protein or polypeptide-bound serine but not of the free amino acid. The observations of SANGER and HOCQUARD (1962) using hen oviduct as an ovalbumin-synthesizing system are also consistent with the concept that phosphorylation of the serine residues of phosphoproteins occurs after incorporation of serine into the polypeptide chain.

We, therefore, have assayed several connective tissues for protein phosphokinase activity. Enzymatic activity which catalyzed the phosphorylation of casein and partially dephosphorylated phosvitin was found in all of the tissues examined including bone, cartilage, skin, tendon, muscle and enamel organ (KRANE *et al.*, 1965). It was possible to purify the enzymatic activity from acetone powders of several of these tissues approximately 45-fold by ammonium sulfate fractionation, Sephadex and DEAE resin column chromatography. These enzymes, as well as one purified from hog kidney by similar procedures, catalyzed the transfer of the terminal phosphoryl from ATP to enamel matrix protein, whereas the enzyme purified from brewers' yeast was inactive towards this substrate. The reaction was measured using the transfer of label from ATP-$\gamma^{32}P$. At the end of the reaction, 90% of the ^{32}P which was transferred to the protein was released as inorganic orthophosphate in 1 N NaOH, 100° for 1 hour whereas only 5% of the ^{32}P was liberated in 1 N HCl, 100° for 10 minutes. The alkali lability and acid stability are characteristic of polypeptide-bound phosphoserine. Furthermore, ^{32}P-labeled phosphoserine was identified in partial acid hydrolysates.

More recently we have tested this reaction using collagens and gelatins purified from several sources as substrates in the phosphokinase reaction. The results of representative experiments are shown in Tab. 2. In these experiments, the reaction was stopped by heating at 65 °C for 15 minutes and the reaction mixture transferred to a 30×2 cm column of Sephadex G-25 equilibrated with a pyridine-acetic acid buffer, pH 4.4, and eluted with the same buffer. The fractions containing the protein were pooled and the protein precipitated by the addition of trichloroacetic acid to a final concentration of 13%. The protein was collected by centrifugation, dissolved in water and reprecipitated twice with trichloroacetic acid. It is seen that small amounts of ^{32}P were transferred to the protein in the presence of protein phosphokinase. Since the amounts transferred are small the labeled site has not yet been identified. It is also not certain whether the phosphoryl group is transferred to previously unphosphorylated residues or if an exchange reaction between ATP and protein-bound phosphorus occurs.

Table 2. *Gelatins as phosphoryl acceptors in protein phosphokinase reaction*

Experiment	Sample	P transferred mμ moles
I	KCNS bone gelatin (10 mg)	
	1. Complete	0.809
	2. No enzyme	0.062
	3. No gelatin	0.092
II	Bone gelatin, α_2 (3 mg)	
	1. Complete	0.0060
	2. No enzyme	0.0039
III	Rat tail tendon gelatin (2 mg)	
	1. Complete	0.024
	2. No enzyme	0.003
	3. No gelatin	0.008

Incubation: 37°, pH 8.0, 30 min.

The enzymes used in these experiments were different preparations from hog kidney and contained variable amounts of acceptor protein activity. Therefore each experiment must be considered in relation to the control values obtained.

The data reported here further support our hypothesis that matrix-bound organic phosphorus plays an important role in the initial phases of the calcification process.

Acknowledgments

Supported by research grants of the USPHS, N.I.H. (AM-3564, AM-06375). The John A. Hartford Foundation, Inc., the Easter Seal Research Foundation and the USAEC (AT(30-1)2183). This is publication number 387 of the Robert W. Lovett Memorial for the Study of Diseases Causing Deformities. S. M. K. is an Established Investigator of the Helen Hay Whitney Foundation.

References

BLOMBÄCK, B., M. BLOMBÄCK, R. F. DOOLITTLE, B. HESSEL, and P. EDMAN: On the properties of a new human fibrinopeptide. Biochim. biophys. Acta **78**, 563 (1963).

BURNETT, G., and E. P. KENNEDY: The enzymatic phosphorylation of proteins. J. biol. Chem. **211**, 969 (1954).

FLAVIN, M.: The linkage of phosphate to protein in pepsin and ovalbumin. J. biol. Chem. **210**, 771 (1954).

Glimcher, M. J., C. J. Francois, L. Richards, and S. M. Krane: The presence of organic phosphorus in collagens and gelatins. Biochim. biophys. Acta **93**, 585 (1964).
—, and S. M. Krane: Studies of the interactions of collagen and phosphate. In Radioisotopes and Bone. Lacroix, P., and A. M. Budy (eds.). Oxford: Blackwell Scientific Publications 1962, p. 393.
— — The incorporation of radioactive inorganic orthophosphate as organic phosphate by collagen fibrils *in vitro*. Biochemistry **3**, 195 (1964 a).
— — The identification of serine phosphate in enamel proteins. Biochim. biophys. Acta **90**, 477 (1964 b).
Krane, S. M., M. J. Stone, and M. J. Glimcher: The presence of protein phosphokinase in connective tissues and the phosphorylation of enamel proteins *in vitro*. Biochim. biophys. Acta **97**, 77 (1965).
Mellander, O.: Phosphopeptides: Chemical properties and their possible role in the intestinal absorption of metals. In The Transfer of Calcium and Strontium Across Biological Membranes. Wasserman, R. H. (ed.). New York: Academic Press 1963, p. 265.
Perlmann, G. E.: Enzymatic dephosphorylation of phosphoproteins and the nature of phosphorus linkages. In Phosphorus Metabolism, Vol. II. McElroy, W. D., and B. Glass (eds.). Baltimore: The Johns Hopkins Press 1952, p. 167.
Rabinowitz, M., and F. Lipmann: Reversible phosphate transfer between yolk phosphoprotein and adenosine triphosphate. J. biol. Chem. **235**, 1043 (1960).
Sanger, F., and E. Hocquard: Formation of dephospho-ovalbumin as an intermediate in the biosynthesis of ovalbumin. Biochim. biophys. Acta **62**, 606 (1962).
Schlueter, R. J., and A. Veis: The macromolecular organization of dentine matrix collagen. II. Periodate degradation and carbohydrate crosslinking. Biochemistry **3**, 1657 (1964).
Veis, A., and R. J. Schlueter: The macromolecular organization of dentine matrix collagen. I. Characterization of dentine collagen. Biochemistry **3**, 1650 (1964).

The Relationship between Swelling of Hard Tissue Collagen in Acid and Alkali and the Presence of Phosphate Cross-links

W. M. McKernan, S. D. Dailly

Research and Development Department, Gelatine Division, British Glues and Chemicals Ltd., London, England

While the swelling characteristics of soft tissue collagens have been extensively studied (Bowes and Kenten, 1950 a, b) only recently has attention been directed to similar studies of hard collagenous tissue. This latter work has arisen from the observation that the solubility of dentine collagen is very much less than that of corium collagen and this has been attributed to differences in the type or extent of intermolecular stabilisation in these two materials (Veis and Schlueter, 1963). More recently (Veis and Schlueter, 1964; Schlueter and Veis, 1964) it has been proposed that specific phosphate diester bonds are involved in cross-linking dentine collagen and that these esters are attached to the polypeptide chains through serine.

Bovine bone collagen is, in many respects, similar to dentine collagen particularly with regard to its physical organisation and the difficulty with which soluble components can be extracted. Comparative chemical analyses show, however, that purified bone collagen has a very much lower phosphorus content than dentine collagen and it was, therefore, of interest to determine whether bone collagen follows a similar pH-swelling relationship to dentine collagen and, if so, whether the intermolecular stability could be attributable to similar phosphate diester covalent cross-links.

Experimental

Raw material

The inside portion of dehaired, defleshed bovine hide was intensively washed in distilled water to remove all traces of lime salts and was blotted dry.

Bovine bone collagen was isolated from fresh cattle bones which were thoroughly degreased with water (Chayen and Ashworth, 1953) and the mineral matter removed by extensive demineralisation in N hydrochloric acid with several changes of acid. This treatment was continued until a constant value of phosphorus content was obtained for the bone collagen. Residual acid was removed by thorough washing and the collagen was blotted dry.

Swelling curves

Swelling curves were determined over a relatively short time period at pH 2.3 (the maximum acid swelling pH for corium collagen) and at pH approx. 14.0. Bowes and Kenten (1950 a) have shown that the swelling of collagen in sodium hydroxide solution increases progressively with increase in pH and shows no pH maximum corresponding to that occurring in acid solution.

10 g. samples of the purified collagens were suspended in 50 ml. 1.0 N sodium hydroxide or hydrochloric acid solution (pH 2.3) for varying periods of time up to 24 hours at room temperature. At various intervals samples were removed and weighed. In all experiments swelling was taken as the amount of solution retained expressed as a percentage of the weight of the original collagen.

Phosphorus

After determination of the swelling factor the collagen was washed and dried overnight at 105 °C and a known weight ashed at 550 °C. Phosphorus was determined as the molybdovanado-phosphate complex using a slight modification of the method of Michelson (1957). Potassium dihydrogen phosphate was used for the determination of the calibration curve.

Results and discussion

The effects of time on the swelling of collagen in solutions of sodium hydroxide and hydrochloric acid are shown in Fig. 1 and Fig. 2 for bone collagen and corium collagen respectively. In the series of experiments carried out in acid solution the curves obtained for purified bone collagen are similar to those described by Veis and Schlueter (1964) for dentine collagen and confirm the lack of swelling properties of this type of hard tissue. Extension of the swelling time from 24 hours to several days did not result in any increase in the swelling factor.

In contrast, in alkali, bone collagen behaves similarly to corium collagen, exhibiting a rapid uptake of solution during the 24 hour period. Extension of the swelling period beyond this time leads to rapid disintegration of the collagen.

A series of experiments was also carried out whereby purified bone collagen was removed from alkali after a swelling period of 9 hours, thoroughly washed and re-suspended in hydrochloric acid at pH 2.3. Further swelling investigations were carried out at this pH as shown in Fig. 1. No further increase in swelling was observed although the phosphorus content of the bone collagen had been reduced by approximately 80% during the 9 hour alkaline treatment (Fig. 3). The series of experiments carried out in acid solution showed no reduction in phosphorus content over the period of swelling investigated whereas the alkaline series exhibited a dramatic reduction in phosphorus as swelling progressed.

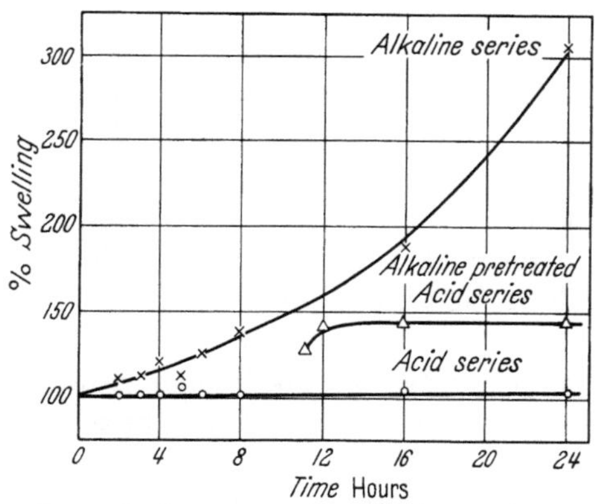

Fig. 1. Swelling curves of purified bone collagens: x, experiments carried out in 1.0 N NaOH; o, experiments in HCl, pH 2.3; Δ, collagens swollen for 9 hours, in 1.0 N NaOH, washed and replaced in HCl, pH 2.3

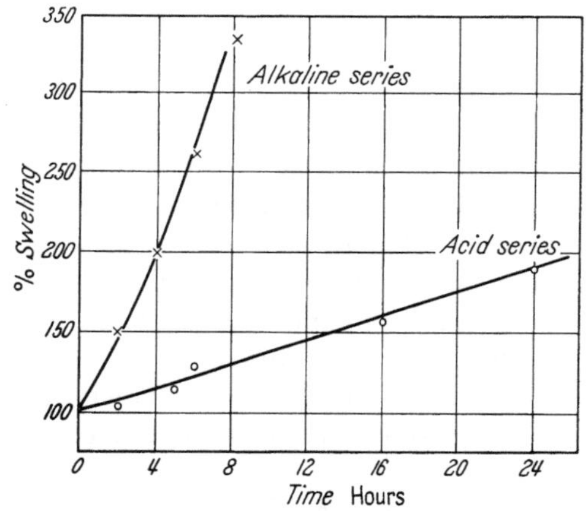

Fig. 2. Swelling curves of purified corium collagens: x, experiments carried out in 1.0 N NaOH; o, experiments in HCl, pH 2.3

The resistance of bone collagen to swelling in acid solution and the comparative ease of swelling in alkali is consistent with the presence of inter-molecular cross-linkages as proposed for dentine collagen. The relatively small content of phosphorus present in bone collagen would not, however provide sufficient phosphate ester linkages to confer on this material the demonstrated stability in acid solution. The phosphorus content noted here is equivalent to only 0.006 per cent of phosphate residues (HPO_3) by weight. In contrast, dentine collagen has been shown to contain 0.4% HPO_3 on a similar basis. This contention is supported by the series of experiments whereby the phosphorus content of bone collagen was reduced by alkali pretreatment and subsequent acid treatment provided no increase in swelling. The presence of a few phosphate-mediated cross-links in bone collagen is suggested by the release of phosphorus during swelling in alkaline solution. The acid stability must, however, be attributed to the presence of alternative cross-links which exhibit similar lability in alkali. SCHLUETER and VEIS (1964) have discussed the types of cross-links common to dentine and corium collagens and suggest that dentine contains in addition to phosphate cross-links "extra" cross linkage sites which are not present in corium collagens. This view is consistent with our findings on bone collagen and

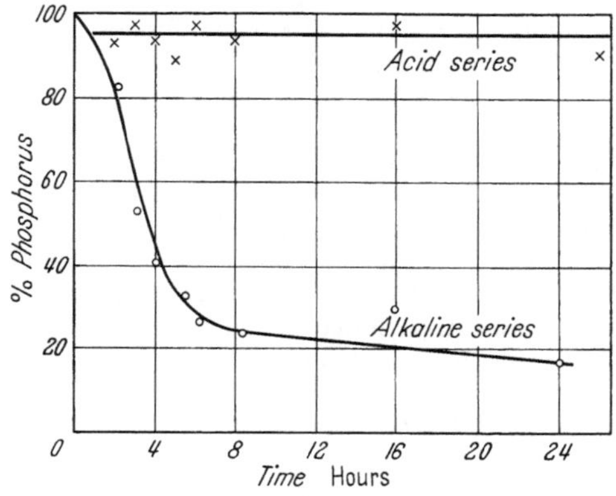

Fig. 3. Phosphorus release during swelling of purified bone collagen in acid, pH 2.3 (x) and alkali, 1.0 N NaOH (o)

would suggest that the "extra" cross-links are responsible for the structural acid stability of both bone and dentine collagens. The nature of these cross-links has yet to be elucidated but current information on the role of hexoses in cross-linking collagen and their stability to oxidation suggest that such structures are likely to be involved.

Summary

1. The swelling behaviour of purified bone collagen and corium collagen has been investigated under both acid and alkaline conditions.

2. In alkali both collagens show progressive swelling increases with time and, in the case of bone collagen, there is a simultaneous release of phosphorus. In acid solution no release of phosphorus was observed for bone collagen and no swelling occurred. In contrast, corium collagen swelled by a factor of approximately 700% under the same conditions.

3. The results are consistent with the presence of acid-stable, alkali-labile cross-links in bone collagen but not to the participation of phosphate cross-links in the acid stability.

4. The presence of additional, unidentified, cross-links which may well be common to both dentine and bone collagens is proposed.

Acknowledgments

The authors wish to express their gratitude to the Directors of British Glues and Chemicals Ltd. for permission to publish this paper.

References

Bowes, J. H., and R. H. Kenten: The swelling of collagen in alkaline solutions. I. Swelling in solutions of sodium hydroxide. Biochem. J. **46**, 1 (1950 a).

— — The swelling of collagen in alkaline solutions. II. Swelling in solutions of univalent bases. Biochem. J. **46**, 524 (1950 b).

Chayen, I. H., and D. R. Ashworth: The application of impulse rendering to the animal-fat industry. J. appl. Chem. **3**, 529 (1953).

Michelson, O. B.: The determination of small concentrations of phosphate by ultraviolet spectrophotometry. Analyt. Chem. **1**, 60 (1957).

Schlueter, R. J., and A. Veis: The macromolecular organisation of dentine matrix collagen. II. Periodate degradation and carbohydrate cross-linking. Biochemistry **3**, 1657 (1964).

Veis, A., and R. J. Schlueter: Presence of phosphate-mediated cross-linkages in hard tissue collagens. Nature (Lond.) **197**, 1204 (1963).

— — The macromolecular organisation of dentine matrix collagen. I. Characterisation of dentine collagen. Biochemistry **3**, 1650 (1964).

Microradiographic and Histological Observations in Primary Vitamin D-resistant Rickets

R. STEENDIJK, J. JOWSEY, A. VAN DEN HOOFF, H. K. L. NIELSEN

Departments of Paediatrics and Orthopaedic Surgery and Histological Laboratory, University of Amsterdam, The Netherlands;
Section of Surgical Research, Mayo Clinic, Rochester, Minn., U. S. A.

Impaired mineralisation of bone in primary vitamin D-resistant rickets (familial or essential hypophosphataemia) is not limited to the presence of wide osteoid bands covering the trabeculae of spongious bone or lining the central canals of growing osteones. There also is a conspicuous lack of mineral around many osteocyte lacunae and their canaliculi as shown by microradiography of undecalcified bone (ENGFELDT *et al.*, 1956; JOWSEY, 1964). Ordinary histological examination of decalcified bone has hitherto failed to demonstrate any abnormality in the organic matrix at these sites. No exhaustive studies have yet been published and a more detailed investigation into the structural and histochemical characteristics of the perilacunar matrix was, therefore, indicated.

Material and methods

Diaphyseal bone from the fibulae of 2 young adult patients with vitamin D-resistant rickets was removed in the course of orthopaedic procedures. Appropriate pieces were fixed in 70% ethanol for subsequent embedding in methyl-methacrylate and microradiography. Similar pieces were fixed in 10% formalin, or in a mixture of formalin, mercuric chloride and picric acid for subsequent decalcification in EDTA or in nitric-picric acid and embedding in paraffin. From the latter material 6 μ sections were cut and treated with various histological stains (see "Results"). Some of the EDTA-decalcified material was cut in the frozen state at 20 μ and used unstained for phase-contrast microscopy, or stained with a modified Schmorl-method (0.01% azure II in water at pH 9.0, followed by 20 ml saturated picric acid in 200 ml of water). Sections from the same blocks were treated with Bodian's silver stain.

Results

The pattern of uptake of the azure II-picric acid stain in decalcified bone from the rachitic patients appeared disturbed in a specific way. In addition to its normal distribution along the walls of the lacunae and canaliculi, the stain was concentrated in the vicinity of many osteocyte lacunae, i. e. at the sites where microradiographs of undecalcified sections revealed a subnormal degree of mineralisation. The localisation was not strictly perilacunar, but rather extending from the lacunae toward the center of the osteone, along the centripetal canaliculi (Fig. 1). Careful inspection of the microradiographs disclosed that the lack of bone mineral was also predominant on that side of the lacunae (Fig. 2). At high magnifications of the stained sections, it appeared that neither lacunae nor canaliculi were enlarged and that the matrix had taken up the stain in a globular fashion (Fig. 3). Similar pictures were obtained after Bodian's silver impregnation technique. By phase-contrast microscopy of 20 μ decalcified unstained sections, the abnormal pattern of the matrix was visible as a conglomeration of small globules, interrupting the normal lamellar architecture of the osteone (Fig. 4). Non-mineralised osteoid, at the inner aspects of growing Haversian systems, did not take up these stains and did not exhibit an abnormal pattern under phase-contrast. The van Gieson-, Mallory-, PAS-, and Sudan-black-

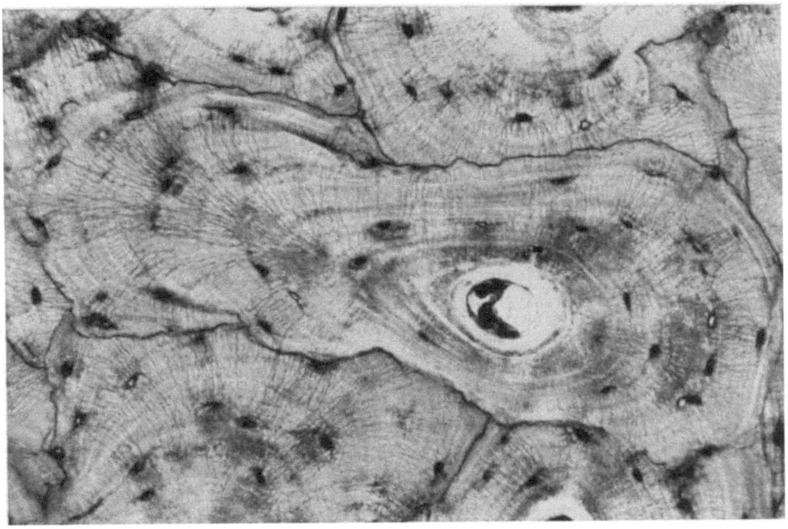

Fig. 1. Azure II — picric acid stained, 20 μ thick section from decalcified bone from the fibula of a 22-year-old man with primary vitamin D-resistant rickets (× 190)

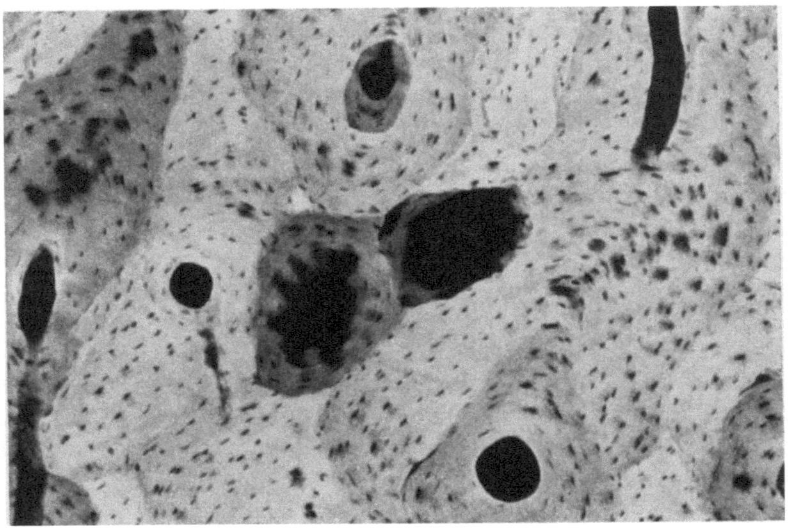

Fig. 2. Microradiograph from a 100 μ thick undecalcified cross-section from the same fibula as in Fig. 1. (× 100)

stains failed to reveal anything abnormal. A slight affinity for alcian blue at these sites was observed only very occasionally; with haematoxylin the perilacunar regions were discernible with difficulty and inconsistently by a slightly darker hue. Prior digestion of the sections with pepsin or trypsin did not interfere with the pattern as revealed by azure II; the acrolein-Schiff reaction for protein (VAN DUYN, 1961) failed to demonstrate the lesion.

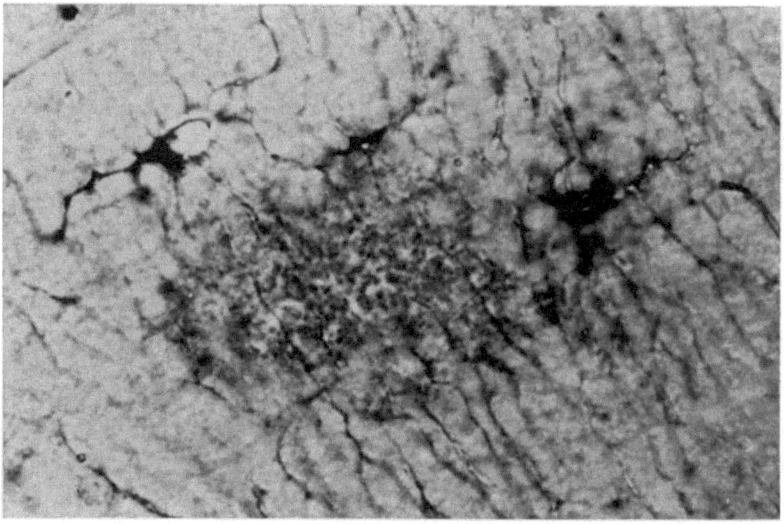

Fig. 3. Azure II — picric acid stained, 6 μ thick section from the same bone as in Fig. 1. (× 1200)

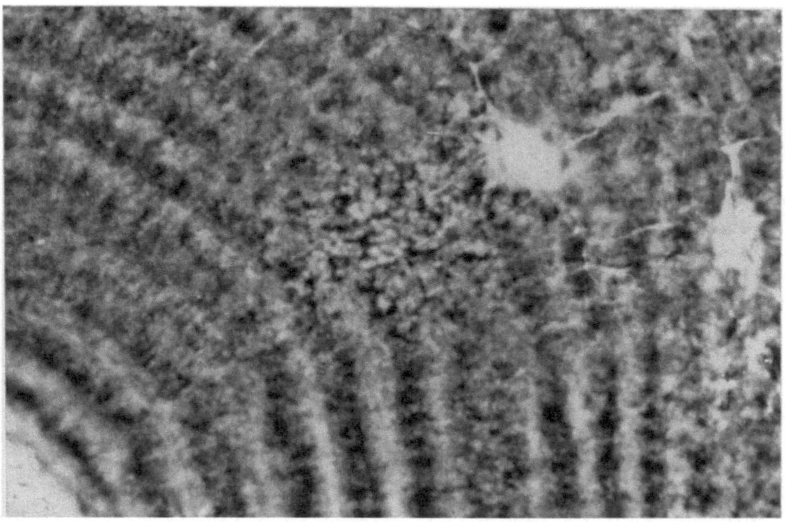

Fig. 4. Phase-contrast photomicrograph of an unstained, 20 μ thick section from the same bone as in Fig. 1. (× 1200)

Discussion

The findings described above favour the hypothesis that a structural change rather than a chemically defined abnormality of the matrix is responsible for the observed affinity for azure II. As far as the authors know, this particular type of lesion has not been described before. It may be of interest, however, that SHELDON and ROBINSON (1961), using the electron-microscope, found in osteoid from rachitic rats an abnormal, random orientation of the collagen fibrils surrounding osteocytes.

The causal relationship between the matrix lesion and the concurrent lack of bone mineral can only be speculated upon. As has been mentioned before (ENGFELDT *et al.*, 1956; JOWSEY *et al.*, 1964), it is not known whether the lack of mineral in the immediate vicinity of osteocytes is the result of a failure of mineralisation or of removal of mineral from calcified tissue. It is conceivable that a structural change of the matrix is involved in either of these processes.

Recently one of the authors pointed out that osteocytes probably are capable of controlling the composition of the adjacent tissue in terms of mineral and matrix (JOWSEY *et al.*, 1964). The peculiar localisation of the lesion — predominantly on one side of the lacunae — indicates that, at least under certain circumstances, the effect of this controlling capacity is not evenly distributed. The significance of this finding as regards osteocyte metabolism is not known at present.

Summary

By histological examination of decalcified bone from patients with vitamin D-resistant rickets it was found that the bone matrix in perilacunar regions, which were characterised by a subnormal degree of mineralisation, had an abnormal affinity for certain stains, in particular for azure II — picric acid. These findings are discussed. It is pointed out that the observed abnormality probably is structural rather than chemical in nature.

References

DUYN, P. VAN: Acrolein-Schiff, a new staining method for proteins. J. Histochem. Cytochem. 9, 234 (1961).

ENGFELDT, B., R. ZETTERSTRÖM, and J. WINBERG: Primary vitamin D-resistant rickets III; Biophysical studies of skeletal tissue. J. Bone Jt Surg. **38 A,** 1323 (1956).

JOWSEY, J.: Variations in bone mineralization with age and disease. In Bone Biodynamics. FROST, H. M. (ed.). Boston: Little, Brown 1964, p. 461.

—, B. L. RIGGS, and P. J. KELLY: Mineral metabolism in osteocytes. Proc. Mayo Clinic **39,** 480, (1964).

SHELDON, H., and R. A. ROBINSON: Studies in rickets I; The fine structure of uncalcified bone matrix in experimental rickets. Z. Zellforsch. **53,** 671 (1961).

Therapeutic Response and Effect on the Kidney of 100 Units Vitamin D Daily in Osteomalacia after Gastrectomy

D. B. MORGAN, C. R. PATERSON, C. G. WOODS, C. N. PULVERTAFT, P. FOURMAN

Departments of Chemical Pathology and Pathology, Leeds University Medical School; and the York County Hospital, England

The Peptic Ulcer Clinic in York follows 1443 persons who have had an operation for ulcer during the last 22 years. To establish the prevalence of osteomalacia after gastrectomy we have surveyed 1228 of these persons. Patients with osteomalacia were given a minute dose of vitamin D.

Of the patients surveyed, 6 had classical osteomalacia. The incidence of osteomalacia among patients with a Polya gastrectomy was 1 per cent for men and 3 per cent for women. There were 2 other patients not drawn from the survey with osteomalacia after gastrectomy. These 8 patients all had bone pain; 4 had LOOSER's nodes; all had a raised serum alkaline phosphatase activity; all had extensive osteoid seams in a bone biopsy.

Table 1 shows the prevalence of a raised alkaline phosphatase and of a low calcium concentration in the serum of 975 of the patients in the survey with the more common operations compared with 185 patients with peptic ulcer who did not have an operation. Many operated patients had a raised alkaline phosphatase but so did many unoperated patients. While this abnormality is more common in the operated patients, it is misleading to estimate the prevalence of osteomalacia after gastrectomy from the number of patients with a raised alkaline phosphatase (JONES *et al.*, 1962; CLARK *et al.*, 1964). A low serum calcium was more frequent in patients who had had an operation than in those who had not. A low plasma protein concentration accounted for about half of the low values for the serum calcium in the operated patients. The meaning of the low serum calcium in the remainder is not yet clear.

Table 1. *Prevalence of raised alkaline phosphatase and of low serum calcium concentration in the serum of 975 patients after gastric surgery and 185 patients with peptic ulcer who had not had an operation*

		No. pts	Serum alkaline phosphatase > 12 K. A. units per 100 ml.		Serum Calcium < 9.1 mg per 100 ml	
			No.	%	No.	%
Men	Peptic ulcer	128	8	6.3	7	5.4
	VGE or V. Ant'y	190	16	8.4	18	9.4
	Polya Gast'y	599	74	12.3	91	15.2
Women	Peptic ulcer	57	4	7.0	0	0
	VGE or V. Ant'y	67	7	10.4	5	7.4
	Polya Gast'y	119	18	15.1	15	12.6

VGE = Vagotomy and gastroenterostomy V. Ant'y = Vagotomy and antrectomy
Gast'y = Gastrectomy

103 operated patients had a bone biopsy. In the patients with a raised alkaline phosphatase or a low serum calcium who did not have bone pain the biopsies were seldom abnormal. There was an excess of osteoid in about one-sixth of these biopsies but the seams were narrow, with no more than three laminae, and they covered less than 30% of the trabecular surface. There was little cellular reaction. The biopsies of the patients with osteomalacia selected for this report had broad osteoid seams with 3—12 laminae; the seams covered the trabeculae completely. Osteoblasts covered part of the surface but there was remarkably little osteoclastic activity.

The final confirmation of a diagnosis of osteomalacia depends on the response to treatment with vitamin D. Simple deficiency of vitamin D should respond to small doses. In 7 patients we tried the effect of 130 units daily given as a weekly injection of 1,000 units. Three patients also had calcium 2 g daily. The bone pains disappeared within 3 to 12 weeks. Some Looser's nodes healed. Fig. 1 shows that the alkaline phosphatase in the serum, remarkably constant before treatment, nearly always changed greatly and significantly after treatment but the direction of the change varied. In 3 patients it fell to near normal after 3, $3^1/_2$ and 5 months. In 3 patients it rose, from 30 to 40, from 32 to 45 and from 42 to 90 K.A. units per 100 ml. In one patient it did not change at all. Changes in the serum calcium and phosphorus were small and inconsistent. Two patients had a second biopsy after 4 and 5 months of treatment. In one who had had calcium the broad osteoid seams had disappeared; in the other, who had not had calcium, they were beginning to calcify. It is clear that these patients had responded to 1,000 units weekly of vitamin D 2.

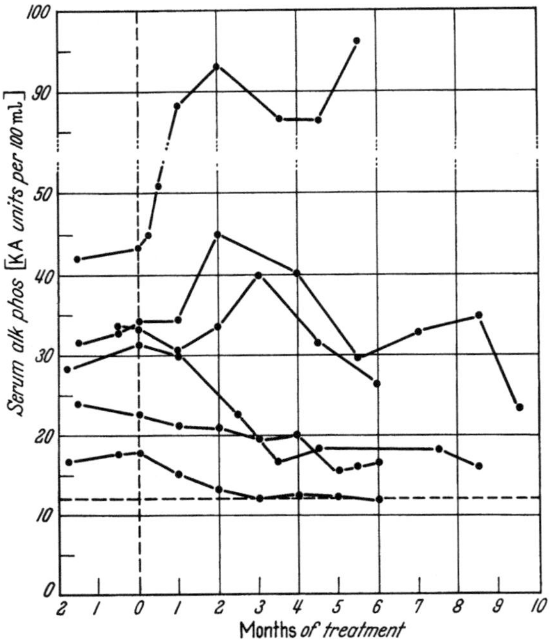

Fig. 1. Changes in serum alkaline phosphatase of 6 patients with osteomalacia treated with weekly injections of 1000 units vitamin D 2. In one patient the serum alkaline phosphatase did not change and these data have been omitted from the figure

We have studied in more detail the immediate response to vitamin D.

Dr. Ph. Bordier had suggested to us that a fall in the phosphate clearance is the most sensitive sign of response to vitamin D in patients with osteomalacia. Because it is difficult to measure the rate of urine excretion accurately, it is difficult to measure clearances accurately and we have therefore resorted to the use of the ratio phosphate clearance/creatinine clearance $\frac{C_p}{C_{cr}}$ which is independent of the urine volume.

It may be recalled that the $\frac{C_p}{C_{cr}}$ is related to the tubular reabsorption of phosphorus according to the formula $TRP = 1 - \frac{C_p}{C_{cr}}$ where TRP is the net proportion of phosphorus reabsorbed from the glomerular filtrate by the renal tubule. $\frac{C_p}{C_{cr}}$ is said to be high in osteomalacia (Nordin and Fraser, 1956), supposedly as a result of parathyroid compensation.

The $\frac{C_p}{C_{cr}}$ was measured in 3 of the patients with osteomalacia and in two patients without osteomalacia (Fig. 2). In two of the patients with osteomalacia it was more than 0.2 and it fell during the four days' treatment with vitamin D. In the third patient with osteomalacia and in the two without it was less than 0.2 and it did not fall. One of the patients who responded to 100 units of vitamin D daily had not responded to 50 units of vitamin D. Fig. 3 shows the relation between the changes in the $\frac{C_p}{C_{cr}}$ and the changes in the serum calcium and serum phosphorus in one patient with severe osteomalacia. When the $\frac{C_p}{C_{cr}}$ fell the serum calcium fell; the serum phosphorus hardly changed. We draw 3 conclusions from these and other studies we have made:

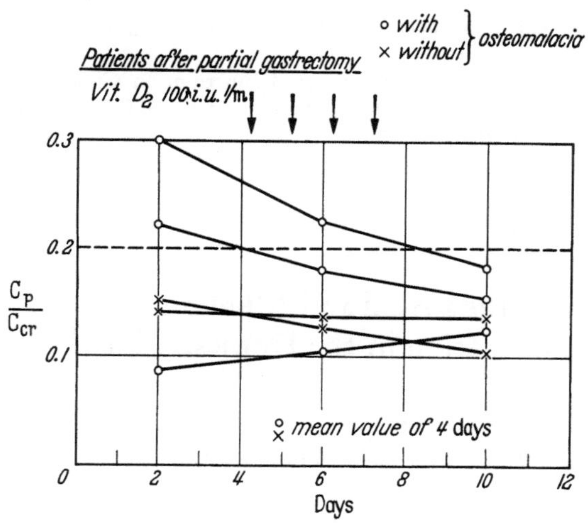

Fig. 2. Effect of daily injections 100 units vitamin D 2 on C_p/C_{cr} in 3 patients with osteomalacia and 2 patients without osteomalacia

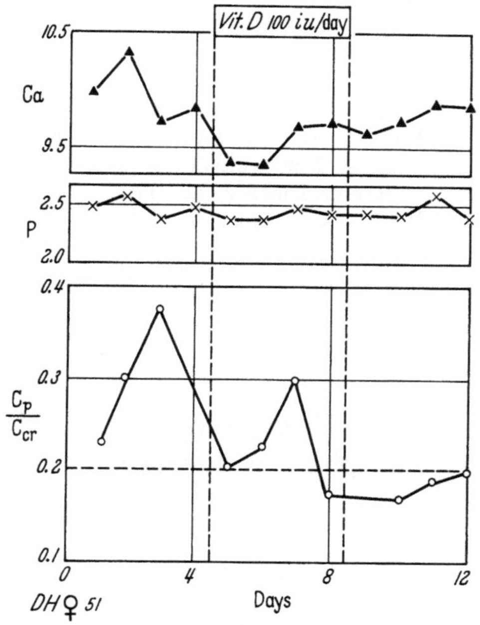

Fig. 3. The serum calcium, phosphate and C_p/C_{cr} in a patient with osteomalacia treated with four daily injections of 100 units vitamin D 2

1. The $\frac{C_p}{C_{cr}}$ may not be raised in osteomalacia.

2. When it is raised it may fall with the administration of 100 units of vitamin D_2 daily for 4 days.

3. In the patient whose serum calcium fell, the fall in $\frac{C_p}{C_{cr}}$ could not be attributed to a suppression of the parathyroid activity. The data suggest that a small dose of vitamin D may directly influence the tubular reabsorption of phosphorus in patients with osteomalacia.

Conclusion

Patients with osteomalacia after gastrectomy get better with a dose of vitamin D_2 equivalent to 130 units daily. While we do not suggest that this dose produces an optimal rate of healing, the clinical and biochemical response to this minute dose shows that these patients have a simple deficiency of vitamin D. The factors contributing to this deficiency have not been discussed. They involve both the patients' dietary intake which can be very small, and the patients' ability to absorb vitamin D, which may be impaired.

Acknowledgements

We are indebted to Miss JUDITH METCALFE and Miss JANET STANLEY for their assistance; and to Messrs Sandoz Products Ltd for their help. The work was supported by grants from the Medical Research Council to P. FOURMAN and to C. G. WOODS.

References

CLARK, C. G., J. CROOKS, A. A. DAWSON, and P. E. G. MITCHELL: Disordered calcium metabolism after Polya gastrectomy. Lancet i, 734 (1964).

JONES, C. T., J. A. WILLIAMS, E. V. COX, M. J. MEYNELL, W. T. COOKE, and F. A. R. STAMMERS: Peptic ulceration: some haematological and metabolic consequences of gastric surgery. Lancet ii, 425 (1962).

NORDIN, B. E. C., and R. FRASER: The indirect assessment of parathyroid function. In Ciba Foundation Symposium on Bone Structure and Metabolism. WOLSTENHOLME, G. E. W., and C. M. O'CONNOR (eds.). London: Churchill 1956, p. 222.

Changes in the Activities of Plasma Acid and Alkaline Phosphatases during Egg Shell Calcification in the Domestic Fowl

T. G. TAYLOR, A. WILLIAMS, J. KIRKLEY

Department of Physiological Chemistry, The University, Reading, England

The calcium metabolism of the laying bird is probably more intense than that of any other organism. The laying hen, for example, secretes on the egg shell 1.6—2.4 g calcium, in the form of the carbonate, in a period of 20 hours or so, most of it during the last 16 hours of the shell-calcification process. The total plasma volume of an average hen is 100 ml and the average level of total plasma calcium is 25 mg/100 ml and it may thus be calculated that a weight of calcium equal to the total amount in circulation at any one instant is removed from the blood every 10—15 minutes during the main period of the formation of the egg shell. When the rate of calcium absorption from the gut is less than the rate at which calcium is deposited on the shell the balance is derived from the skeleton, and during the early hours of the morning the bulk of calcium is supplied from the latter source.

During the laying period the marrow cavities of the majority of the bones of female birds contains a system of secondary bone which grows out from the endosteal surface in the form of fine interlacing spicules, and it is this bone (known as medullary bone) which is mobilized during the process of shell formation, and rebuilt when shell calcification is not in progress. The phase of bone-destruction is characterized by the presence of large numbers of osteoclasts and in the bone-forming phase osteoblasts predominate, and the cell population thus undergoes cyclic changes during the formation of the egg.

Because of the rapid changes in cellular activity which the medullary bone undergoes, the laying hen is a most useful species for the study of bone metabolism and in the present work the changes in the activities of acid and alkaline phosphatases in the plasma during critical stages of laying cycle have been studied. The overall pattern of the changes in the activities of these enzymes has already been reported (TAYLOR *et al.*, 1965), and these changes are shown in Fig. 1.

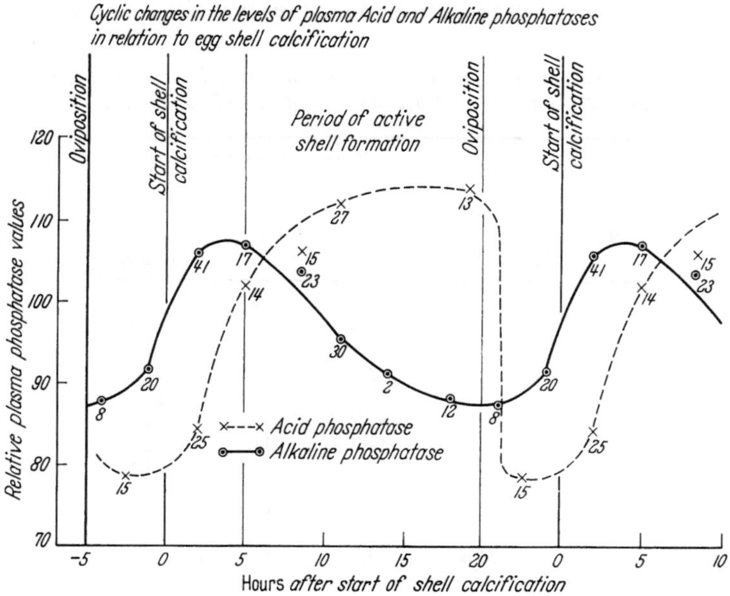

Fig. 1. Cyclic changes in the levels of plasma acid and alkaline phosphatases in relation to the eggshell calcification process. The points represent mean corrected values for each particular stage of shell formation and the number of individual values from which the means are derived are given below each point

Experimental

Ten laying hens were bled at the following times:

Sample A – at the time the egg entered the shell gland (determined by regular palpation).

Sample B – 4 hours after A, when maximum alkaline phosphatase activity was expected.

Sample C – 18 hours after A, when maximum acid phosphatase activity was expected.

Sample D – 2 hours after oviposition.

Samples A, B and C were assayed for alkaline phosphatase and samples A, C and D for acid phosphatase.

The acid phosphatase was determined by the method of BELL and SILLER (1962) using 0.2 M acetate buffer at pH 4.9 and the alkaline phosphatase according to BELL (1960). Both methods employ disodium p-nitrophenyl phosphate as substrate and the units of activity were calculated in terms of μM substrate hydrolysed per minute per litre plasma.

Results

The activities of plasma acid and alkaline phosphatase obtained for the individual birds at the 3 stages of the laying cycle are given in Tables 1 and 2 respectively. The marked increase observed in the acid phosphatase values from the time the egg entered the shell gland (A samples) to the time 18 hours later when shell calcification was almost completed (C samples), and the sharp fall during the subsequent 4 hour period confirmed the results obtained previously (Fig. 1). The expected fall in the level of plasma alkaline phosphatase during shell calcification from the peak observed 4 hours after the start of shell formation (B samples) was also confirmed.

Table 1. *Activities of plasma acid phosphatase for individual hens at 3 stages of the laying cycle expressed as μM p-nitro-phenol phosphate hydrolysed per minute per litre plasma*

	Stages of shell calcification		
	A	C	D
Hours after start of shell calcification	0	18	22 (2 hr after laying)
	12.5	19.3	18.3
	14.3	75.4	14.2
	17.7	20.8	19.4
	7.9	22.9	14.6
	15.6	21.1	16.1
	12.7	30.8	14.5
	18.7	24.5	21.9
	15.2	23.9	18.1
	12.3	17.7	15.4
	15.1	17.3	11.0
Mean	14.2	27.4	16.4

Table 2. *Activities of plasma alkaline phosphatase for individual hens at 3 stages of the laying cycle expressed as μM p-nitrophenyl phosphate hydrolysed per minute per litre plasma*

	Stages of shell calcification		
	A	B	C
Hours after start of shell calcification	0	4	18
	125.3	124.1	90.7
	95.2	120.7	88.3
	88.1	126.2	81.3
	111.0	135.6	91.2
	110.0	108.1	73.9
	89.2	95.5	74.0
	103.4	118.1	85.0
	105.3	122.0	63.7
	114.3	105.5	86.8
	98.8	92.0	68.2
Mean	104.1	114.8	80.3

Discussion

The time of maximal alkaline phosphatase activity in the plasma (Fig. 1) corresponded very closely to the time in the egg cycle at which STRINGER (1962) observed peak osteoblastic activity in the medullary bone (3.5 hours after the start of shell calcification) and the subsequent decline in enzyme activity paralleled the reduction in osteoblast population. A similar parallelism occurred between the increasing level of plasma acid phosphatase which was observed as shell formation advanced and the increasing osteoclast activity in the medullary bone reported by BLOOM *et al.* (1958) and STRINGER (1962).

The presence of acid phosphatase in regions of osteoclastic resorption has been demonstrated histochemically by SCHAJOWICZ and CABRINI (1958) and since bone trabeculae which are undergoing active ossification are rich in alkaline phosphatase (SIFFERT, 1951; HELLER-STEINBERG, 1951; PRITCHARD, 1952), it may be inferred that osteoblasts liberate this enzyme. It is not known, however, whether bone cells secrete phosphatases when they are actively carrying out their normal metabolic functions, whether these enzymes leak passively out of the cells or whether they are liberated only when the cells degenerate.

There is no direct evidence that the phosphatases studied in this experiment originated in the bone but the fact that the changes in the plasma levels observed during shell calcification did not occur in the absence of shell formation (TAYLOR *et al.*, 1965), point to the skeleton as the most likely source, and the remarkable manner in which changes in the cell population of the medullary bone during shell calcification were reflected in changes in the levels of plasma acid and alkaline phosphatase suggests that the osteoclasts and osteoblasts release their respective phosphatases during their active metabolic phases.

Acid phosphatase is one of the most active of the enzymes found in the lysosomes and a study of other lysosomal enzymes in the plasma of laying hens might be expected to shed light on the possible role of these enzymes in the activity of the osteoclast. Mr. K. M. L. MORRIS working in this Department has recently shown that there is a sharp fall in the level of β-glucuronidase following oviposition in the fowl.

References

BELL, D. J.: Tissue components of the domestic fowl. 4. Plasma alkaline phosphatase activity. Biochem. J. **75**, 224 (1960).

—, and W. G. SILLER: Cage layer fatigue in Brown Leghorns. Res. Vet. Sci. **3**, 219 (1962).

BLOOM, M. A., L. V. DOMM, A. V. NALBANDOV, and W. BLOOM: Medullary bone of laying chickens. Amer. J. Anat. **102**, 411 (1958).

HELLER-STEINBERG, M.: Ground substance, bone salts and cellular activity in bone formation and destruction. Amer. J. Anat. **89**, 347 (1951).

PRITCHARD, J. J.: A cytological and histochemical study of bone and cartilage formation in the rat. J. Anat. **86**, 259 (1952).

SCHAJOWICZ, F., and R. L. CABRINI: Histochemical localization of acid phosphatase in bone tissue. Science **127**, 1447 (1958).

SIFFERT, R. S.: The role of alkaline phosphatase in osteogenesis. J. exp. Med. **93**, 415 (1951).

STRINGER, D. A.: The chemistry and physiology of bone, with special reference to medullary bone in the fowl. THESIS. University of Reading 1962.

TAYLOR, T. G., A. WILLIAMS, and J. KIRKLEY: Cyclic changes in the activities of plasma acid and alkaline phosphatases during eggshell calcification in the domestic fowl. Canad. J. Biochem. **43**, 451 (1965).

Calcium Exchanges in the Aorta of the Rat

J. C. STOCLET, Y. COHEN

Laboratoire de Pharmacodynamie, Faculté de Pharmacie, Paris, France

The present experiments were carried out to study the chemical dynamics of aorta mineral of the non-treated rat. Calcium exchanges were measured *in vivo* with ^{45}Ca and the data interpreted by comparison with extracellular ions diffusion spaces: ^{82}Br and ^{24}Na.

The marked sensitivity of the wall of the aorta to calcification has been reported in arteriosclerosis (LANSING *et al.*, 1950) and after treatment by vitamine D or dihydrotachysterol (SELYE and RENAUD, 1959) but until now no quantitative data have been reported on calcium exchange reactions inside the aorta maintained in a physiological state.

Methods

The experiments were carried out on male Wistar rats. Their weight averaged 200 g and they were between 60 and 70 days old. All animals were freely fed on an equilibrated diet (calcium 1 per cent, inorganic phosphate 0.8 per cent, vitamin D 1,270 i. u. per Kg) and tap water.

High specific activity $^{45}Ca\,Cl_2$ (15 μCi-, 0.02 mg of calcium in 0.25 ml of isotonic NaCl solution) was given intravenously to 50 rats. Groups of five animals each were killed by bleeding under ether anesthesia at varying intervals ranging from one minute to 48 hours after injection. The thoracic and abdominal aorta were dissected out, carefully and rapidly cleaned of adhering tissue and weighed (un-washed, wet weight about 40 mg). Total calcium (SOLOMON *et al.*, 1946) and ^{45}Ca (COMAR *et al.*, 1951) were determined in blood plasma and aorta samples after wet ashing by nitro-perchloric mixture and addition of 50 μg of Ca.

^{24}Na and ^{82}Br spaces have been measured on two groups of five rats each, killed twenty minutes after intravenous injection of 5 μCi of one of the radioisotopes ($^{24}NaCl$ or $Na^{82}Br$). Tissue samples were dissolved in concentrated OHNa solution (40 per cent). The volume was adjusted to 1.5 ml and the radioactivity was counted directly.

For each group of rats the result was expressed as the mean of experimental determinations plus or minus standard error of the mean multiplied by t 0.05 (fiducial limits at a probability of 95 per cent).

The kinetic study of specific activity of plasma and aorta calcium permits measurement of size and exchange rates of different compartments in which aorta calcium is distributed. It is assumed that calcium concentration does not vary in the aorta and in blood plasma during the course of the experiment.

For further details on the collection of samples, analytical methods, counting and calculations, see STOCLET (in press).

Results

The wall of the aorta is surprisingly high in calcium. We found $19.2 \pm 2.5\ \mu M$ per gram of wet aorta, instead of 2.7μ M/ml in blood plasma and 1.5 μM/g in skeletal muscles.

The decrease with time of the specific activity of plasma calcium in the same rats as presently used has been described previously by one of us (STOCLET, 1964) and has been shown to correspond to the scheme shown in Fig. 1. ^{45}Ca once intro-

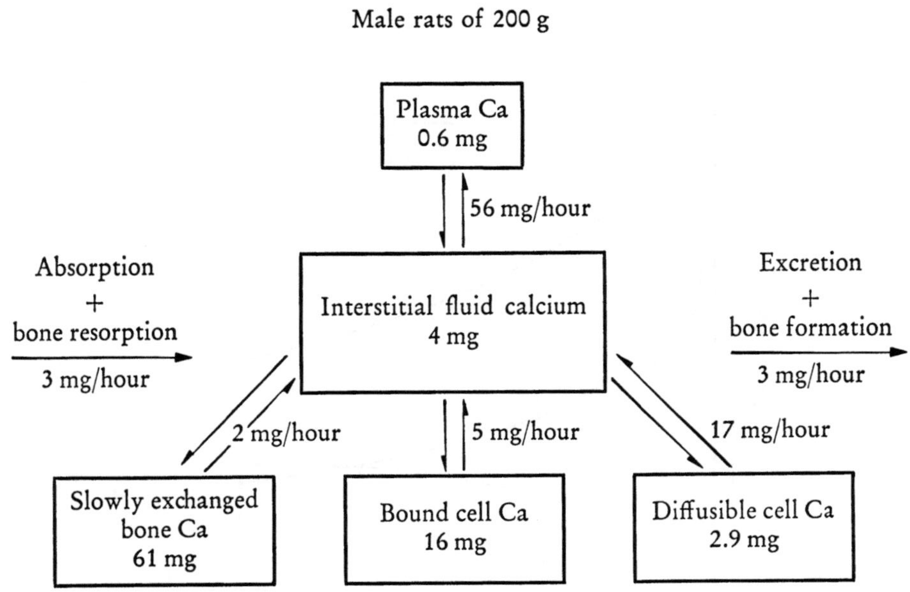

Fig. 1. Scheme of calcium distribution and dynamics in the 200 g male rat

duced into the blood plasma rapidly exchanges with "interstitial calcium" located in interstitial fluid and connective tissue. Interstitial calcium is itself submitted to much slower exchange reactions with tissue calcium and is continuously renewed by unidirectional processes; resorption from bone and absorption supply calcium which is lost by deposition in bone and excretion. Non-extracellular tissue calcium is distributed in three compartments in which the exchange rates are very different i.e. diffusible calcium, bound calcium and slowly exchangeable bone calcium. Diffusible and bound calcium have been identified in soft tissues (smooth and striated muscle) but the corresponding compartments shown in Fig. 1 are larger than the calcium content of the soft tissues of the whole rat. In growing rats some of the exchangeable fractions of bone calcium are included in diffusible and bound compartments since their exchange rates are respectively equal to the one of diffusible and bound cellular calcium (STOCLET and COHEN, 1963).

The specific activity of calcium contained in each compartment has been calculated at the different experimental times and compared with the specific activity of aorta calcium at the same time. Fig. 2 shows the variations with time of the specific activity of calcium in the aorta (R. S.a), in "interstitial" rapidly exchangeable compartment (R. S.) and in slowly exchangeable compartment (R. S. 4). The plain line represents the calculated curve for the following distribution of aorta calcium: rapidly exchangeable (extracellular) 3.5 μM per g, slowly exchangeable (like bone calcium) 6.7 μM per g and non-exchangeable calcium 9.0 μM per g. This calculated curve has been plotted from ^{45}Ca radioactivity in the aorta at two minutes and four hours and it fits all other experimental determinations. The corresponding rates of exchange are 2.8 μM/min/g for the rapid exchange and 0.012 μM/min/g for the slow exchange.

We found a ^{82}Br space of 650 ± 15 μl and a ^{24}Na space of 830 ± 350 μl per gram of aorta.

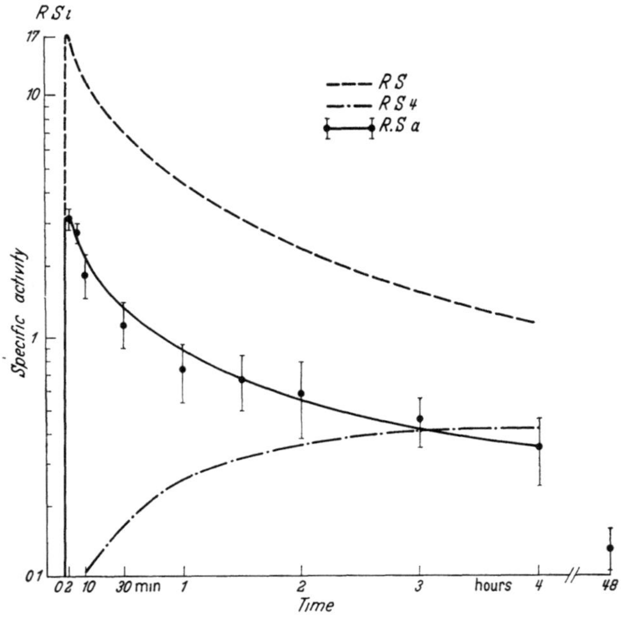

Fig. 2. Variations with time of the specific activity of aorta calcium (R. S. a), rapidly exchangeable ("interstitial") calcium (R. S.) and slowly exchangeable calcium (R. S. 4) after intravenous injection of $^{45}CaCl_2$ to the male rat of 200 g: calculated curves and mean of experimental measures (fiducial limits at a probability of 0.95)

Discussion

The wall of the aorta is made up mainly of elastic membranes which are known to be very sensitive to calcification in pathological or extraphysiological conditions. It seems reasonable to admit that the high calcium content of the aorta in the physiological state is characteristic of non-degraded elastic tissue. It could represent the first of the three steps in calcification of elastic tissue recently described by Urist *et al.* (1964). This high calcium content masks the cellular calcium of the smooth muscle fibers of the aorta. We did not find any diffusible or bound calcium.

The kinetics of aorta calcium are very similar to those of bone calcium since we found the same three compartments in the aorta as are usually found in bone. We should like to emphasize two points: 1. The aorta is the only soft tissue of the rat (amongst several striated and smooth muscles) where slowly exchangeable and non-exchangeable calcium have been found *in vivo*. 2. Rapidly exchangeable calcium is usually located in extracellular fluids where calcium concentration is about the same as in a plasma ultrafiltrate. The situation is different in the aorta but reminds the one of bone. Although its extracellular space (^{82}Br) is high (65 per cent of the wetweight), the aorta also contains "extra" sodium and rapidly exchangeable calcium.

Summary

The kinetics of calcium have been analysed in the wall of the aorta of the living rat. The calcium content of the aorta in the physiological state is surprisingly high (19.2 μM/g). It exchanges with blood calcium according to the same modalities as bone calcium and includes three fractions: rapidly exchangeable (3.5 μM/g), slowly exchangeable (6.7 μM/g) and non exchangeable calcium (9.0 μM/g).

References

Comar, C. L., S. L. Hansard, S. L. Wood, M. P. Plumlee, and B. F. Barrentine: Use of calcium 45 in geological studies. Nucleonics **8/3**, 19 (1951).

Lansing, A. I., M. Alex, and T. B. Rosenthal: Calcium and elastin in human arteriosclerosis. J. Geront. **5**, 112 (1950).

Selye, M., and S. Renaud: Participation of various electrolytes in the production of heart lesions by dihydrotachysterin. Z. Kreisl.-Forsch. **48**, 237 (1959).

Solomon, K., B. W. Gabrio, and C. F. Smith: A precision method for quantitative determination of calcium in blood plasma. Arch. Biochem. **11**, 433 (1946).

Stoclet, J. C.: Etude des mouvements du calcium dans l'organisme du Rat. C. R. Soc. Biol. **158**, 1208 (1964).

— Mouvements du calcium dans le muscle au repos et en activité chez le Rat *in vivo*. J. Physiol. (in press).

—, et Y. Cohen: L'élution plasmatique du ^{45}Ca injecté au Rat, analysée en fonction du sexe et le l'âge. Ann. Nutr. **17 B**, 193 (1963).

Urist, M. R., M. J. Moss, and J. M. Adams, Jr.: Calcification of tendon. Arch. Path. **77**, 594 (1964).

Estimation of the 24 Hour Exchangeable Calcium Pool in Children Using ^{48}Ca

G. D. McPherson

The Hospital for Special Surgery — Affiliated with the New York Hospital — Cornell University Medical College, New York City, U.S.A.

Stable ^{48}Ca is now produced in enrichments sufficiently high in relation of its low natural abundance to permit its use as a non-radioactive tracer in dilution studies of calcium metabolism. Changes in the abundance of ^{48}Ca may be determined precisely by either mass spectrometry or neutron activation analysis.

The ten milligram samples of calcium required for ^{48}Ca abundance estimation by neutron activation analysis are isolated from timed urine collections by oxalate precipitation. Sodium, which is an important source of interference in activation analysis of biological samples, is removed to a considerable extent by the simple isolation procedure. The induced ^{24}Na does not interfere with the counting of ^{49}Ca because of the high energy of ^{49}Ca (3.1 MeV). As the specific activity of urine and serum are similar, the abundance of a stable tracer in samples of calcium isolated from urine collections reflects the specific activity of the isotope in serum.

This report describes the use of stable ^{48}Ca in the estimation of the 24 hour exchangeable calcium pool in children.

Methods

Methods are described in detail elsewhere (McPherson, 1965). The ten cases studied are listed in Table 1. Except for cases H3 and H5, all were active children

Table 1. *Children studied using ^{48}Ca as a tracer*

Case No.	Age (years)	Sex	Weight (kg)	Ideal Weight (kg)	Diagnosis
H-3	12.25	F	26.9	38.3	Osteogenesis imperfecta tarda; healing fracture of the femur; confined to bed.
H-4	10.0	F	49.	31.9	Meningomyelocoele; soft tissue surgery of feet.
H-5	7.5	M	30.5	25.9	Bilateral Legg-Perthes disease; confined to bed.
H-6	12.6	M	37.5	42.2	Post-polio paresis of leg; soft tissue surgery.
H-7	10.8	F	44.5	35.7	Mild spastic paraplegia; soft tissue surgery.
H-8	7.25	M	37.2	24.5	Mild spastic paraplegia; soft tissue surgery.
H-9	8.2	F	19.2	26.4	Congenital hypoplasia of leg muscles possibly post-polio; soft tissue surgery.
H-10	8.2	F	31.	26.4	Mild spastic paraplegia; soft tissue surgery.
H-11	10.2	M	22.7	31.9	Mild spastic hemiplegia; soft tissue surgery.
H-12	8.5	F	42.2	27.7	Mild spastic quadriplegia; soft tissue surgery.
Mean ± S. D.	(9.5 ± 1.9)		(34.1±8.8)	(31.1 ± 6.)	

without evidence of metabolic bone disease. Following the collection of a control urine sample for determination of the pre-injection abundance of ^{48}Ca, each child received an intravenous injection of 4 milligrams of ^{48}Ca as $CaCl_2$ in 2 cc. of sterile water. At the 39.7% enrichment level used, the total dose of element was 10 mg; it was injected slowly over one minute. Following the injection period, timed urine samples were collected at the normal voiding times of the children and pooled to give six to twelve hour collections in the first three days followed by 24 hour collections for up to ten days.

Calcium was isolated from each urine sample by double oxalate precipitation followed by ashing to give calcium carbonate. Approximately 25 milligrams of calcium carbonate from each sample were placed in a small sealed polyethelene capsule and exposed to a neutron flux of 3×10^{13} neutrons/cm²/sec. for a period of one or two minutes at the Union Carbide Research Reactor, Tuxedo Park, New York. Five minutes after irradiation the ^{49}Ca in the samples was measured by gamma scintillation spectrometry and related to the ^{49}Ca content of standards irradiated under the same conditions. After a one week delay to reduce activity, the samples were dissolved in 1. N HCl and the total calcium content of each sample and standard was determined by a direct recorded EDTA titration method. The abundance of ^{48}Ca in each sample was expressed as a percentage of the normal abundance in standards. Increased abundance levels in each sample were related to the total dose of ^{48}Ca to give specific activity as percent dose ^{48}Ca per gram calcium.

Results

In all cases ^{48}Ca specific activity fell rapidly following injection so that normal abundance levels were reached within one week. A typical pattern of ^{48}Ca abundance change following injection is shown in Fig. 1. When plotted logarithmically the

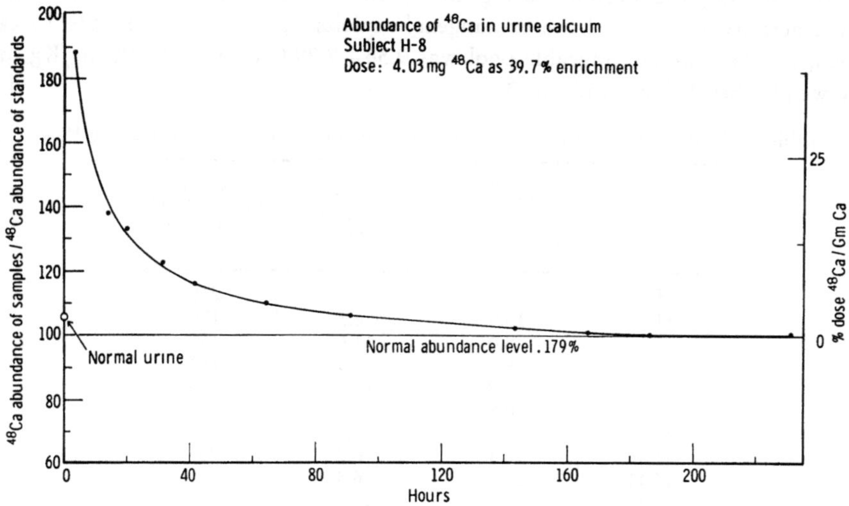

Fig. 1

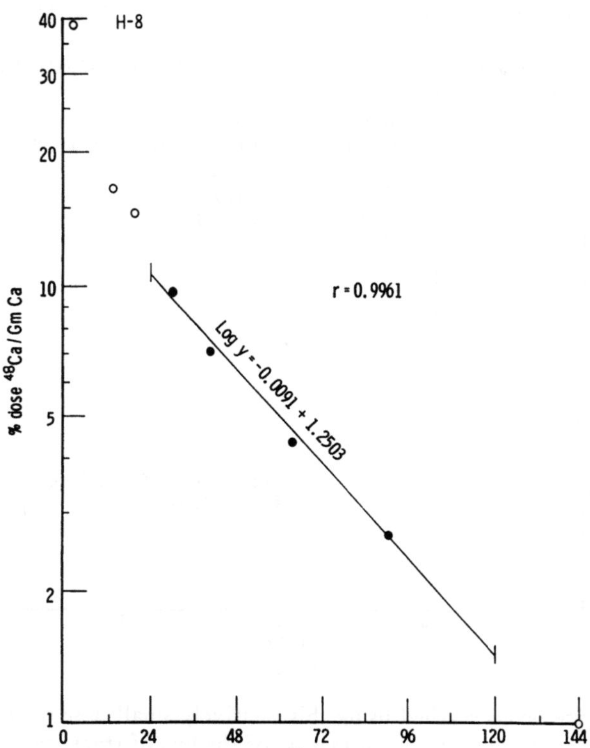

Fig. 2

specific activity appeared to fall on a straight line during the period from 24 to 120 hours as shown in Fig. 2. The ^{48}Ca specific activity at 24 hours was considered to represent that of the exchangeable calcium pool. The values for specific activity between 24 and 120 hours were treated by least squares analysis to derive an equation representing the decline during this period. The reciprocal of the 24 hour specific activity represented the exchangeable calcium pool in Gms. In the 10 cases studied, the 24 hour exchangeable pool was 9.34 + 2.29 Gms or 307 + 95 mg/Kg ideal body weight. See Table 2 and Fig. 3.

Table 2. *Estimation of 24 hour exchangeable calcium pool in children using* ^{48}Ca

Case No.	24 hour Specific Activity (% dose ^{48}Ca/Gm. Ca)	24 hour Exchangeable Ca Pool (Gm)	24 hour Ca Pool (mg.) Ideal Weight (kg.)
H-3	10.5	9.5	248
H-4	15.9	6.3	196
H-5	8.6	11.6	450
H-6	8.4	11.9	283
H-7	8.8	11.4	319
H-8	10.8	9.3	380
H-9	12.5	8.0	304
H-10	16.1	6.2	236
H-11	15.8	6.4	198
H-12	7.8	12.8	460
Mean ± S.D.	(11.5 ± 3.34)	(9.34 ± 2.29)	(307 ± 95)

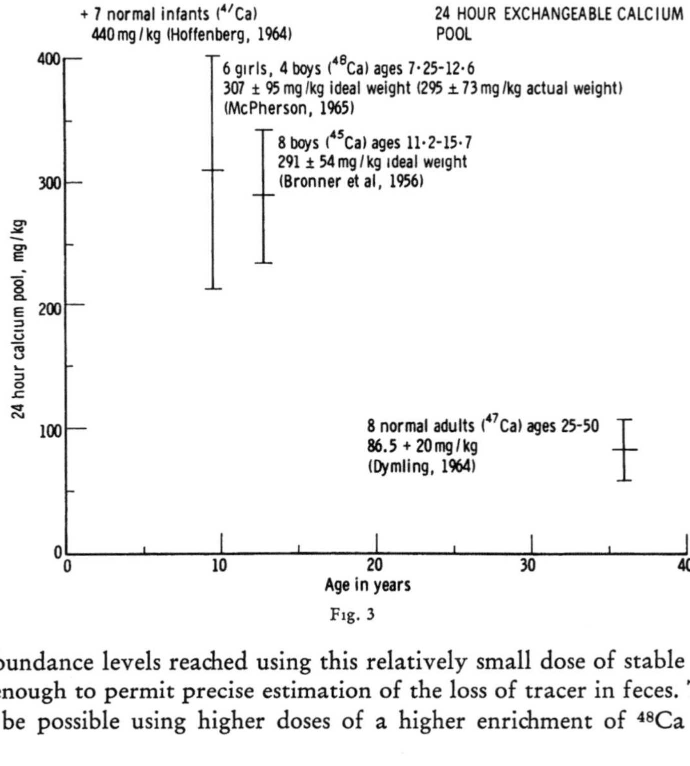

Fig. 3

The abundance levels reached using this relatively small dose of stable tracer were not high enough to permit precise estimation of the loss of tracer in feces. This would, however, be possible using higher doses of a higher enrichment of ^{48}Ca and would permit further analysis of the disappearance curve in terms of both accretion and excretion.

In the cases studied, the ^{48}Ca abundance in pre-injection urine Ca as well as in samples at the end of the experiment was similar to the abundance of the standards used. There was no evidence of biological fractionation of ^{48}Ca.

Discussion

Because of a reluctance to employ radioactive tracers in young children-particularly normal children, little is known about the kinetics of calcium metabolism in young normal subjects. Calculation of the 24 hour exchangeable calcium pool based upon the 24 hour specific activity of radioactive calcium isotopes gave a value of 440 mg/Kg in seven normal one-year-old infants studied by HOFFENBERG *et al.* (1964) using ^{47}Ca. Data from BRONNER *et al.* (1956) on eight adolescent boys using ^{45}Ca gave a pool size of 291 ± 54 mg/Kg ideal weight. Eight normal adults under age 50 years (mean age 36 years) studied by DYMLING (1964) with ^{47}Ca had a 24 hour exchangeable calcium pool of 86.5 ± 20 mg/Kg. The relation of these values to the data from this study is shown in Fig. 3.

Conclusions

Stable ^{48}Ca in enriched form may be used as a tracer in dilution studies of calcium kinetics in young children and other rádiosensitive subjects. In the 10 cases studied, the 24 hour exchangeable calcium pool relative to body weight was three to four times as high as in normal adults.

References

BRONNER, F., R. S. HARRIS, C. J. MALETSKOS, and C. E. BENDA: Studies of calcium metabolism: the fate of intravenously injected radiocalcium in human beings. J. clin. Invest. **35**, 78 (1956).

DYMLING, J.-F.: Calcium kinetics in osteopenia and parathyroid disease. Acta med. scand. Suppl. Vol. **175** (1964).

HOFFENBERG, R., F. HARRIS, and E. BACK: Ca^{47} in the investigation of rickets. Medicals uses of Ca^{47}. Second Panel Rep. IAEA, Tech. Rep. Ser. 32 Vienna 1964.

MCPHERSON, G. D.: Stable calcium isotopes as tracers in studies of mineral metabolism. Acta orthop. scand. Suppl. **78** (1965).

Transfert du calcium intestinal chez l'homme dans les maladies déminéralisantes de l'os

L. MIRAVET, D. HIOCO

Centre du métabolisme phospho-calcique, Hôpital Lariboisière, Paris, France
(Groupe Recherches I.N.S.E.R.M.)

Pour explorer le transfert du calcium intestinal chez l'homme, nous avons effectué, en utilisant la technique simplifiée d'AUBERT et MILHAUD (1960), 218 explorations chez 5 sujets normaux et 182 sujets atteints des maladies suivantes: 39 ostéoporoses communes, 29 ostéoporoses idiopathiques, 2 maladies de Lobstein, 7 ostéomalacies d'apport (5 fois sans traitement et 4 fois sous calciférol), 9 ostéomalacies par diabète phosphoré

(4 fois sans traitement, 5 fois sous calciférol et 3 fois après calciférol), 10 hyperparathyroïdies avant intervention et 8 après adénomectomie, 3 hypoparathyroïdies, 4 spasmophilies normocalcémiques, 2 hyperthyroïdies, 2 hypothyroïdies, 5 acromégalies, 2 syndromes de Cushing, 13 affections traitées par les corticoïdes, 5 insuffisances rénales, 9 diabètes calciques, 2 lithiases rénales, 5 gastrectomies dont 3 avec une ostéoporose, 8 maladies de Paget, 15 néoplasies dont 13 cancers secondaires du sein, 9 maladies de Kahler, 1 maladie de Waldenströem.

Nous avons exploré dans chaque maladie le pourcentage absorbé (α %) du calcium ingéré et la quantité de calcium qui est éliminée par voie digestive et qui n'est pas réabsorbée (Caf); nous avons essayé de préciser si l'intestin est une voie d'élimination calcique et s'il existe un rapport entre l'élimination calcique digestive et l'élimination rénale.

1. Variation du pourcentage d'absorption du calcium (α %)

Il est calculé par la formule suivante:

$$\frac{(\text{CaI} + \text{Caf}) - \text{CaF}}{\text{CaI}} \times 100 = \alpha\ \%\ [1].$$

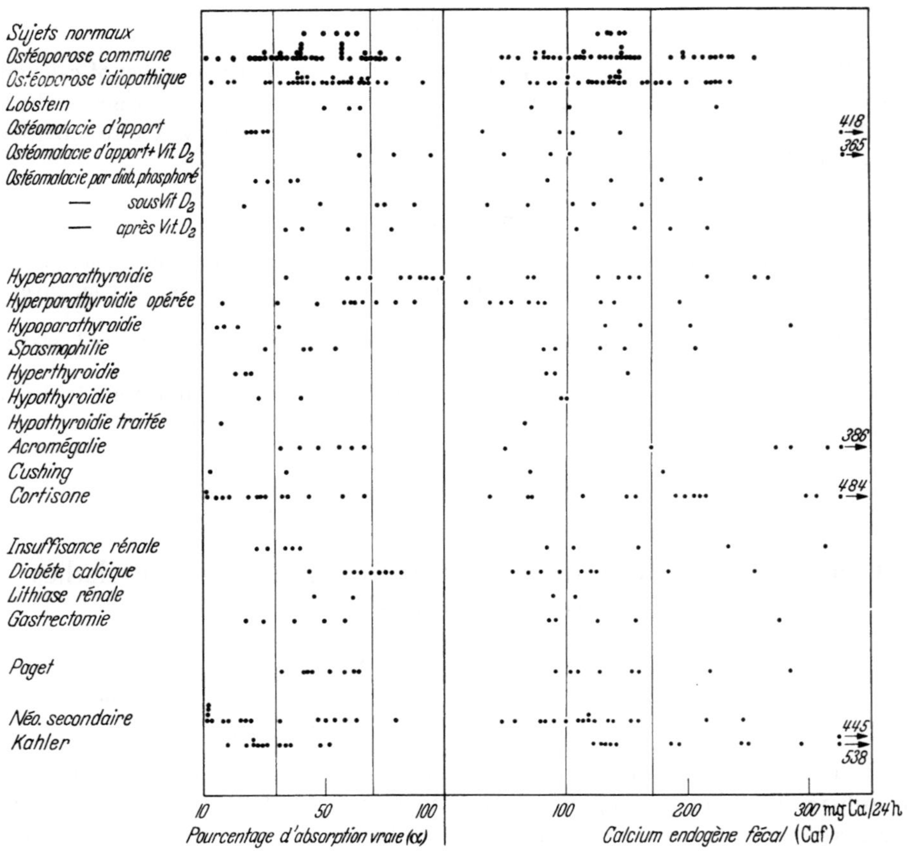

Fig 1

[1] CaI = Calcium ingéré; CaF = Calcium fécal total; Caf = Calcium fécal endogène.

— Les résultats sont indiques dans la Figure 1.

— Chez le normal (5 sujets), nous trouvons 53%.

— Nous n'avons trouvé d'hyperabsorption (> 70%) que dans l'hyperparathyroïdie 7 fois sur 10 (dans les 3 autres cas, d'absorption normale, il existait une insuffisance rénale), dans les ostéomalacies traitées par la vitamine D, dans quelques ostéoporoses communes (5 sur 40) et idiopathiques du sujet jeune (3 sur 29), enfin dans les diabètes calciques (4 sur 9).

— Par contre, l'hypoabsorption est très fréquente; nous l'avons trouvée dans les ostéomalacies d'apport (5 fois sur 5) et dans certaines ostéomalacies par diabète phosphoré (2 fois sur 4), chez les sujets traités par les corticoïdes (11 fois sur 14) ou atteints de maladie de Cushing (2 fois sur 2), l'insuffisance rénale (2 fois sur 5), l'hypoparathyroïdie (4 fois sur 4), quelquefois dans la spasmophilie (2 fois sur 5) et dans l'hyperthyroïdie (3 fois sur 3). L'hypoabsorption est aussi observée dans un nombre important d'ostéoporoses (ostéoporoses communes 14 fois sur 40, ostéoporoses idiopathiques du sujet jeune, 5 fois sur 29) et elle est très fréquente dans des néoplasies secondaires (11 fois sur 17) et la myélomatose (10 fois sur 12).

En revanche dans la maladie de Lobstein, l'acromégalie et la maladie de Paget, l'absorption est normale.

Ainsi, le pourcentage d'absorption du calcium est modifié au cours de certains états pathologiques étudiés et parfois même caractéristique de la maladie considérée (Milhaud *et al.*, 1961).

2. Variations du calcium fécal endogène et ses corrélations avec le pourcentage d'absorption

Le calcium excrété par voie digestive et non réabsorbé par l'intestin (Caf) a été calculé d'après la formule suivante:

$$\mathrm{Caf} = \mathrm{T}\frac{\mathrm{RF}}{\mathrm{Ri}}\left(\frac{1}{1-e^{-at}}\right)\frac{t_6}{t_1}\,[1].$$

La quantité calculée chez le sujet normal est de 135 mg/j; la moyenne des 218 études réalisées est de 149 ± 80 mg/j. Si l'on supprime les chiffres nettement supérieurs aux $2\,\sigma$ (6 malades se répartissant ainsi: 2 ostéomalacies, 1 acromégalie, 1 sujet traité par les corticoïdes, 2 maladies de Kahler), la moyenne est de 141 ± 65 mg/j et nous pouvons constater que Caf est très variable à l'intérieur d'un même groupe de malades.

Heaney et Skillman (1964) ont trouvé une corrélation entre α, CaI et Caf; en effet, cette corrélation semble exister pour les absorptions extrêmes (< 20% ou > 70%), les Caf suivent cette règle, sauf pour quelques exceptions. Mais, en fait, les deux valeurs sont liées par la technique de calcul elle-même; il est donc surprenant d'observer que, lors de certaines maladies, cette relation ne soit plus suivie, notamment: dans l'hyperparathyroïdie (Fig. 1) où l'on trouve α extrêmement élevé (moy.: 76%), tandis que Caf est normal, voire même augementé (moy.: 146 mg/j) et dans l'acromégalie (Fig. 1) où un α normal (moy.: 51%) est accompagné d'un Caf extrêmement élevé (moy.: 243 mg/j).

[1] T = turnover; RF = radioactivité fécale totale, Ri = radioactivité injectée; t = jours.

Contrairement à ce que l'on pourrait croire d'après les variations importantes du Caf dans un même groupe de malades, Caf paraît être lié à l'état pathologique des sujets puisqu'il est en rapport avec α et que α est en relation avec la maladie.

3. Relations entre la calciurie (CaU) et le calcium fécal endogène (Caf)

Chez l'individu normal, le rapport CaU/Caf est voisin de 1; ce rapport est conservé dans quelques maladies, lorsque la calciurie reste dans les limites de la normale. Il peut se modifier fortement quand il se produit des variations extrêmes de la calciurie, soit une diminution comme dans l'ostéomalacie ou les insuffisances rénales, soit une élévation comme dans le diabète calcique, l'hyperparathyroïdie, l'hyperthyroïdie, l'acromégalie, les lyses osseuses.

4. Facteurs qui modifient α et Caf

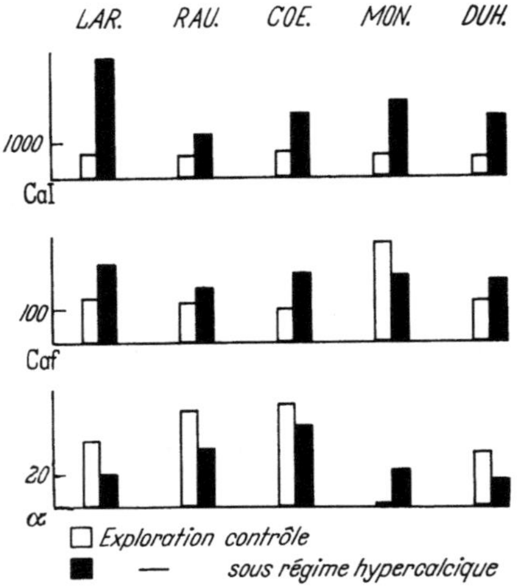

Fig. 2

a) Variation du régime calcique (5 cas)

Lorsqu'on fait varier l'ingestion calcique de façon importante (en passant d'un régime normal contenant en moyenne 656 mg/j à au régime riche en calcium: 2160 mg/j), on voit que α diminue et que le calcium endogène fécal augmente (Fig. 2).

b) Effet de la vitamine D_2 dans l'ostéomalacie (4 cas)

Quand on administre du calciférol, l'effet contraire se produit: α augmente dans les 4 cas étudiés, Caf diminue 3 fois sur 4 (Fig. 3).

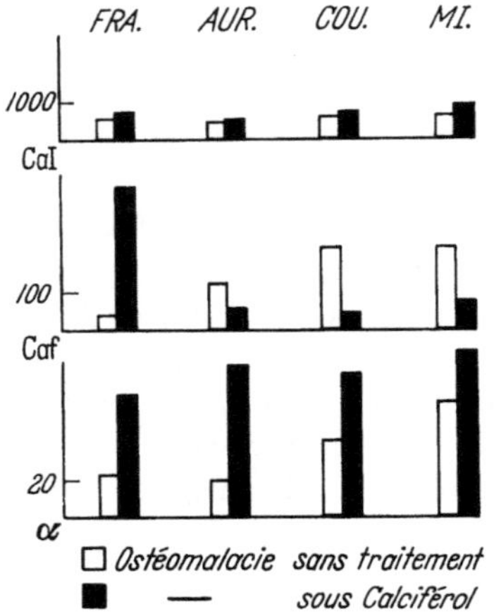

Fig. 3

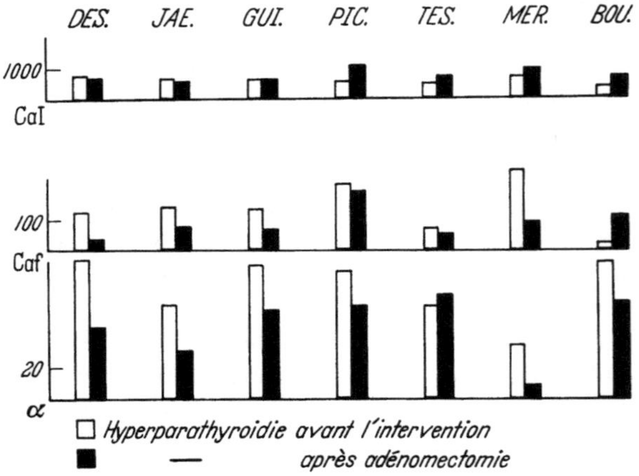

Fig. 4

c) Effet de l'adénomectomie chez 7 hyperparathyroïdiens

Après l'extirpation de l'adénome, le coefficient d'absorption, élevé au départ, diminue presque régulièrement; mais, contrairement à ce que l'on pouvait escompter, le calcium fécal endogène diminue aussi (Fig. 4).

Discussion

1. L'hyperabsorption est rare

Nous avons trouvé une hyperabsorption calcique dans les hyperparathyroïdies et les ostéomalacies traitées par le calciférol, bien en accord avec l'importance de ces deux régulateurs, hormone parathyroïdienne et vitamine D, dans le métabolisme du calcium. Mais, fait important à signaler, l'hyperabsorption calcique existe aussi dans certains diabètes calciques et paradoxalement dans quelques ostéoporoses. Dans ces derniers cas, il peut exister soit un trouble de réceptivité à la vitamine D ou à l'hormone parathyroïdienne. En outre, diabète calcique et ostéoporose ont d'autres traits communs qui peuvent faire penser qu'il y a une parenté entre eux (Hioco *et al.*, 1964).

Quant à l'hypoabsorption, elle est très fréquente: elle existe non seulement dans les hypoparathyroïdies et les ostéomalacies où manquent les régulateurs bien connus de l'absorption, mais encore dans de très nombreuses maladies. Il est vraisemblable que tout trouble du fonctionnement digestif puisse entraver l'absorption du calcium.

La rareté des hyperabsorptions plaide en faveur d'un processus actif dans l'absorption calcique qui ne peut être augmentée que dans des circonstances bien précises.

2. Relations entre le calcium fécal endogène et le coefficient d'absorption

Bien qu'il semble exister une relation entre Caf et α, les variations de Caf dans notre série sont très importantes, probablement parce que le calcium apporté par les sécrétions digestives n'est pas absorbé (pour une part importante au moins) dans les mêmes conditions que le calcium alimentaire. La grande fréquence des troubles du transit intestinal peut expliquer des larges variations de Caf. Celui-ci est dans l'ensemble relativement bas lorsque α est inférieur à 20%; ceci est peut-être la conséquence d'une diminution des sécrétions digestives et, de ce fait, du calcium apporté par ces sécrétions. Le cas inverse se produit dans l'acromégalie où une augmentation des sécrétions digestives serait responsable du Caf élevé.

3. Relation entre la calciurie et le calcium fécal endogène

Apparemment, il n'existe pas de relation, mais en fait celle-ci est peut-être masquée par l'existence de variations de la calciurie plus larges et plus étroitement liées à l'état pathologique que les variations du calcium fécal. La calciurie est fortement diminuée dans l'insuffisance rénale, alors que le Caf est irrégulièrement augmenté. Malgré ces limites, dans certains cas et dans une certaine mesure, l'intestin peut devenir une voie d'élimination du calcium, complémentaire de la voie rénale, mais probablement cette compensation est limitée par suite de la variabilité de la quantité des sécrétions digestives d'un sujet à l'autre et d'une maladie à l'autre.

4. Facteurs qui modifient α et Caf (Bronner, 1964)

Les cas étudiés sous régime riche en calcium ou sous calciférol montrent que ces deux facteurs ont un effet contraire sur le coefficient d'absorption et sur le calcium endogène fécal. Par contre, l'adénomectomie des hyperparathyroïdiens provoque une diminution paradoxale de Caf en même temps que le coefficient α diminue; ceci fait penser que, dans ces cas, la variation de concentration calcique provoquée par la chute importante de la calcémie peut diminuer l'élimination de calcium par voie digestive.

Bibliographie

Aubert, J.-P., et G. Milhaud: Méthode de mesure du métabolisme calcique chez l'homme. Biochim. biophys. Acta **39**, 22 (1960).

Bronner, F.: Dynamics and function of calcium. In Mineral Metabolism. Comar, C. L., and F. Bronner (eds.). New York: Academic Press 1964, p. 341.

Heaney, R. P., and T. Skillman: Secretion and excretion of calcium by the human gastrointestinal tract. J. Lab. clin. Med. **64**, 29 (1964).

Hioco, D., L. Miravet, and P. Bordier: Physiopathology and treatment of osteoporosis in younger men. In Bone and Tooth. Blackwood, H. J. J. (ed.). Oxford: Pergamon Press 1964, p. 365.

Milhaud, G., J.-P. Aubert et J. Bourrichon: Etude du métabolisme du calcium chez l'homme à l'aide du Ca^{45}. I: Absorption du calcium au cours de la digestion. Path. et Biol. 9, 1761 (1961).

Absorption of Calcium in Man: Effect of Disease, Hormones and Vitamin D*

L. Lutwak

Clinical Nutrition Unit, Graduate School of Nutrition, Cornell University, Sage Hospital, 512 East State Street, Ithaca, N. Y., U.S.A.

The kinetics of the absorption and retention of calcium were calculated from measurements *in vitro* of isotope content of the forearm by counting in a large volume liquid scintillation counter after the oral administration of ^{47}Ca (Lutwak and Shapiro, 1964). The fecal excretion of unabsorbed tracer, and the urinary excretion of absorbed isotope were also followed. These measurements permitted an estimate of the rates of transfer of calcium from the gut to the arm during the initial absorptive phase and the subsequent turnover of tracer calcium retained during the first phase.

After the oral administration of the tracer dose of ^{47}Ca of between four and eight microcuries admixed with 100 mgm. of stable calcium, in the form of skim milk or calcium gluconate, the radioactivity appearing in the patient's forearm counted *in vivo* is followed at three minute intervals for the first five to six hours and thereafter twice a day. Blood samples were obtained at 15 minute to half hour intervals over the course of the first four hours to monitor the procedure. Maximum levels of blood radioactivity are seen in most of our patients between two and four hours after the ingestion of the tracer, and thereafter fall quite rapidly. Assuming a value for extracellular fluid in the forearm of approximately 150—200 ml., between 20 and 40% of the radioactivity appearing in the forearm in the first three of four hours can be attributed to radioactivity in the blood, and remainder being that which has been taken up by bone.

* This paper was prepared with the support of grant number AM-07451 from the National Institutes of Health.

Typical curves for the first four hours of observation are presented in Fig. 1. There are two separate studies of the same individual, a normal 21 year old male, plotted on the graph; the studies were performed approximately six weeks apart. Excellent reproducibility of observations was achieved.

In all patients there was a lag period of 10 to 30 minutes after ingestion before any discernible radioactivity above background could be measured in the forearm. Thereafter, there was a relatively rapid increase, persisting for about two hours in most subjects. From this point on, the increase was more gradual, levelling off in about for to six hours. The maximum activity in the forearm was usually present at between 24 and 36 hours after administration of the dose and thereafter, fell gradually.

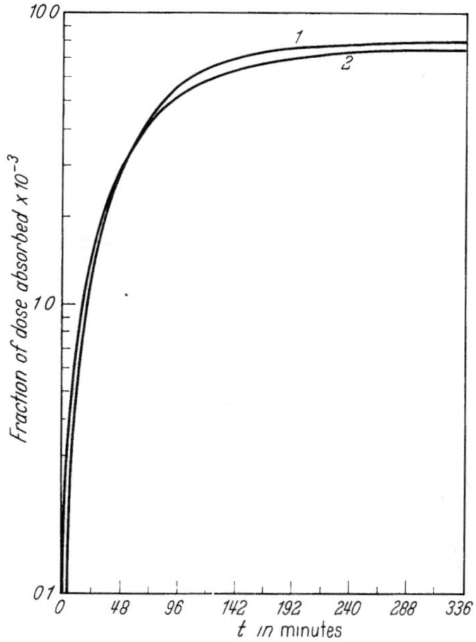

Fig. 1. Empirical Arm Counts Normal 21 year old male. Two oral ^{47}Ca studies, six weeks apart. Ordinate, arbitrary units. absciss, minutes

Attempts have been made to correlate values for apparent absorption obtained from direct stool measurements with various numerical parameters of the arm count curves. Numerical analysis of the plot indicated that four numbers could be readily calculated to describe the semi-logarithmic plot of data: "k_1", representing the initial slope; "k_2", representing the slope of the last portion; "a_1", representing the intercept of the first portion; and "a_2", representing the intercept of the last portion. Statistical correlations were made between each of these four parameters and the net absorption calculated from stool recoveries. Absorption was directly related to "a_2", the intercept value for the asymptotic horizontal portion of the curve and to "k_1". The correlations obtained, however, were of the order of 0.6 with a probability of less than 0.001 that these were due to chance. Because of the low correlation values for individual observations, it was concluded that while absolute absorption of calcium could not be ascertained from this type of study, considerable information could be derived from sequential studies in the same patient under various modes of therapy and from comparisons of groups of patients with different diagnoses.

Fig. 2 shows four curves obtained from studies of a patient with idiopathic hypoparathyroidism. Curves 1 and 2 represent studies approximately a month apart when the patient was without any treatment other than a dietary regimen of high calcium, low phosphate. The shape of this curve is similar to that obtained in the study of the normal subject, but the maximum value achieved is considerably lower. Curve 3 was measured while the patient was receiving 400 units daily of parathyroid extract injected intramuscularly. It can be seen that the maximum value attained was markedly increased in comparison with the baseline studies. Curve 4 was determined after the patient had been receiving 10,000 units daily of vitamin D_2 for a period of several weeks. This curve begins to resemble the normal pattern described previously. The values obtained were approximately twice as high as those when the patient was untreated.

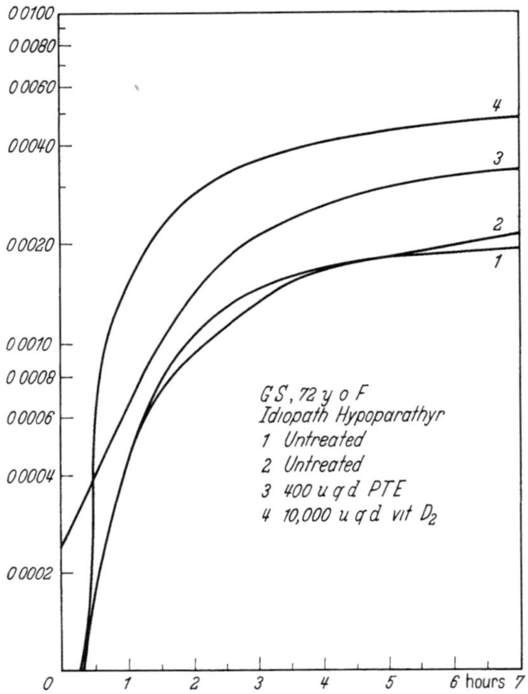

Fig. 2. ^{47}Ca Arm Counts. 72 year old female, idiopathic hypoparathyroidism. 1, 2: untreated. 3: 400 units parathyroid extract daily. 4: 10,000 units vitamin D daily. Ordinate, fraction of administered dose; abscissa, hours

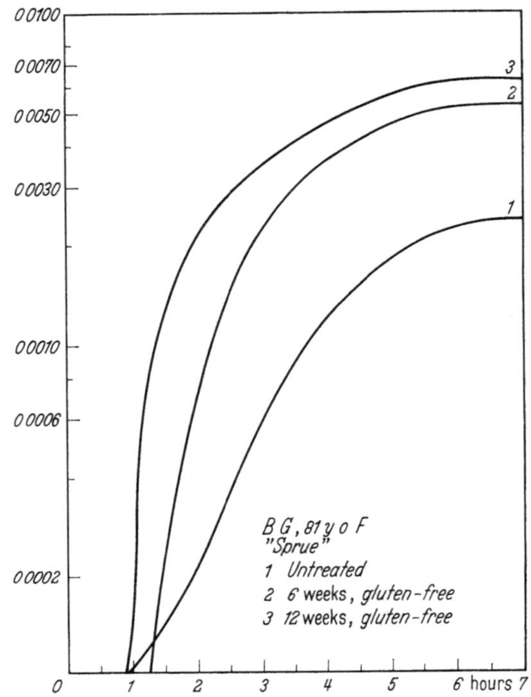

Fig. 3. ^{47}Ca Arm Counts. 81 year old female, sprue. 1: untreated. 2: 6 weeks on gluten-free diet. 3: 12 weeks, gluten-free diet. Coordinates as in Fig. 2

Fig. 3 shows results obtained in an 81 year old woman with a malabsorption syndrome, diagnosed as sprue. Curve 1 was measured when the patient was untreated and was passing four to six fat-containing, foul smelling, watery stools daily. The maximum value achieved is very similar to that seen in the previous patient with idiopathic hypoparathyroidism, but even more striking, is the very gradual, slow slope of the first portion of the curve. No detectable counts were obtained until approximately an hour and a half after the ingestion of the isotope. Curve 2 was obtained six weeks after the patient had been on a gluten-free diet. The values now approximated a normal pattern in terms of the maximum level reached and the increased rate of the first portion of the curve. The third curve was obtained during a follow-up admission, after the patient had been on a gluten-free diet for 12 weeks, and this is even closer to normal. Note, however, that the point of first appearance of significant counts was still markedly delayed, occurring approximately one hour after ingestion.

Table 1 summarizes the estimates of "k_1" and "a_2", as well as percent apparent absorption calculated from stool excretion, in a series of patients who have been studied by this technique. It should be noted that there was no significant difference in any of these parameters between patients with radiologically diagnosed osteoporosis, both male and female, and a small group of apparently normal individuals. Therefore, the normal and all of the osteoporotics were grouped for statistical purposes in Group IV.

Significantly decreased "k_1", and "a_2" and apparent percent absorption values were obtained in three patients with malabsorption syndrome (Group V). On treatment with gluten-free diet, in two of these patients (Group VI), the "k_1" value still remained abnormal and was not significantly different from that in the initial studies. The only value which changed significantly was that for percent apparent absorption.

Group VII, the two patients with hypoparathyroidism, showed significantly decreased "k_1" values but no significant change in either of the other two measurements. When these patients were treated with adequate dosages of vitamin D (Group VIII), the "k_1" value became normal and was significantly different from the untreated state. The change in "a_2", although quite marked, was not significant because of the small number of patients. The change in percent apparent absorption is of interest in that it decreased on vitamin D. The next group (IX) consists of three

Table 1

Group	Diagnosis	N	k_1				a_2				% A			
			mean	s. d.	vs.	†P	mean	s. d.	vs.	†P	mean	s. d.	vs.	†P
I	"Normal"	4	0.0487	0.0011			0.00628	0.00062			33.6	22.1		
II	Female osteoporosis	8	0.0492	0.0264	I	N. S.	0.00629	0.00136	I	N. S.	38.1	11.0	I	N. S.
III	Male osteoporosis	8	0.0453	0.0213	I	N. S.	0.00602	0.00161	I	N. S.	35.7	16.4	I	N. S.
IV	Normal + all osteoporosis	20	0.0475	0.0207			0.00618	0.00131			36.1	15.1		
V	Malabsorption	3	0.0157	0.0055	IV	*****	0.00185	0.00008	IV	*****	0.0	0.0	IV	*****
VI	Treated Malabsorption	2	0.0254	0.0050	IV	****	0.00333	0.00208	IV	N. S.	30.0	0.0	IV	*
					V	N. S.			V	N. S.			V	*****
VII	Hypoparathyroid	2	0.0221	0.0039	IV	*****	0.00333	0.00287	IV	N. S.	30.8	0.3	IV	N. S.
VIII	Hypoparathyroid + Vitamin D	2	0.0488	0.0064	IV	N. S.	0.00513	0.00314	IV	N. S.	24.1	0.1	IV	****
					VIII	**			VIII	N. S.			VIII	*****
IX	Psoriasis	3	0.0382	0.0128	IV	N. S.	0.00582	0.00065	IV	N. S.	18.4	6.9	IV	****
X	Paget's	2	0.0248	0.0027	IV	*****	0.00484	0.00318	IV	N. S.	25.0	19.7	IV	N. S.
XI	Rheumatoid Arthritis, acute	1	0.0226		IV	*****	0.00434		IV	*****	6.0		IV	*****
XII	Rheumatoid Arthritis, remission	1	0.0660		IV	*****	0.00445		IV	*****	10.0		IV	*****
XIII	Fanconi's	1	0.0119		IV	*****	0.00719		IV	****	19.8		IV	*****
XIV	Vitamin D — Resistant Rickets	1	0.0578		IV	**	0.00420		IV	*****	12.0		IV	*****

†P, N. S. = not significantly different, * = < 0.1, ** = < 0.05, *** = < 0 02, **** = < 0.01, ***** = < 0.001.

patients with generalized psoriasis who had extensive exfoliation and, consequently, loss of calcium through the skin. None of the parameters of absorption measured were significantly different from normal. In Group X, two patients with Paget's disease showed significantly decreased values for "k_1" but no significant changes in any of the other measurements. In one patient with acute rheumatoid arthritis all of the values were significantly decreased. When the patient was in remission on treatment with salicylates and intramuscular gold, the measured "k_1" and percent absorption increased, but still were significantly lower than normal subjects. The last two groups shown here consist of a single patient each with Fanconi's syndrome and with vitamin D resistant rickets. In Franconi's syndrome the value for "k_1" and for percent apparent absorption were markedly lower than normal and the value for "a_2" was greater than normal. In the patient with vitamin D resistant rickets the "k_1" value was greater than normal and both the "a_2" and percent apparent absorption were less than normal.

From these studies it has been tentatively postulated that the value for "k_1" is related to the phenomenon of absorption from the gastrointestinal tract and "a_2" is related both to absorption and to the avidity of the bones in the forearm for tracer.

A new procedure, based on *in vivo* counting of limb, has been demonstrated to yield data related to mechanism of calcium absorption in man. It has the advantages of obviating the need for blood, urine and stool sampling and of yielding results within three or four hours of observation.

Bibliography

LUTWAK, L., and J. SHAPIRO: Calcium absorption in man: based on large volume liquid scintillation counter studies. Science **144**, 1155 (1964).

Therapeutic Results in Renal Tubular Osteomalacia with Special Reference to Calcium Kinetics

J.-F. DYMLING

Orthopaedic Research Laboratories and the Department of Internal Medicine
Malmö General Hospital, University of Lund, Malmö, Sweden

Introduction

Renal tubular osteomalacia may be defined as a clinical entity characterized by hypophosphatemia, decreased renal tubular reabsorption of inorganic phosphate and vitamin D resistant rickets or osteomalacia: Sporadic and familial occurence has been reported, the probable mode of inheritance being sex-linked, dominant (WILLIAMS *et al.*, 1960).

The pathogenesis is not known. ALBRIGHT *et al.* (1937) postulated a primary defect in the intestinal absorption of calcium, complicated by secondary hyperparathyroidism. FANCONI and GIRARDET (1952) postulated a primary defect in tubular reabsorption of inorganic phosphate leading to hypophosphatemia. A primary skeletal defect was proposed by ENGFELDT *et al.* (1956) and FROST (1958). FRAME *et al.* (1965) proposed a combination of a primary renal defect and a primary skeletal defect. KUHLENCORDT (1958) proposed a general disturbance of phosphorylation. These theories have recently been reviewed by FALKSON and FRAME (1958), WILLIAMS *et al.* (1960), and FRAME *et al.* (1965).

The treatment of choice has generally been vitamin D in massive doses. This treatment has not been entirely satisfactory, since a complete cure is not often accomplished (TAPIA *et al.*, 1964; PIERCE *et al.*, 1964). Addition of calcium supplements has been advocated as has oral supplements of phosphate (LAFFERTY *et al.*, 1964; FRASER *et al.*, 1958; FRAME and SMITH, 1958; KUHLENCORDT, 1958). Three cases are reported here, in which the effect of treatment with oral supplements of inorganic phosphate and phosphate supplements plus vitamin D was investigated with the aid of ^{47}Ca or ^{85}Sr.

Clinical material

The clinical material consists of three cases of renal tubular osteomalacia. The most important clinical findings are found in Table 1.

Table 1. *Laboratory data in three cases of renal tubular osteomalacia. Averages of several determinations*

Case	T. C. Untreated	T. C. Treated	M. B. Untreated	M. B. Treated	J. C. Untreated	J. C. Treated
Height (cm)	158		133		150	
Weight (kg)	57		35		68	
Plasma:						
Ca (mEq/L)	4.7	5.1	4.6	4.6	4.9	4.9
P inorganic (mg%)	2.1	2.0	2.1	2.9	1.6	2.9
Alk. phosphatase (U)	6	6	31	19	6	7
Creatinine (mg%)	0.9	0.8	0.5	0.7	0.6	0.8
Stand. bicarbonate (mEq/L)	23	23	22	23	25	24
Urine:						
Ca (mg/day)	110	190	180	200	120	—
P inorganic (mg/day)	550	1500	500	1350	450	—
Tubular reabsorption of P (%)	51	—	61	—	78	—
Hydroxyproline (mg/day)	—	—	—	54.9	—	47.3
Glucose	Occasionally		None		None	
Aminoacids	Normal		Normal		Normal	
Radiography	Severe osteopenia		Severe osteopenia		Severe osteopenia	

Case T. C. Male, born in 1912. The father and paternal uncle probably suffered from the same disorder. As a child he is said to have had rickets. At the age of 35 he first noted skeletal symptoms. At the age of 48 he was admitted with the fullblown clinical picture of renal tubular osteomalacia. After a detailed study treatment was started with vitamin D plus oral supplements of sodium monophosphate. The dosages were settled at 65.000 I.U. vitamin D_2 and 8 Gm sodium monophosphate.

Case M. B. Female, born in 1944. Family history non-contributory. Skeletal symptoms were first noted at the age of 12. Admitted to several hospitals, and treated with vitamin D_2 in doses amounting to 240.000 I.U. This treatment was sedated 20 months before admission to Malmö General Hospital. At that time, age 18, she presented a clinical picture of severe renal tubular osteomalacia. After a detailed study treatment was started with sodium monophosphate 8 Gm daily. After another study vitamin D_2 was given in addition. The dosages were settled at 6 Gm sodium monophosphate and 675.000 I.U. vitamin D_2.

Case J. C. Male, born in 1908. Family history not possible to trace. Skeletal symptoms were first noted at the age of 25. Admitted to several hospitals, and given a tentative diagnosis of Albright's disease. No treatment before admission to Malmö General Hospital in 1963. At that time he presented a clinical picture of moderately severe renal tubular osteomalacia. After an initial study with ^{85}Sr, he refused treatment, but later he changed his mind and a second study in the untreated state was performed using ^{47}Ca. Treatment was started with sodium monophosphate, 10 Gm daily. After another study vitamin D_2 was given in addition. The dosages were settled at 10 Gm of sodium monophosphate and 65.000 I.U. of vitamin D_2.

Methods

The kinetic studies were performed with ^{47}Ca or ^{85}Sr according to DYMLING (1964).

Results

The results are found in Tables 1 and 2 and Fig. 1.

Case T. C. During treatment there was a slight increase in serum calcium and urine calcium. There was no change in serum phosphate but a striking increase in urine phosphate. After seven months of treatment there was an increase of the accretion rate, which returned to the orginal level after two years of treatment. Radiographically there appeared healing of the pseudofractures and calcification of vertebral osteophytes. The clinical improvement was dramatic and he resumed work as a painter.

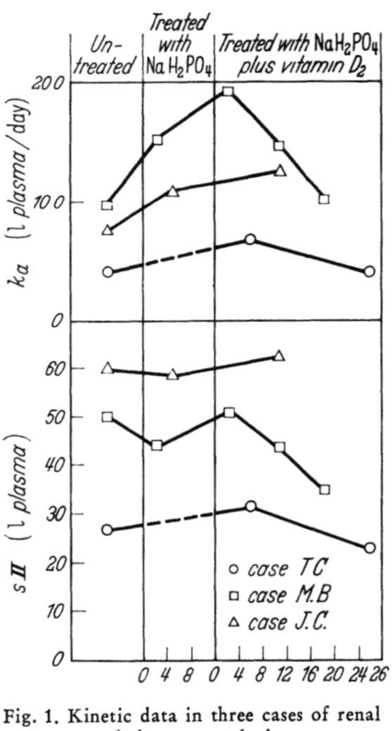

Fig. 1. Kinetic data in three cases of renal tubular osteomalacia

Case M. B. During treatment there were no changes in serum or urine calcium. The serum phosphate rose as did the urine phosphate. The level of alkaline phosphatase decreased. The accretion rate increased on oral supplements of phosphate, and increased further on phosphate supplements plus vitamin D. Having reached a peak value the accretion rate slowly returned to the original value two years after treatment was started. The exchangeable compartment S_{II} remained unchanged during the first six months of treatment but tended to decrease thereafter. Radiographically an increased mineral content was established after two and a half years of treatment. The clinical improvement was very dramatic and she has for the first time in her life been able to work and to take part in out-door life.

Case J. C. The chemical findings during treatment were essentially the same as in case M. B. The accretion rate increased on phosphate supplements and increased furthermore on phosphate supplements plus vitamin D. The clinical improvement

Table 2. *Kinetic data in three cases of renal tubular osteomalacia.* k_a*: accretion rate (1 plasma/day).* S_I *and* S_{II}*: exchangeable compartments (1 plasma).* k_u*: urinary clearance rate (1 plasma/day).* k_f*: endogenous faecal clearance (1 plasma/day)*

Case	Date	Isotope	k_a	S_I	S_{II}	k_u	k_f	Treatment
T.C.	60.12.	^{47}Ca	4.1	23.9	26.8	0.9	2.4	O
	61.07.	^{47}Ca	6.7	32.0	31.3	4.2	0.8	$P + D_2$
	63.03.	^{47}Ca	4.0	23.6	22.5	2.0	0.9	$P + D_2$
M.B.	62.01.	^{47}Ca	9.7	19.5	49.9	2.3	0.03	O
	62.03.	^{47}Ca	15.2	17.4	43.9	1.3	0.1	P
	62.06.	^{47}Ca	19.2	19.2	50.7	1.6	0.1	$P + D_2$
	63.03.	^{47}Ca	14.5	19.2	43.5	2.2	0.1	$P + D_2$
	64.10.	^{47}Ca	10.1	15.1	34.7	2.6	0.1	$P + D_2$
	64.10.	^{85}Sr	10.4	16.8	38.9	5.6	1.0	$P + D_2$
J.C.	63.02.	^{85}Sr	7.5	22.2	60.1	4.1	1.5	O
	63.10.	^{47}Ca	8.9	22.6	53.5	1.5	2.0	O
	64.03.	^{85}Sr	10.9	20.4	58.9	1.4	2.8	P
	65.02.	^{85}Sr	12.4	28.0	62.6	2.0	2.5	$P + D_2$

was less dramatic in this case. However, he felt subjectively better. No radiographic changes have been observed so far.

Discussion

The accretion rate has been found to be high in untreated renal tubular osteomalacia when studied with ^{47}Ca or ^{85}Sr (MELTZER *et al.*, 1960; LAFFERTY *et al.*, 1964). In two children treated with 15.000 I.U. of vitamin D, the accretion rate was normal, studied with ^{32}P (BAUER *et al.*, 1956). In one adult there was almost no new bone formation when studied with tetracycline labelling (FRAME *et al.*, 1965). There was, however, a diffuse deposition of tetracycline in interstitial bone. The conclusion must be that the data observed with ^{47}Ca or ^{85}Sr reflects a diffuse deposition in bone rather than true bone formation. The two children studied with ^{32}P may have had a lower accretion rate in the untreated state.

On treatment with phosphate supplements the accretion rate increased. This contrasts to the decrease of the accretion rate found by LAFFERTY *et al.* (1964) during treatment with calcium supplements. Since an increased mineral deposition rate is the aim of treatment this favours the treatment with phosphate supplements.

On treatment with vitamin D, the accretion rate fell in the case described by MELTZER *et al.* (1960) and after a slight initial increase decreased below the original value after five months of treatment in the case described by LAFFERTY *et al.* (1964). In all the cases presented here the accretion rate increased on treatment with phosphate supplements plus vitamin D. In two cases (M. B. and T. C.) the accretion rate started to decrease after a peak value, but two years after treatment was started, the accretion rate was still not lower than the original value. It may be concluded that this effect is a satisfactory result of treatment. The clinical findings support this conclusion.

Summary

Kinetic studies with ^{47}Ca or ^{85}Sr have been performed in three cases of renal tubular osteomalacia in the untreated state and during oral treatment with sodium monophosphate and sodium monophosphate plus vitamin D. The accretion rates were high in the untreated state. They were increased by phosphate supplements, but even more increased by phosphate supplements plus vitamin D. The kinetic changes have been interpreted as signs of healing, which was supported by the observed clinical and radiographic improvement.

Acknowledgements

Financial support was obtained from the Herman Järnhardt Foundation, Malmö, and from grants to G. C. H. BAUER from the International Atomic Energy Agency and United States Public Health Service grant D-1452.

References

ALBRIGHT, F., A. M. BUTLER, and E. BLOOMBERG: Rickets resistant to vitamin D therapy. Amer. J. Dis. Child. **54,** 529 (1937).

BAUER, G. C. H., A. CARLSSON, and B. LINDQUIST: Bone salt metabolism in human rickets studied with radioactive phosphorus. Metabolism **5,** 573 (1956).

DYMLING, J.-F.: Calcium kinetics in osteopenia and parathyroid disease. Acta med. scand. **175,** suppl. 408 (1964).

ENGFELDT, B., R. ZETTERSTRÖM, and J. WINBERG: Primary vitamin-D resistant rickets. III Biophysical studies of skeletal tissue. J. Bone Jt Surg. **38 A,** 1323 (1956).

FALKSON, G., and B. FRAME: Phosphate diabetes. Henry Ford Hosp. Bull. **6,** 244 (1958).

FANCONI, G., and P. GIRARDET: Familiäre persistierende Phosphatdiabetes mit D-vitamin-resistenter Rachitis. Helv. paediat. Acta **7,** 14 (1952).

FRAME, B., A. R. ARNSTEIN, H. M. FROST, and R. W. SMITH, JR.: Resistant osteomalacia. Amer. J. Med. **38,** 134 (1965).

—, and R. W. SMITH: Phosphate diabetes. A study of osteomalacia. Amer. J. Med. **5,** 771 (1958).

FRASER, D., D. W. GEIGER, J. D. MUHN, P. E. SLATER, R. JAHN, and E. LIU: Calcification studies in clinical vitamin D deficiency and in hypophosphatemic vitamin D-refractory rickets. Amer. J. Dis. Child. **96,** 460 (1958).

FROST, H. M.: Some observations on bone mineral in a case of vitamin D-resistant rickets. Henry Ford Hosp. Bull. **6,** 300 (1958).

KUHLENCORDT, F.: Die glucosurische Osteopathie. Ergebn. inn. Med. Kinderheilk. **9,** 622 (1958).

LAFFERTY, F. W., C. H. HERNDON, and O. H. PEARSON: Skeletal dynamics in vitamin D resistant rickets. In Dynamic Studies on Metabolic Bone Disease. PEARSON, O. H., and JOPLIN (eds.). Oxford: Blackwell Scientific Publications 1964, p. 163.

MELTZER, W., I. LYON, E. D. MENSEN, and R. D. RAY: Radioisotope studies of generalized skeletal disorders. Clin. Orthop. **17,** 269 (1960).

PIERCE, D. S., W. M. WALLACE, and C. H. HERNDON: Long-term treatment of vitamin-D resistant rickets. J. Bone Jt Surg. **46 A,** 978 (1964).

TAPIA, J., G. STEARNS, and I. V. PONSETI: Vitamin-D resistant rickets. J. Bone Jt Surg. **46 A,** 935 (1964).

WILLIAMS, T. F., R. W. WINTERS, and C. H. BURNETT: Familial hypophosphatemia and vitamin D-resistant rickets. In the Metabolic Basis of Inherited Disease. STANBURY, WYNGAARDEN, and FREDRICKSON (eds.). New York: McGraw Hill 1960, p. 1177.

Etude du métabolisme du calcium chez l'homme à l'aide de calcium 45: l'ostéopétrose et l'ostéopsathyrose

G. MILHAUD, J. BOURICHON

Laboratoire des Isotopes, Institut Pasteur, Paris, France

Nous nous sommes proposé de mettre en évidence les perturbations du métabolisme du calcium qui existent dans deux affections héréditaires et rares de l'os, l'ostéopsathyrose ou maladie de Lobstein et l'ostéopétrose ou maladie d'Albers-Schönberg. Nous rapportons les valeurs des principaux paramètres du métabolisme du calcium de deux enfants, un adolescent et deux adultes atteints d'ostéopétrose et d'un enfant et d'une adulte atteints d'ostéopsathyrose.

Techniques

Chez l'adulte ou l'adolescent, la méthode d'analyse du métabolisme du calcium a été exposée précédemment (MILHAUD et AUBERT, 1958; AUBERT et MILHAUD, 1960). Chez l'enfant, nous avons employé une méthode simplifiée comportant 7 prises de sang aux temps 2, 4, 6, 24, 32, 48 et 72 heures. La courbe représentant la variation de la radioactivité spécifique du calcium en fonction du temps est exprimée à l'aide de la somme de deux exponentielles, comme nous l'avons fait pour le rat (MILHAUD *et al.*, 1960 a).

Tableau 1

Sexe	N° d'observation	Age (années)	Poids (kg)	(Ca)	P	V_{0+}	V_{0-}	V_u	V_f	V_i	V_a	α(%)	Δ
				Ostéopétrose									
F	217	51	73	105	4629	954	846	292	90	917	490	53,4	+ 108
F	131	27	51	102	6220	510	142	189	98	998	655	65,6	+ 368
M	59	15	45	90	4467	2429	2123	256	95	995	657	66,0	+ 306
M	236	1,2	7	100	1878	1071	777	5	61	521	360	69,0	+ 294
F	361	0,5	4	90	2059	532	160	9	21	551	402	72,9	+ 372
				Ostéopsathyrose									
F	392	32	42,4	97	3028	420	463	108	123	750	188	25,0	— 43
M	360	1	8,8	100	1098	331	182	11	416	1000	576	57,6	+ 149
				Sujets Normaux									
M	174	52	83	103	5950	581	549	166	138	1083	336	31,0	+ 32
M	104	22	64	100	6530	790	830	190	100	930	250	26,9	— 40
F	303	16	43,5	100	6054	869	612	136	138	905	531	58,6	+ 257
M	287	1,1	10,4	106	1678	1067	799	28	65	904	361	39,9	+ 268
M	385	1	8,7	104	1788	857	636	13	42	739	276	37,3	+ 221
M	384	0,5	6,5	92	1565	972	769	22	26	765	251	32,8	+ 203

Tableau 2. *Action de la cortisone dans l'ostéopétrose* (Cas No 131)

	(Ca)	P	V_{0+}	V_{0-}	V_u	V_f	V_i	V_a	α (%)	Δ
Avant traitement	102	6220	510	142	189	98	998	655	65,6	+ 368
Apres traitement	106	3598	867	824	175	106	858	314	36,5	+ 43

(Ca), calcémie (mg/l); P, fonds commun calcique (mg); V_{0+}, anabolisme osseux (mg/j); V_{0-}, catabolisme osseux (mg/j); V_u, calciurie (mg/j); V_f, calcium endogène fécal (mg/j); V_i, calcium ingéré (mg/j); V_a, calcium absorbé par l'intestin (mg/j); α(%), taux d'absorption, Δ, bilan (mg/j).

Résultats

Les résultats relatifs aux 5 cas d'ostéopétrose, aux 2 cas d'ostéopsathyrose et à 6 sujets normaux d'âge comparable, sont rapportés dans le Tableau 1. Le Tableau 2 rapporte l'effet de l'administration d'un dérivé de la cortisone sur le métabolisme du calcium dans un cas d'ostéopétrose de l'adulte. La triamcinolone a été donnée à raison de 4 mg par jour pendant 18 jours.

Discussion

Ostéopétrose — L'augmentation progressive de la densité de l'os, qui caractérise cette affection, implique que les perturbations du métabolisme du calcium continuent à se manifester à l'âge adulte. Il en résulte que les anomalies devraient être plus faciles à mettre en évidence lorsque la croissance est achevée. Considérons tout d'abord les deux cas d'ostéopétrose de l'adulte (observations N° 217 et 131): ils diffèrent des sujets normaux d'âge comparable par une hyperabsorption du calcium au cours de la digestion et un bilan fortement positif. Les autres paramètres sont soit normaux ou diminués — comme le fonds commun calcique, l'anabolisme osseux et le catabolisme osseux — soit normaux ou augmentés comme la calciurie; de ce fait, leurs variations ne peuvent être considérées comme caractéristiques de l'ostéopétrose.

Si l'on admet que l'augmentation de l'absorption du calcium est constante dans l'ostéopétrose, on peut se demander comment se comporte l'excrétion de calcium endogène par l'intestin.

Chez le sujet normal, il existe une relation linéaire entre la quantité de calcium endogène fécal, V_f, et la quantité de calcium absorbé, V_a, qui est $V_f = 0{,}232\ V_a + 42$ (unités: mg/jour) pour une ingestion moyenne de calcium de 900 mg/jour (Milhaud *et al.*, 1961; Milhaud et Aubert, 1963). La Fig. 1 montre que cette relation est fortement perturbée dans l'ostéopétrose de l'adulte puisque les 2 cas se situent en-dessous de la droite de régression du sujet normal. Ce comportement signifie l'existence dans l'ostéopétrose d'une diminution de l'excrétion de calcium endogène, V_f, par rapport à l'absorption au cours de la digestion, V_a.

Chez l'adolescent normal, l'absorption du calcium au cours de la digestion est élevée, ce qui a pour conséquence de masquer l'hyperabsorption de l'ostéopétrose (obs. N° 59). Dans cette affection, le bilan est plus positif, le fonds commun calcique diminué et l'intensité du métabolisme osseux nettement augmentée.

Enfin, chez le jeune enfant (obs. N° 236 et 361), la quantité moyenne de calcium absorbé est plus élevée que chez le sujet normal (obs. N° 287, 385, et 384), ce qui est d'autant plus frappant que l'ingestion de calcium est plus faible dans les cas d'ostéopétrose.

En ce qui concerne le métabolisme osseux, le fonds commun calcique est du même ordre de grandeur que chez l'enfant normal. L'anabolisme osseux est normal (obs. N° 236) ou diminué (obs. N° 361), le catabolisme est normal dans le premier cas et effondré dans le second.

Correction des perturbations de l'ostéopétrose par la cortisone

La cortisone diminue l'absorption du calcium au cours de la digestion chez le rat (Milhaud *et al.*, 1960 b) et chez l'homme, bien que de façon moins régulière (Milhaud *et al.*, 1961). Il était donc logique de suivre les effets de l'administration de cortisone sur le métabolisme calcique dans l'ostéopétrose.

Ces effets comportent (Tableau 2):

1. une diminution de moitié de la quantité de calcium absorbé au cours de la digestion. — 2. la réduction de la positivité du bilan qui passe de +368 mg/j à +43 mg/j. — 3. une réduction du fonds commun calcique, qui porte particulièrement sur le compartiment osseux. — 4. une augmentation de l'intensité du métabolisme de l'os, qui intéresse l'anabolisme osseux, V_{0+}, et surtout le catabolisme osseux, V_{0-}, dont la valeur sextuple. — 5. la calciurie et la quantité de calcium endogène fécal ne sont pas modifiées. Enfin, la cortisone corrige la perturbation de la relation V_a, V_f de l'ostéopétrose: après traitement, le point correspondant au cas 131 se situe sur la droite du sujet normal (Fig. 1).

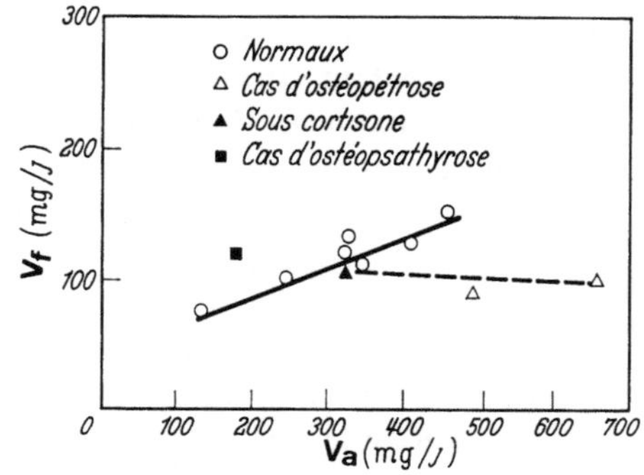

Fig. 1. Relation entre la quantité de calcium excrété, V_f, et la quantité de calcium absorbé par l'intestin, V_a, chez l'homme normal, dans l'ostéopétrose et l'ostéopsathyrose de l'adulte

On peut conclure de ce qui précède que la diminution du catabolisme osseux n'est pas la lésion primaire de l'ostéopétrose puisque si l'on diminue par la cortisone la quantité de calcium absorbé au cours de la digestion, on observe une augmentation considérable de l'intensité du catabolisme osseux. L'effondrement du catabolisme osseux serait donc la conséquence de l'hyperabsorption.

Hérédité de l'ostéopétrose

En ce qui concerne l'aspect héréditaire de l'ostéopétrose, une étude récente fait état de 12 sujets touchés en 4 générations (Lievre *et al.*, 1962); le N° 131 fait partie de cette famille.

Ostéopétrose animale

Les anomalies du squelette de la souris microphtalmique ressembleraient à celles de l'ostéopétrose humaine. L'étude du métabolisme du calcium de ces animaux a été faite à l'aide de ^{45}Ca et de ^{85}Sr; elle a montré une diminution très nette de la vitesse du catabolisme osseux (Adams et Carr, 1965). L'affection humaine diffère de l'affection animale puisque le catabolisme osseux peut être normal et même dans le cas où il est effondré, il peut redevenir normal si l'on diminue l'absorption intestinale par de la cortisone.

Ostéopsathyrose

Les perturbations du métabolisme du calcium liées à cette affection, caractérisée par un amincissement et une grande fragilité des os, apparaissent avant la naissance ou peu de temps après. Elles peuvent donc être étudiées commodément chez le jeune enfant. A propos du cas N° 360, on constate, par rapport aux deux enfants normaux: 1. une réduction du fonds commun calcique de plus de 30%; 2. une diminution de l'anabolisme et du catabolisme osseux respectivement au 1/3 et au 1/4 de la normale; 3. une augmentation considérable de l'excrétion fécale de calcium endogène; 4. une hyperabsorption du calcium au cours de la digestion; 5. un bilan moins positif que chez l'enfant normal.

Chez l'adulte, cas N° 392, on observe une diminution du fonds commun calcique, de l'anabolisme et du catabolisme osseux. L'absorption du calcium au cours de la digestion est à la limite inférieure de la normale. La relation V_a, V_f est déséquilibrée dans le sens d'une augmentation de l'excrétion fécale, V_f, par rapport à l'absorption, V_a (Fig. 1). Enfin, le bilan est légèrement négatif.

En résumé, l'enfant atteint d'ostéopsathyrose a une entéropathie avec déperdition de calcium (MILHAUD et VESIN, 1964), et l'adulte, un déséquilibre de la relation calcium endogène fécal-calcium absorbé. Il n'est pas possible avec un cas de savoir si l'entéropathie avec déperdition de calcium est un facteur pathogénique important ou accidentel de l'ostéopsathyrose.

LEE (1965) a mesuré la formation de l'os fémoral à l'aide de la tétracycline chez deux enfants atteints d'ostéopsathyrose; il conclut à une augmentation de la vitesse de déposition du calcium osseux par unité de masse d'os. Ce résultat, qui concerne un os isolé, ne s'accorde pas avec nos constatations qui portent sur l'ensemble du squelette et montrent une diminution très importante de l'anabolisme osseux. Ce désaccord tient au mode d'expression utilisé par LEE, qui ne tient pas compte de la diminution de la masse totale de l'os dans l'ostéopsathyrose.

Conclusion

L'étude cinétique du métabolisme du calcium met en évidence dans l'ostéopétrose, une hyperabsorption du calcium au cours de la digestion et dans un cas d'ostéopsathyrose, une entéropathie avec déperdition de calcium, qui peuvent contribuer à expliquer la pathogénie des lésions osseuses.

Bibliographie

ADAMS, P. J. V., and T. E. F. CARR: Some observations on the calcium and strontium metabolism in the microphthalmic mutant of the mouse. In Calcified Tissues. RICHELLE, L. J., and M. J. DALLEMAGNE (eds.). Liège: Université de Liège 1965, p. 145.

AUBERT, J. P., et G. MILHAUD: Méthode de mesure des principales voies du métabolisme calcique chez l'homme. Biochim. biophys. Acta **39**, 122 (1960).

LEE, W. R.: A quantitative microscopic study of bone formation in a normal child and in two children suffering from osteogenesis imperfecta. In Calcified Tissues. RICHELLE, L. J., and M. J. DALLEMAGNE (eds.). Liège: Université de Liège 1965, p. 451.

LIEVRE, J. A., G. MILHAUD, et J. P. CAMUS: Ostéopétrose, étude d'une famille comportant 12 sujets touchés en 4 générations; étude métabolique à l'aide du calcium radioactif. Rev. Rhum. **29**, 258 (1962).

MILHAUD, G., et J. P. AUBERT: Exploration des principales voies du métabolisme calcique chez l'homme. Colloque Biophysique. Bordeaux: Soc. Edit. Enseig. Sup. 1958, p. 209.

—, W. REMAGEN, A. GOMES DE MATOS, et J. P. AUBERT: Etude du métabolisme du calcium chez le rat à l'aide de calcium 45: le rachitisme expérimental. Rev. Franç. Etud. clin. biol. **5**, 254 (1960 a).

— — — — Etude du métabolisme du calcium chez le rat à l'aide du calcium 45: action de la cortisone. Rev. Franç. Etud. clin. biol. **5**, 354 (1960 b).

MILHAUD, G., J. P. AUBERT, et J. BOURICHON: Etude de métabolisme du calcium chez l'homme à l'aide de calcium 45: l'absorption du calcium au cours de la digestion. Path. et Biol. 9, 1761 (1961).
— — L'absorption du calcium au cours de la digestion chez l'homme. Ann. Nutr. **17 B**, 181 (1963).
—, et P. VESIN: Entéropathies avec pertes de protéines et métabolisme du calcium. In Protides of the Biological Fluids. PEETERS, H. (ed.). Amsterdam: Elsevier 1964, p. 239.

Calcium Clearance and Re-absorption in Patients with Osteoporosis, Renal Stone and Primary Hyperparathyroidism

D. A. SMITH, J. C. MACKENZIE

University Department of Medicine, Gardiner Institute, Western Infirmary, Glasgow, Scotland

Introduction

Hypercalciuria is known to occur in patients with hyperparathyroidism and in about 30% of patients with renal stone disease. It is not yet known for certain whether there is any difference in calcium reabsorption by the tubules in these conditions. KLEEMAN *et al.* (1958) reported that there was decreased clearance of calcium in normal subjects following the administration of parathyroid hormone during calcium infusion. LOKEN and GORDAN (1959), and GORDAN *et al.* (1962) reported that calcium clearance was in fact increased in patients with primary hyperparathyroidism and decreased in patients with hypoparathyroidism. BERNSTEIN *et al.* (1963) showed a decreased calcium clearance in patients with hypoparathyroidism given parathyroid hormone during calcium infusion. They also pointed out the importance of associating the calcium clearance with the level of the plasma diffusible calcium. Since some doubt remained, it was decided to investigate this further.

Patients studied

Three groups of patients were studied. Firstly, eight patients with osteoporosis and normal renal function; secondly, nine patients with recurrent renal stone with normal parathyroid function and creatinine clearances; thirdly, eight patients with hyperparathyroidism with normal creatinine clearances.

Methods

The calcium: creatinine clearance ratios, and the calcium reabsorbed per 100 ml of filtrate, were estimated in all the patients with renal stone disease and those with osteoporosis before and during the infusion of 10% calcium gluconate in physiological saline. 22.5 mg of calcium/kg was infused over 6 hours in six of the osteoporotic patients and eight patients with renal stone disease. In the remaining two osteoporotic subjects, and one patient with renal stone disease, 15 mg/kg of calcium was infused over 4 hours. Two patients with primary hyperparathyroidism were studied in a similar manner each being given 15 mg of calcium/kg over 4 hours. Urine samples were collected over one hour periods, and blood samples were taken at the midpoints of the urine collections. In a further six patients with primary hyperparathyroidism, the calcium:creatinine clearance ratios and re-absorption of calcium per 100 ml of filtrate were estimated during two hour urine collections, a blood sample being taken at the midpoint of the collection.

Calcium was estimated in plasma, ultrafiltrate and urine by a modification of the Autoanalyzer technique (MACFADYEN *et al.*, 1965). Creatinine was estimated by the standard Autoanalyzer technique (Technicon Instruments Limited). Ultrafiltration was performed on fresh serum, transferred to cellophane tubing without exposure to the atmosphere and centrifuged at 37 °C for one hour at 2,000 g in tubes similar to those devised by TORIBARA *et al.* (1957).

Results

The calcium:creatinine clearance ratios are seen to be directly related to the plasma ultrafilterable calciums in all three groups of patients. In Fig. 1 it can be seen that the calcium:creatinine clearance ratios in patients with [1] primary hyperpara-

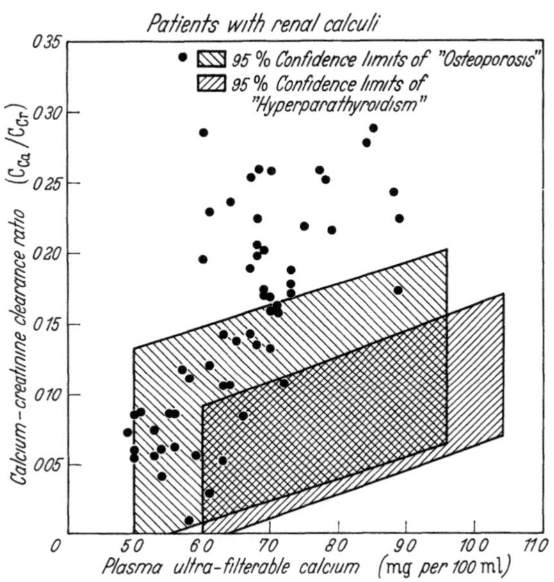

Fig. 1. This shows the relation of calcium; creatinine clearance ration to plasma ultrafilterable calcium in patients with osteoporosis (y = 0.016x — 0.019±0.068; r = .47, P < .0001), primary hyperparathyroidism (y = 0.018 — 0.065±.050; r = .66, P < .001) and renal stone (dots)

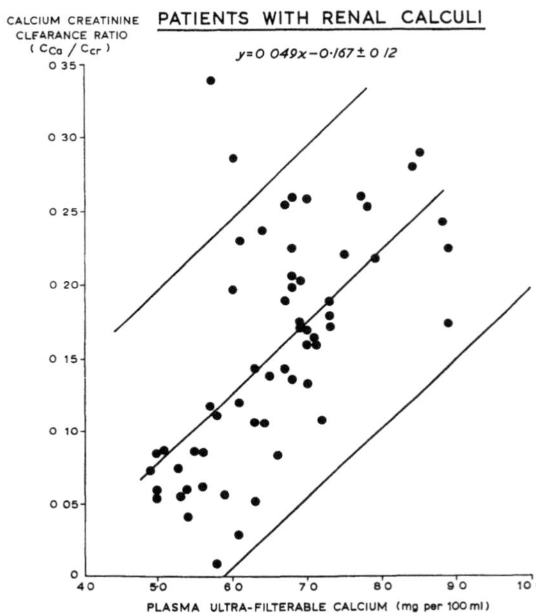

Fig. 2. The relation between the calcium: creatinine clearance ratio and plasma ultrafilterable calcium in patients with renal stone (r = .63, P < .001)

thyroidism are lower than the clearance ratios in the osteoporotic patients, the 95% confidence limits of the data being shown by the cross-hatched areas. The differences between the clearances of ultrafilterable calciums between 6 and 9.5 mg% are highly significant (P < .001). In the patients with renal stone disease, the calcium:creatinine clearance ratios are significantly higher than in the patients with primary hyper-

[1] The data obtained during calcium infusion and the results from the 2 hour urine collections and mid point blood samples were tested seperately but found not to differ significantly and the date therefore pooled.

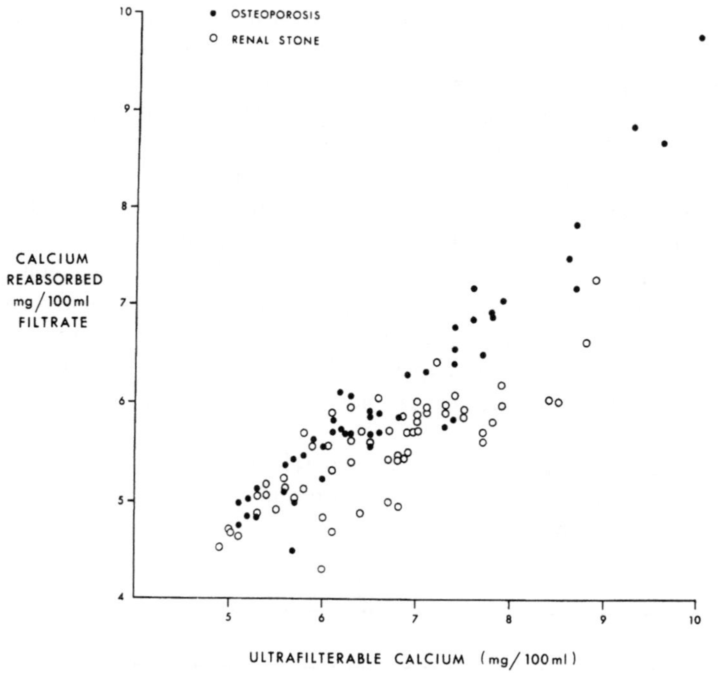

Fig. 3. The relation between re-absorption of calcium per 100 ml. filtrate and plasma ultrafilterable calcium in patients with renal stone and osteoporosis

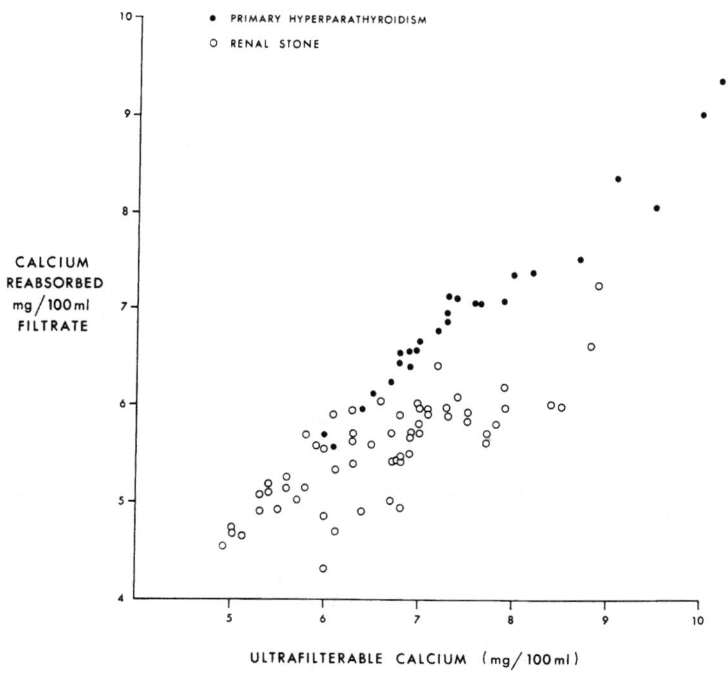

Fig. 4. The relation between re-absorption of calcium per 100 ml. filtrate and plasma ultrafilterable calcium in patients with osteoporosis and primary hyperparathyroidism

parathyroidism and those with osteoporosis, this being more apparent at higher levels of ultrafilterable calcium. Fig. 2 shows the distribution of the data obtained in the patients with renal stone disease with the 95% confidence limits.

In Fig. 3 the re-absorption of calcium per 100 ml of filtrate is related to the plasma ultrafilterable calcium in patients with osteoporosis and renal stone. The re-absorption of calcium in patients with renal stone is significantly lower than in the osteoporotic group, especially at the higher levels of plasma ultrafilterable calcium. It is also evident that the maximum tubular re-absorption of calcium is approached only in the patients with renal stone, and this occurs at about a value of 6 mg per 100 ml of glomerular filtrate. Fig. 4 shows the tubular re-absorption in the osteoporotic and hyperparathyroid patients. The tubular re-absorption is slightly higher in patients with primary hyperparathyroidism. It is evident that a maximum tubular re-absorption of calcium has not been reached in the hyperparathyroid patients.

The percentage re-absorption of calcium falls in all three groups of patients as the plasma calcium rises during calcium infusion, a typical example being shown from each group in Table 1.

Table 1

Patient	Diagnosis	% Reabsorption of calcium
A. M.	Osteoporosis	95.9
		94.6
		92.7
		90.6
		90.2
		87.2
		85.8
A. S.	Renal stone disease	91.2
		91.3
		87.3
		85.6
		84.0
		74.0
		77.0
H. C.	Primary hyperparathyroidism	95.5
		94.0
		90.0
		87.0
		85.6

Discussion

The lowered calcium clearance and slightly raised calcium re-absorption in patients with primary hyperparathyroidism would tend to support the evidence of KLEEMAN *et al.* (1958) and BERNSTEIN *et al.* (1963). The increased calcium clearance and decreased re-absorption in patients with renal stone disease has not been described before, and strongly suggests a specific tubular resorptive defect for calcium. In contrast to the findings of MCPHERSON (1959), it is only in this group that a Tm for calcium was approached. Since the calcium clearance and re-absorption is so different in patients with renal stone disease and primary hyperparathyroidism, it is suggested that the estimation of càlcium clearance during a calcium gluconate infusion might help to establish the diagnosis in those patients in whom the diagnosis remains in some doubt. The importance of relating clearance or re-absorption to the level of plasma ultrafilterable calcium is stressed as the percentage re-absorption falls in all three groups of patients as the plasma ultrafilterable calcium rises. If this is not taken into consideration an apparently lower tubular re-absorption of calcium will be seen in patients with primary hyperparathyroidism as they have a higher ultrafilterable calcium than normal subjects.

References

BERNSTEIN, D., C. R. KLEEMAN, and M. H. MAXWELL: The effect of calcium infusions, parathyroid hormone and vitamin D on renal clearance of calcium. Proc. Soc. exp. Biol. **112**, 353 (1963).

GORDAN, G. S., H. F. LOKEN, A. BLUM, and J. S. TEAL: Renal handling of calcium in parathyroid disorders. Metabolism **11**, 94 (1962).

KLEEMAN, C. R., R. E. ROCKNEY, and M. H. MAXWELL: The effect of parathyroid extract (PTE) on the renal clearance of diffusible calcium. J. clin. Invest. (Abstract) **37**, 907 (1958).

LOKEN, H. F., and G. S. GORDAN: Renal mechanisms in the production of hypercalcaemia in hyperparathyroidism and breast cancer. J. clin. Invest. (Abstract) **38**, 1021 (1959).

MACFADYEN, I. J., B. E. C. NORDIN, D. A. SMITH, D. J. WAYNE, and S. L. RAE: Effect of variation in dietary calcium on plasma concentration and urinary excretion of calcium. Brit. med. J. **1**, 161 (1965).

MCPHERSON, G. D.: Regulation of plasma calcium in man. Thesis. University of British Columbia 1959.

TORIBARA, T. Y., A. R. TEREPKA, and P. A. Dewey: The ultrafilterable calcium of human serum. I. Ultrafiltration methods and normal values. J. clin. Invest. **40**, 738 (1957).

Bony Targets of Non-"skeletal" Hormones

G. NICHOLS, JR.

Harvard Medical School, Department of Medicine, Boston, Mass., U.S.A.

Even the most superficial review of the older literature in endocrinology quickly reveals that there was a time when skeletal changes were considered to be among the important features expected in any endocrine disorder. It seemed obvious, for example, that changes in skeletal growth should be a prominent if not central feature of disturbances of pituitary function and growth hormone secretion. Thus, as the effects of other endocrine glands — thyroid, adrenal, gonads — began to be explored it was not surprising that the list of organ systems examined almost always included the skeleton. Thanks to this broad view a considerable number of empiric observations about hormonal effects on bone gradually accumulated (SILBERBERG and SILBERBERG, 1956; ASLING and EVANS, 1956). In some instances this search for skeletal effects was richly rewarded, as in the case of the parathyroids. In others, the effect could only be clearly shown in certain species as for example the marked influence of female sex hormones on avian bone (KYES, 1934). In still another group — the thyroid and adrenals are good examples — while effects on the skeleton were seen these were far less dramatic than the effects observed in other organs and systems.

The inevitable result of these early discoveries of different degrees of organ response to various humeral agents was the development of the concept of target organs or systems for each hormone. The classic example of this idea, of course, was its application to the anterior lobe of the pituitary. Once the secretion by the hypophysis of trophic hormones for other endocrine organs had been shown, several things happened. First, there was an enormous surge forward in understanding the systems for the control of body processes. Not only could endocrinologists use this concept in "reverse" to predict the existence of trophic hormones for each endocrine gland, but in addition it provided the necessary background for the development of the whole theory of feed-back control — a control system now recognized as one of the most fundamental in all living systems.

However, this target organ concept had another, perhaps less desirable, outgrowth. Attention became so closely focused on the effects of each hormone on what appeared to be its particular target that interest in its effects in other areas tended to wane. On the positive side this resulted in the learning of all sorts of details concerning the nuances of the action of each hormone. On the negative side, so many details were learned that the study of each hormone's action on its chief target threatened to become a field of specialization in itself while the broader biological influences of these agents tended to be forgotten.

Two phenomena combined to rescue the field of endocrinology from a limbo of ultimate reductionism. First, as the focus of experimental approaches to endocrine effects improved a number of inconsistencies and even contradictions in the apparent actions of hormones were revealed. These not only further complicated the field but convinced many that a number of effects long accepted as primary were in reality only secondary reflections of effects on more fundamental processes. Second, biochemists and cellular physiologists having described a number of metabolic pathways and having found them to be common to many types of cells began to become interested in hormones as potential controls for these processes.

The outcome of all this has been the development of a new phase in endocrinology — one in which the old complexities are beginning to be set aside in favor of concepts of more universal application. Hormones are being classified in terms of chemical structure, and hormone effects are being sought at the molecular rather than the tissue or organ system level. Although so far attention has remained focused largely upon effects on specific target organs, the fact that the systems which are being examined are common to many cells suggests that similar effects are going to be found in many other tissues — even bone. Thus a variety of hormones once thought important in the control of bone metabolism and then ignored in the face of the more dramatic effects of others with clearer skeletal effects promise to become again the subject of fruitful investigation.

My purpose in this discussion will be to review some of the ideas about cell physiology and general biochemistry upon which this new phase of endocrinology is based and indicate how they can be used to formulate and test hypotheses regarding sites and mechanisms of hormone action. In so doing I shall use bone and bone cell physiology as my model — not because in most cases such effects have even been considered in bone — but rather because it is the tissue of ultimate interest in this symposium and can be used advantageously to indicate how widely these ideas can be applied. At the end I will attempt to indicate how far these ideas have actually been carried with respect to skeletal physiology. While little material of this sort has been available the situation should be very different after this session.

The first step needed to develop these concepts is to review the anatomy and physiology of a cell in order to identify potential sites for hormone action. To this end the chief physiological systems of a bone cell have been drawn schematically in Fig. 1. Clearly this is a biochemist's cell, since all the processes carried on by a variety of bone cell types have been confined inside a single cell wall! However, despite the obvious violation of anatomical truth, this diagram can serve to illustrate the important points.

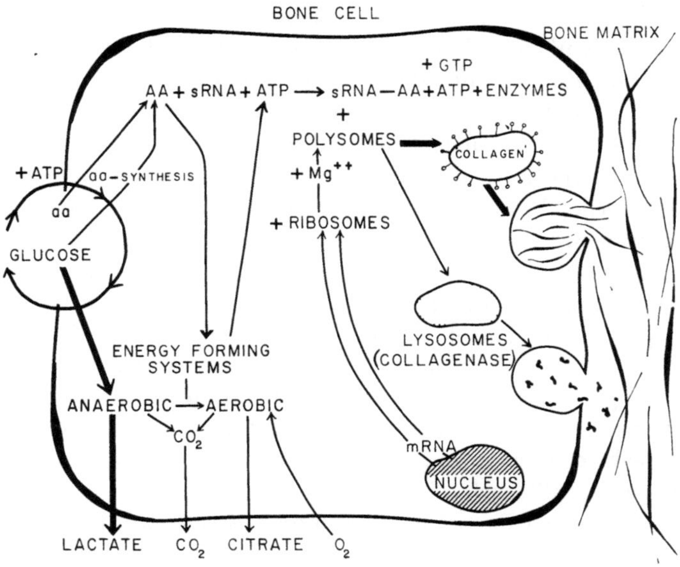

Fig. 1. A biochemist's view of a bone cell (see text for details)

Three general schemes of metabolism are shown which represent the 3 major functions of bone cells: a scheme for the biosynthesis, storage, and release of a structural protein, collagen, which is, of course, the matrix upon which the mineral phase is ultimately deposited (GLIMCHER, 1960); a scheme illustrating the biosynthesis, storage and release of an enzyme, collagenase, which is specifically required for the resorption of bone matrix (NICHOLS, 1963; WOODS and NICHOLS, 1963; WOODS and NICHOLS, in press); and a scheme representing the systems which produce the chemical energy to drive these processes (BORLE *et al.*, 1960). Although these represent only a fraction of the metabolic paths present they are sufficient to remind us of the major features of the systems available for hormonal control.

All 3 begin with the transfer of substrates across the cell membrane. This can occur by diffusion, illustrated by the passage of O_2; by transport, which, when requiring energy, leads to intracellular concentration of substrates as shown here for glucose and amino-acids (FLANAGAN and NICHOLS, unpublished studies) or by the process of pinocytosis. Similar membrane transfer systems, responsible for maintenance of normal intracellular concentrations of salts and water, have been omitted for simplicity.

Once inside, substrates can be used for a variety of purposes. Glucose and amino-acids have both been shown to serve as fuel for energy producing systems. These, we know, follow the same general scheme in bone as in all tissues — hexoses are degraded in step-wise fashion through the glycolytic pathway to pyruvate. Unlike most tissues, however, the majority of this pyruvate is used in bone to form lactate which is excreted from the cell while only about 10 per cent goes on through the tricarboxylic acid cycle. Thus ATP is produced both anaerobically and aerobically (presumably via mitochondrial oxidative phosphorylation) with the release of chiefly "non-volatile" acid end products — lactic and citric acids — which seem likely to play an important role in bone resorption and calcium homeostasis (NICHOLS, 1963).

Amino-acids (FLANAGAN and NICHOLS, 1962), concentrated in the cell sap by active transport or synthesized intracellularly from carbohydrate precursors (FLANAGAN and NICHOLS, 1964), are used chiefly in the biosynthesis of proteins. In the diagram a single common pathway for protein synthesis is shown because only one is believed to exist — the particular amino-acid sequence characteristic of each protein being determined by the particular messenger RNA upon which the polysome which makes it is assembled. The messenger RNA is represented as being derived from the nucleus — a notion whose application to bone cells is supported by recent experiments (SIMMONS and NICHOLS, 1964; STEINBERG and NICHOLS, unpublished studies). Current belief, of course, holds that at least part of this nuclear RNA is a complementary copy of a section of a DNA chain in which is encoded the necessary information for specifying the structure of the protein whose synthesis is guided by the RNA "messenger". The arrow representing the transfer of messenger RNA to the polysomes has been made double to remind us that the differences between the systems which make collagen on the one hand and collagenase on the other probably lie at this "informational" level.

One other point about these 2 bone cell products is shown. Both are thought to be stored in membrane bounded vacuoles before being released into the extracellular space (PORTER, 1964; WOODS and NICHOLS, in press). Although the apparent intermittency of collagen deposition under certain conditions (TANZER, 1964) suggests that this feature might be important in the control of new bone matrix synthesis, no evidence on this point is yet available. However, recent evidence (ASHER and NICHOLS, 1965) suggests that the storage of collagenase in such intracellular bodies may offer an important means of controlling bone resorption.

Having refreshed our memory regarding the main features of bone cells and their physiology we can examine these schemes and current biochemical knowledge for likely hormone targets. Three general areas where hormones might act form the 3 main headings of Fig. 2. Possible mechanisms of action at the molecular level under each heading are listed below it — predictions which are based on what is commonly known about the biochemistry, biophysics, and fine structure of cells. The fact that these mechanisms occur in more than one area is indicated by repetitions and the arrows between headings.

The extraordinary prominence of membranes in the structure of all cells suggests that the rates of cellular metabolic processes could readily be controlled by regulating the passage of materials across these boundaries, as indicated by the first heading. Three general modes of transfer across membranes are known: 1) *diffusion* whose rate depends on the physical characteristics of the membrane and an electrochemical gradient; 2) *pinocytosis* — the name currently given to the active engulfing of materials by cells through invaginations of the plasma membrane; and 3) the *processes of transport* under which name all cell membrane transfer systems involving the concept of a carrier have been grouped.

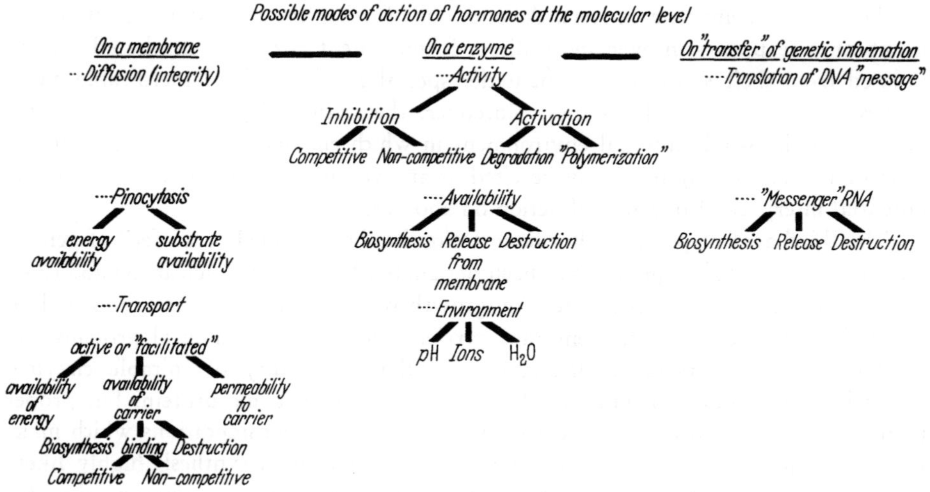

Fig. 2.

The rate of transfer of a substance by any of these methods depends on a variety of factors potentially amenable to modification by hormones. Even the rate of transfer by diffusion (the simplest case) depends on pore size, charge, bound ions etc. while the 2 more complex processes are often coupled to cell metabolic activity and potentially depend on a host of items. Thus pinocytosis, which clearly involves cell movement and new membrane synthesis, must depend at least on the availability of pools of energy and appropriate substrate. In the case of transport, besides energy to drive the system, a carrier must be supplied whose movement in the membrane (real or apparent) depends on some of the same factors as diffusion. The availability of this carrier to transport a given molecular species will, in turn, depend on its rate of biosynthesis, its rate of destruction, and the degree to which it is bound — either to the material under study or some competitive molecule. While this analysis obviously could be carried further enough has been said to indicate the general line of reasoning which can be pursued.

Clearly, the processes of transport, pinocytosis and even diffusion must ultimately depend on enzymes and their activity. Thus potential effects of hormones on enzymes form the second major area which must be considered in any survey of molecular mechanisms which might be affected by these substances.

A direct effect of a hormone on an enzyme or enzyme system could occur in 3 ways: through direct modification of its action on its substrate, through changes in the total quantity of enzyme available, or through changes in the local environment in which it has to act. As in the case of potential effects on membrane transfer systems, possible modes of action each worthy of investigation are suggested for each category by current knowledge. It is noteworthy that when these are examined the only wholly novel possible actions which present themselves in this area are those related directly to enzyme activity through inhibition — competitive or non-competitive — or activation by degradation of a zymogen or polymerization of inactive subunits. When enzyme *availability* is considered, relative rates of synthesis and destruction which must depend in turn on the availability and activity of still other enzymes offer potential controls very reminiscent of the factors controlling the availability of membrane carriers. As one looks further the potential importance of membranes reappears in even more direct form. Potent enzymes may be effectively isolated from their substrates except under special conditions by impermeable membranes as is the case in lysosomes. Moreover, the critical dependence of the composition of the whole internal environment in which enzymes act on the activity of membrane transport systems may be cited as an even more dramatic example of the potential interplay of one area of action on another.

The third area of potential hormone action has been termed "transfer" of genetic information but could equally have been designated "control of nuclear metabolism". In any case its inclusion is a direct outgrowth of the notion that the rates of biosynthesis and destruction of membrane carriers, membranes, structural proteins and metabolic energy depend fundamentally on the availability of suitable enzymes which in turn implies not only synthesis of the proper enzyme proteins but proper guidance and integration of the entire system as well — considerations which make the metabolic processes by which cell nuclei control protein synthesis highly likely targets for hormonal influence. Once this view is entertained numerous sites for hormone action suggest themselves ranging from selection of the DNA "message" to be "transcribed" through the steps involved in the biosynthesis, release, transport, utilization and destruction of "messenger" RNA. Each of these steps, it must be remembered, probably involves in its turn enzymes and thus protein synthesis etc. — even the veiling and unveiling of genetic loci on DNA strands may depend on protein formation and interaction if JACOB and MONOD's (1961) concepts of repression and de-repression can be proven applicable in animal systems. Finally, the factors which affect transfer of substances across membranes, in this case the nuclear membrane, again must be considered. Thus when this third area of possible hormone activity is reviewed the same handful of mechanisms seem to be the ones available for mediation of hormone influences on metabolism.

These thoughts lead inevitably to the view that only 3 modes of action of hormones at the molecular level seem possible — *effects on membrane structure* yielding changes in permeability; *direct inhibition or activation of enzyme activity;* and effects on the cell nucleus resulting in qualitative or quantitative changes in the *transcription of genetic information* which are reflected by changes in messenger RNA and protein synthesis. The next step is to see how well present evidence of hormonal action at the molecular level appears to fit these predictions. The few examples which follow have been selected from the many available to illustrate that hormone effects on each of the 3 basic mechanisms postulated have now been demonstrated.

The first of these — a direct effect on membrane structure and permeability — is well illustrated by the increase in the bulk flow of water across the toad's bladder induced by vasopressin. Fig. 3 taken from HAYS and LEAF's (1962) original paper clearly indicates that the flux of water across this membrane under a variety of osmotic gradients is several fold greater when vasopressin is added *in vitro*, apparently because of an increase in the effective size of the pores in the membrane. Moreover, later studies (FRAZIER and LEAF, 1964) indicate that increases in the permeability of the mucosal surface of the bladder epithelial cells to sodium account for the increased active transport of his ion which is similarly induced. Thus the rate of an active transport system as well as the more obvious passive flow of water across the bladder epithelium can be controlled by changes in membrane permeability.

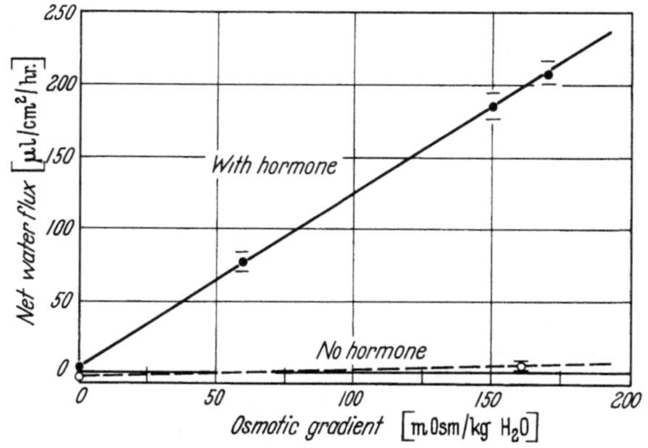

Fig. 3. The increased flux of water through the isolated toad bladder at various osmotic gradients which is induced by vasopressin *in vitro*. (From HAYS and LEAF 1962, reproduced with the permission of the authors.)

Other instances of hormone effects on membrane transfer such as the effects of growth hormone on cellular amino-acid uptake (KNOBIL and HOTCHKISS, 1964) and the apparent stimulation of pinocytosis by insulin (BALL and BARNETT, 1960) might also be cited as examples. However, in neither case has the ultimate molecular mechanism been as clearly demonstrated.

One other hormone mediated membrane effect should be mentioned because of its possible importance in bone resorption. This is the effect of certain steroids upon the stability of the lipid membranes which confine the hydrolases of lysosomes. WEISSMAN'S (in press) intriguing observations of the contrasting effects of neutral steroids depending on their steric form suggest that these agents can become incorporated into lipid membranes and thereby alter their structure in a significant way.

Turning to the second postulated molecular mode of action of hormones — direct action on an enzyme — a number of examples of apparent hormone effects on enzyme binding of substrates or cofactors including effects of gonadal, adrenal, thyroid and pituitary secretions have recently been cited in a review by a number of authors (LITWACK and KRITCHEVSKY, 1964). However, the observations of TOMPKINS *et al.* (1963) regarding the effects of certain steroids on glutamic dehydrogenase activity provide a model of another kind of effect whose precision of definition compels me to use it as my example. In these experiments the rate of oxidation of glutamate by crystalline enzyme from liver was followed by the reduction of DPN in the presence of various concentrations of several different estrogenic steroids. As shown in Fig. 4 taken from a recent publication (TOMPKINS and YIELDING, 1964) all inhibited the reaction although to different degrees. Subsequently these workers have shown that this effect is secondary to reversible steroid-induced dissociation of the protein subunits which make up the enzyme. The fact that the dissociated subunits turn out to have increased alanine dehydrogenase activity provides an added embellishment to these experiments which so elegantly demonstrate this hormonal effect on an enzyme's structure.

The third and final molecular target proposed — the transcription of genetic information — has become such a popular site in which to seek the basic action of one's favorite hormone that it is difficult to settle upon a suitable example! The one I have selected, drawn from some experiments by WIDNELL and TATA (1963), concerns the action of triiodothyronine *in vivo* on metabolic activities in fractions of liver

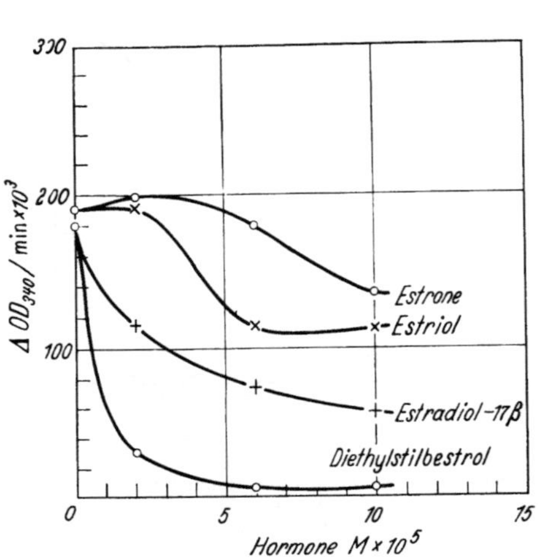

FIG. 4. Inhibition of glutamic dehydrogenase activity by various estrogenic steroids, measured as the change in O.D. due to reduction of DPN, 2×10^{-4} M, present in the system. (From TOMPKINS and YIELDING 1964, reproduced with the permission of the publishers.)

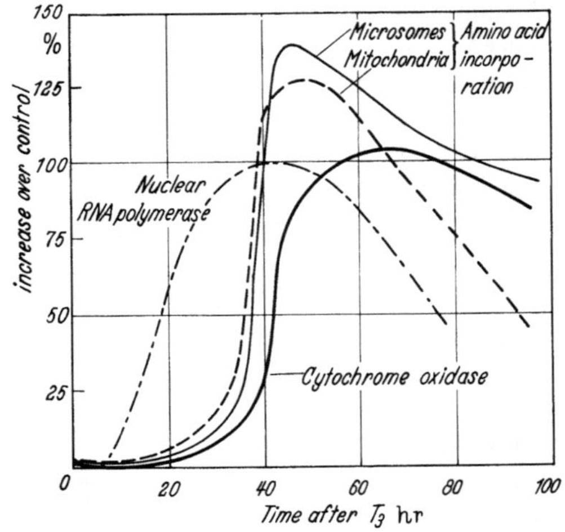

FIG. 5. An idealized diagram showing the sequential changes in activity of various nuclear and cytoplasmic metabolic processes in liver at various times after a single injection of triiodothyronine into thyroidectomized rats. (From TATA 1964, reproduced with the permission of the publisher.)

taken from thyroidectomized rats. Fig. 5 was selected (TATA, 1964) because it shows so clearly the time sequence involved — from the earliest effect on nuclear RNA polymerases through the synthesis of new protein and the availability of additional cytochrome activity to the final disappearance of each change. Moreover, these experiments emphasize that the place where such hormonal effects should be sought is at the earliest point in the metabolic system — in this case the transcription of information from DNA by RNA synthesis. Evidence (often derived from studies with various metabolic inhibitors) of similar sorts of effects produced by steroids, insulin, and various trophic hormones is rapidly becoming available (LITWACK and KRITCHEVSKY, 1964; TOMPKINS and MAXWELL, 1963).

Before leaving this area one more point should be made. While current fashion tends to dictate that an effect on the "interpretation" of DNA is the ultimate in "molecular" endocrinology behind which it is not necessary to look for earlier or more basic effects, it must be remembered that such changes — be they qualitative or quantitative — must involve changes in enzyme activity and hence perhaps protein synthesis. Which came first, change in DNA or change in protein may well be a question, therefore, which is far from being solved!

The present status, then, can be summarized quite simply: Knowledge of cell physiology, structure, and metabolic pathways permits the prediction of sites and modes of action of hormones on purely theoretical grounds — a process which leads to the conclusion that hormones act in only 3 ways at the molecular level. Moreover, the application of these ideas to studying the effects of a variety of hormones on several tissues has already supplied abundant evidence of the validity and usefulness of these concepts. What remains to be done is to examine how far these ideas have been applied to studies of the effects of the "non-skeletal" hormones on the potential targets in bone.

Here the field of investigation remains largely untouched. Although a number of laboratories have been actively engaged in exploring effects of parathyroid hormone on skeletal metabolism the only available data with respect to other hormones are only just sufficient to indicate that profound and highly important effects will be found when someone undertakes to search for them. The kinds of biochemical studies so far available are illustrated in the last 3 diagrams.

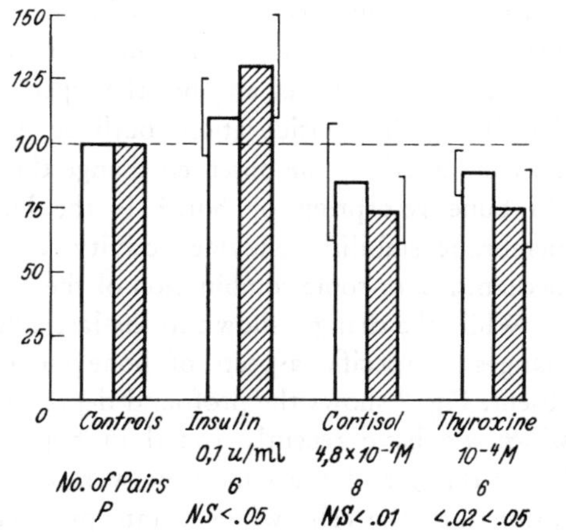

Fig. 6. *In vitro* effects of insulin, cortisol, and thyroxine on glycine-1-^{14}C incorporation into CO_2 (open bars) and organic matrix (shaded bars) of metaphyseal bone from normal rats. Substrates were glucose and glycine. (From Vaes and Nichols 1962, reprinted with permission of the editor.)

Fig. 6 although originally published by Dr. Vaes and me in 1962 remains, to my knowledge, the only demonstration of its kind in the literature. The choice of hormones was determined by information suggesting that insulin enhanced protein synthesis and amino-acid uptake in diaphram while cortisol and thyroxine were examined because of the bony lesions which seem to occur with excesses of each. Significant stimulation of glycine uptake by insulin and inhibition by both thyroxine and cortisol were observed in the experiments with rat bone — effects which in the case of cortisol, at least, seemed to fit with available information regarding bony changes in hyperadrenocortical states. Nothing further was done at that time, but recently we have begun some further experiments using pigs to explore the details of these effects. To our surprise, only the effects of insulin have been possible to confirm. Both cortisone and thyroxine appear to stimulate rather than to inhibit aminoacid uptake and collagen synthesis in this species (Nichols, unpublished experiments). While the reasons for these differences are not clear they indicate clearly the importance of variations between species and tissues in determining the nature of hormone effects even at the molecular level!

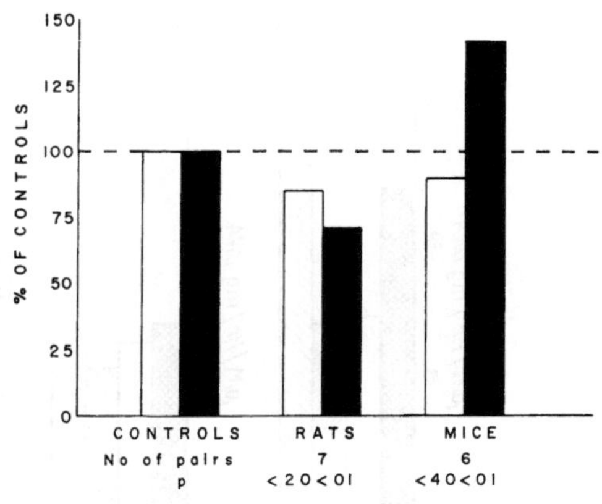

Fig. 7. Contrasting effects of estradiol treatment on the incorporation of glycine-1-^{14}C into CO_2 (clear bars) and organic matrix (shaded bars) of metaphyseal bone from male rats and mice. Rats received estradiol valerate in oil s.c., 2.0 mg. in 4 doses 6 days apart, mice 2 mg. in 4 doses 6 days apart. Controls received oil s.c. only. (Recalculated from data of Vaes and Nichols 1962.)

This species' variability may be even better illustrated by the difference in the uptake of glycine into male rat and mouse bone following estradiol treatment. As shown in Fig. 7 (VAES and NICHOLS, 1962) incorporation into bone was *depressed* by estradiol in rats while *stimulated* in mice. These findings, which confirmed histologic observations, indicate that in rats estrogens *inhibit* bone resorption while in mice they *stimulate* new bone formation. Thus the accumulation of cancellous bone in the marrow cavities of the long bones which results in both species occurs for entirely different reasons. Clearly, these observations show the need to explore hormone effects in depth if understanding is to be obtained sufficient to predict actions in other tissues and in other species — predictions which are so important in the clinic. The considerations outlined earlier indicate the kind of question which must be asked: Is the observed change the result of changes in new bone synthesis or old bone resorption or both? Is the hormone affecting membrane permeability, membrane stability, enzyme activity, the biosynthesis of proteins through nuclear mechanisms, or some combination of these factors?

While the changes shown in the last 2 diagrams were relatively small, very marked changes in specific aspects of bone metabolism occur when certain hormones are absent. Fig. 8 shows the profound depression in the rate of bone collagen biosynthesis which we have recently found in hypophysectomized and thyroidectomized rats. Lesser changes of the same type were also found in O_2 uptake and proline incorporation into the cells while lactate production was not significantly changed. Interestingly none of these effects were reproduced by parathyroidectomy alone. Again the details remain to be explored, but the relation of these observations to the growth failure noted in animals and patients deprived of pituitary or thyroid secretions during the growth phase seems clear.

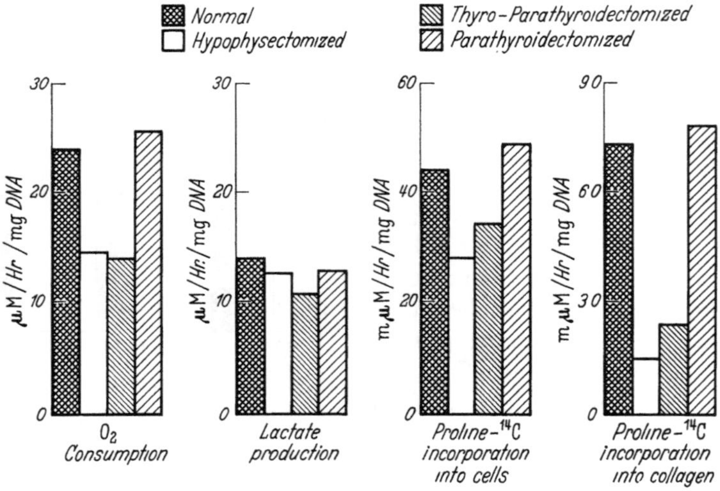

Fig. 8. Changes in several *in vitro* metabolic indices induced in rat bone by removal of various endocrine organs 10 days before sacrifice

One other indication of the importance of these hormones in the control of bone cell metabolism has recently been pointed out by JOHNSTON and DEISS (1965). The presence of an intact pituitary seems to be necessary for the development of some of the late effects of parathyroid extract on bone metabolism — an example of "permissive" effects of these hormones in bone which appears to be confirmed by recent experiments in our laboratory.

In closing a few general remarks seem in order. Clearly the whole subject of effects of "non-skeletal" hormones on bone while once popular has been passing through a period of partial eclipse during which only the clinician, faced as he always is with the need to aleviate the distresses of the sick, has maintained an interest in how these substances may modify skeletal behavior. During the same time new views in endocrinology, based in biochemistry and cellular physiology, have been developing which provide new insights into the fundamental modes of action of many hormones. While these have yet to be applied systematically to bone, the need to do so is obvious; the way to pursue such studies seems clear; and all that is needed now is to get to work.

Acknowledgements

Unpublished work quoted in this communication was supported by grants from the National Institutes of Health, USPHS. The technical assistance of H. Alstrup, N. Steinberg, S. Ault and R. Smith is gratefully acknowledged.

References

Asher, J. D., and G. Nichols, Jr.: Heparin stimulation of bone collagenase activity. Fed. Proc. (Abstract) **24**, 211 (1965).

Asling, C. W., and H. M. Evans: Anterior pituitary regulation of skeletal development. In The Biochemistry and Physiology of Bone. Bourne, G. H. (ed.). New York: Academic Press 1956, p. 671.

Ball, E. G., and R. J. Barnett: Insulin and pinocytosis. Diabetes **9**, 70 (1960).

Borle, A. B., N. Nichols, and G. Nichols, Jr.: Metabolic studies of bone *in vitro*. I. Normal bone. J. biol. Chem. **235**, 1206 (1960).

Flanagan, B., and G. Nichols, Jr.: Metabolic studies of bone *in vitro*. IV. Collagen biosynthesis by surviving bone fragments *in vitro*. J. biol. Chem. **237**, 3686 (1962).

— — Metabolic studies of bone *in vitro*. V. Glucose metabolism and collagen biosynthesis. J. biol. Chem. **239**, 1261 (1964).

Frazier, H. S., and A. Leaf: Cellular mechanisms in the control of body fluids. Medicine **43**, 281 (1964).

Glimcher, M. J.: Specificity of the molecular structure of organic matrices in mineralization. In Calcification in Biological Systems. Sognnaes, R. F. (ed.). Washington: Amer. Ass. Advanc. Sci. 1960, p. 421.

Hays, R., and A. Leaf: Studies of the movement of water through the isolated toad bladder and its modifications by vasopressin. J. gen. Physiol. **45**, 905 (1962).

Jacob, F., and J. Monod: On the regulation of gene activity. Cold Spring Harbor Symp. on Quant. Biol. **26**, 193 (1961).

Johnston, C. C., jr., and W. P. Deiss, jr.: Some effects of hypophysectomy and parathyroid extract on bone matrix biosynthesis. Endocrinology **76**, 198 (1965).

Knobil, E., and J. Hotchkiss: Growth hormone. Amer. Rev. Physiol. **26**, 47 (1964).

Kyes, P., and T. S. Potter: Physiological marrow ossification in female pigeons. Anat. Rec. **60**, 377 (1934).

Litwack, G., and D. Kritchevsky: Actions of Hormones on Molecular Processes. New York: John Wiley and Sons. 1964.

Nichols, G., jr.: *In vitro* Studies of bone resorptive mechanisms. In Mechanisms of Hard Tissue Destruction. Sognnaes, R. F. (ed.). Washington: Amer. Ass. Advanc. Sci. 1963, p. 557.

Porter, K. R.: Cell fine structure and biosynthesis of intracellular macromolecules. In- Connective Tissue: Intracellular Macromolecules. Proc. Symp. Sponsored by the New York Heart Assoc. Boston: Little, Brown 1964, p. 167.

Silberberg, M., and R. Silberberg: Steroid hormones and bone. In The Biochemistry and Physiology of Bone. Bourne, G. H. (ed.). New York: Academic Press 1956, p. 623.

Simmons, D., and G. Nichols, Jr.: Diurnal variations in the metabolic activity of bone and cartilage. Argonne National Laboratory, Radiological Physics Div., Summary Report. ANL-6938, July 1963 — June 1964, p. 179.

Tanzer, M. L., and J. Gross: Collagen metabolism in the normal and lathyric chick. J. exp. Med. **119**, 275 (1964).

Tata, J. R.: Biological action of thyroid hormones at the cellular and molecular levels. In Actions of Hormones on Molecular Processes. Litwack, G., and D. Kritchevsky (eds.) New York: John Wiley and Sons 1964, p. 58.

Tompkins, G. M., and E. S. Maxwell: Some aspects of steroid hormone action. Ann. Rev. Biochem. **32**, 677 (1963).

—, and K. L. Yielding: Action of steroid hormones on glutamic dehydrogenase. In Action of Hormones on Molecular Processes. Litwack, G., and D. Kritchevsky (eds.). New York: John Wiley and Sons 1964, p. 209.

— —, N. Tolol, and J. F. Curran: Protein structure and biological regulation. Cold Spring Harbor Symp. on Quant. Biol. **28**, 461 (1963).

Vaes, G., and G. Nichols, jr.: The metabolism of glycine-l-C^{14} by bone *in vitro;* effects of hormones and other factors. Endocrinology **70**, 890 (1962).

Weissman, G.: Studies on lysosomes. VI. The effect of neutral steroids and bile acids on lysosomes *in vitro*. Biochem. Pharmacol. (in press).

Widnell, C. C., and J. R. Tata: Stimulation of nuclear RNA polymerase during the latent period of action of thyroid hormones. Biochim. biophys. Acta. **72**, 506 (1963).

Woods, J. F., and G. Nichols, Jr.: Collagenolytic activity in mammalian bone. Science **142**, 386 (1963).

— — Collagenolytic activity in rat bone cells: characteristics and intracelleluar location. J. cell. Biol. **26**, 747 (1965).

Hormones and Calcium Metabolism

B. E. C. Nordin

Mineral Metabolism unit, the General Infirmary, Leeds, England

Introduction

The literature on the effects of hormones on bone and calcium metabolism is so large that it is impossible to review it adequately. All this paper will attempt to do is to report selected papers which appear to the writer to shed significant light upon the action of hormones on calcium and bone metabolism in man. Parathyroid hormone and calcitonin have been deliberately omitted.

Thyroid hormone

Thyrotoxic bone disease had been recognised for a long time when Aub *et al.* (1929) first noted the increased excretion of calcium in the urine and faeces which is a feature of hyperthyroidism. The nature of this bone disorder was not defined until much later, however, when Albright and Reifenstein (1948) recognised it as a form of osteoporosis which they attributed to malnutrition resulting from an increased requirement of protein and vitamins. This brought thyrotoxic bone disease into line with their protein matrix hypothesis for osteoporosis.

This concept that thyrotoxic osteoporosis was connected in some way with the negative nitrogen balance which is a feature of hyperthyroidism was accepted (perhaps rather uncritically) until KRANE *et al.* (1956), showing that the calcium balance might be negative even when the nitrogen balance was positive, challenged it. COOK *et al.* (1959) also failed to find any correlation between calcium and nitrogen balance in hyperthyroidism and PUPPEL *et al.* (1945) had previously shown that oral administration of calcium alone could produce a positive calcium balance in patients with hyperthyroidism.

The protein matrix concept had previously been questioned at the histological level. As early as 1933 ASKANAZY and RUTISHAUSER had shown that the histology of thyrotoxic bone disease resembled that of osteitis fibrosa, and this was subsequently confirmed by FOLLIS (1953) in a paper which has become a classic. These observations showed that the osteoporosis was probably caused by increased bone destruction rather than diminished formation.

The present view is undoubtedly that the effect of hyperthyroidism on calcium metabolism is to increase rather than decrease the rates of bone formation and destruction. KRANE *et al.* (1956) were the first to use radiocalcium to demonstrate accelerated bone turnover in thyrotoxicosis, and this observation was subsequently confirmed by FRASER *et al.* (1960) with stable strontium. The *in vitro* uptake of radiophosphorus by bone powder has been shown by HERNBERG (1960) to be increased in thyrotoxicosis and this again is taken to signify an increased rate of new bone formation. The enhancing effect of thyroid hormone on bone resorption has been demonstrated by the elevation of urinary hydroxyproline in thyrotoxicosis which has been reported by KIRIVIKKO *et al.* (1964) and BENOIT *et al.* (1963). Conversely HEANEY and WHEDON (1958) have shown the bone formation rate to be lowe in myxoedema.

It has already been mentioned that early calcium balance studies in thyrotoxicosis showed both the faecal and urinary calcium to be increased. This was amply confirmed by COOK *et al.* (1959) in calcium balances on nine cases. In four of these the urinary calcium exceeded 900 mg. daily and in four the faecal calcium exceeded the dietary intake. This latter observation suggests an increase in the endogenous faecal or digestive juice calcium, but this is not born out by examination of the data of KRANE *et al.* (1956). COOK *et al.* (1959) also found an increased faecal fat in eight of their nine patients, possibly due to intestinal hurry.

Hypercalciuria was also a feature of the hyperthyroid cases described by GREEN and LYALL (1951) and this hypercalciuria was supressed in the one patient to whom they administered alkali. This latter observation is one which we have since confirmed and we have also found (as have HERNBERG and JAKOBSEN, 1964) that the urinary calcium in thyrotoxicosis is a function of the severity of the disease. In our experience, it is correlated with the plasma level of protein bound iodine (NORDIN, 1964) (Fig. 1).

The plasma calcium also tends to rise in hyperthyroidism (HARRISON *et al.*, 1964) and a number of cases of frank hypercalcaemia have been reported (ROSE and BOLES, 1953; PRIBEK and MEADE, 1957; KLEEMAN *et al.*, 1958; GUYER, 1965). In one case (SATALINE *et al.*, 1962) this hypercalcaemia was reversed by cortisone but in another (DAVID *et al.*, 1962) it was not.

In view of the histological changes in the bone and the tendency to hypercalcaemia in thyrotoxicosis, one has to consider the activity of the parathyroid glands. Some cases have in fact been reported of simultaneous hyperthyroidism and

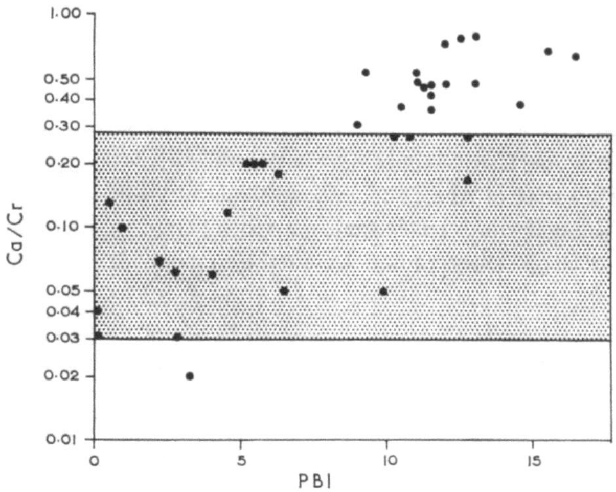

Fig. 1. Relation between plasma protein bound iodine and urinary calcium creatinine ratio in 38 thyrotoxic patients before and after radioactive iodine therapy

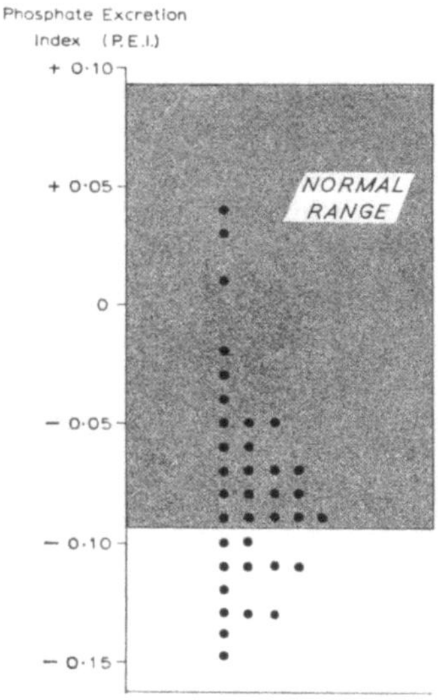

Fig. 2. Phosphate excretion indices in patients with thyrotoxicosis

hyperparathyroidism (BORTZ *et al.*, 1961). Generally, however, parathyroid activity is probably reduced in hyperthyroidism. This at least is the implication of the low phosphate clearances and subnormal response to phosphate loading reported by HARDEN *et al.* (1964) (Fig. 2), and the high Tm phosphate reported by PARSONS and ANDERSON (1964). These changes are unlikely to be due to the thyroid hormone itself.

To summarise, excessive secretion of thyroid hormone has the following effects on calcium metabolism:

It increases the rates of bone formation and resorption.

It raises the plasma and urinary calcium.

It diminishes parathyroid activity as measured by phosphate clearance.

It reduces absorption of calcium, possibly by suppressing the parathyroids.

These effects suggest that the action of the thyroid hormone on calcium metabolism is qualitatively not unlike that of the parathyroid hormone.

The gonadal hormones

It was ALBRIGHT *et al.* (1941) who first drew attention to the apparent relation between osteoporosis and the menopause when they described 42 cases of osteoporosis under the age of 65, 40 of whom were postmenopausal women. Before that time the role of oestrogens in calcium and bone metabolism in birds and mice had been appreciated (GARDNER and PFEIFFER, 1938; PFEIFFER and GARDNER, 1938) but the extension of this to man had not been envisaged.

Albright subsequently extended his concept to embrace both the male and female sex hormones. He pointed out, that osteoporosis was a feature of ovarian agenesis, which may be true (TURNER, 1938), but claimed that it was also a feature of eunuchoidism, which is open to some doubt (LABHART and COURVOISIER, 1950). Since that time, the concept that the gonadal hormones play a part in the pathogenesis of osteoporosis has been questioned by many people and the present position is confusing to say the least.

There is no doubt that the oestrogenic hormones affect calcium metabolism. Disregarding their highly specific effects in birds and mice, which have no counterpart in other species, there is convincing evidence that they inhibit the resorption of metaphyseal bone in rats (LINDQUIST *et al.*, 1960). In humans, there can be no doubt that a fall in bone volume occurs soon after the menopause in women and that a similar though less marked change occurs after the age of 50 in males. We (NORDIN *et al.*, in press) have found a fall in spinal density and metacarpal cortical thickness in women 5 to 10 years after the menopause and (like other workers in the field) we have seen several cases of osteoporosis following an artificial menopause. Moreover, the development of osteoporosis in the iliac crest starts at the age of about 50 (BECK and NORDIN, 1960) particularly in women (SAVILLE, 1962). On a recent visit to Africa, India, Japan, Central America and other countries, I observed that spinal osteoporosis did not appear in any part of the world before middle age in either males or females after which there was a sharp rise in incidence in women and a less marked rise in men (Fig. 3). It is true that DONALDSON and NASSIM (1954) found no relation between osteoporosis and artificial menopause but if one takes all the facts into account it appears probable that reduced sex hormone activity play some part, directly or indirectly, in the development of osteoporosis in women and possibly in men.

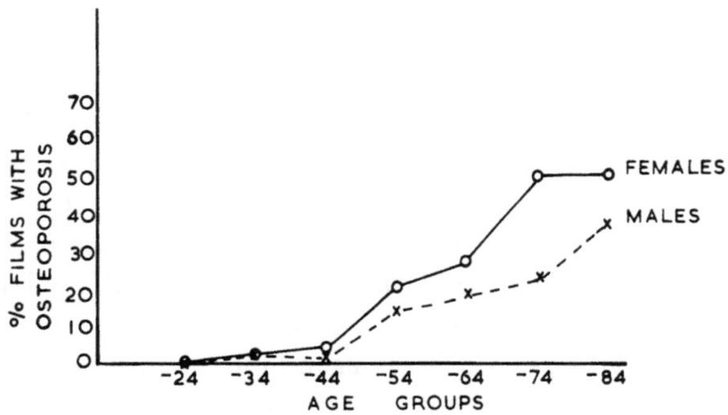

Fig. 3. Mean percentages of osteoporotic films among 373 male and 398 female lumbar spine X-rays examined in United Kingdom, India, Japan, United States and Finland

When it comes to considering the mechanism of action of sex hormones on calcium metabolism in man, one finds that the effect of the oestrogens is better established than that of the androgens. Thus the balance data of ALBRIGHT and REIFENSTEIN (1948) repeatedly demonstrate a fall in urinary calcium on the administration of oestrogenic hormones to cases of osteoporosis, although the changes in feacal calcium are less convincing. ACKERMAN *et al.* (1954) observed a slight fall in urinary calcium in elderly women given oestrogens when in negative calcium balance. HENNEMAN and WALLACH (1957) found that oestrogen therapy had improved the calcium balance in 13 out of 15 published cases. However, the only large changes in balance were those reported by ANDERSON (1950). The most convincing data are those of SHORR (1945) who showed that oestradiol benzoate lowered urinary calcium and raised urinary citrate, an observation which we have recently confirmed (Fig. 4).

The evidence regarding the effect of the androgens on calcium balance is rather scanty. Albright and Reifenstein (1948) were able to demonstrate the good effects of testosterone on several cases of osteoporosis but Ackerman *et al.* (1954) could find no effect at all. Henneman and Wallach (1957) considered that testosterone had some effect in senile men but no effect in women. Bartter (1957) reported an improvement in calcium balance in one case of osteoporosis on testosterone. Lafferty *et al.* (1964) reported that androgens and oestrogens both reduced bone resorption in osteoporosis but that after long administration a secondary decline in bone formation occurred. This is an interesting suggestion but unfortunately their method of calculating bone resorption rate is open to question.

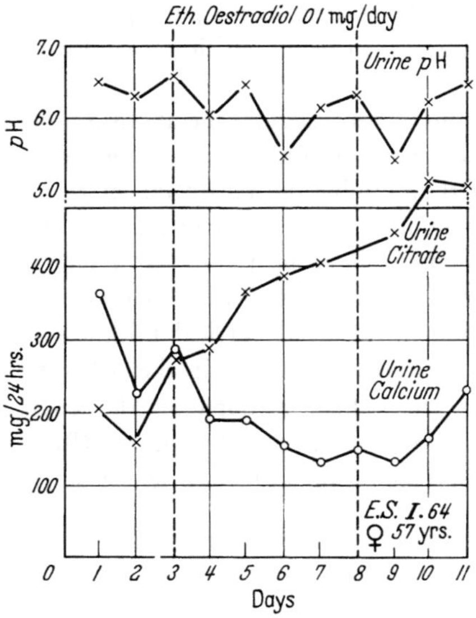

Fig. 4. Effect of ethinyl oestradiol 0.1 mg. daily on urinary pH, citrate and calcium in a 57 year old women

As far as the anabolic steroids are concerned the effect of these compounds on nitrogen balance is well established though it is not certain that the same effect could not be achieved in some instances at least by increased nitrogen intake. The effect on calcium balance is less consistent (Everse and Keep, 1961). There appears to be a fall in faecal calcium and sometimes a fall in urinary calcium but the overall effect on calcium balance is rather small and hardly comparable with that which can be achieved by high calcium feeding (Whedon, 1964). Dymling (1962) found no effect with an anabolic steroid on bone excretion rate and Gordan and Eisenberg (1963) had the same experience. Lund (1963) found at least as many cases of osteoporosis among steroid treated patients given an anabolic compound simultaneously as among those not given such supplementary therapy.

Thus it would appear that reduction of oestrogenic activity (particularly when acute) may precipitate the reduction in bone volume which we call osteoporosis and that administration of oestrogenic hormones reduces urinary calcium, raises urinary citrate and promotes a positive calcium balance. The nature of these actions cannot be explained at present, but they are unlikely to be connected with nitrogen balance on which oestrogens have little if any effect (Albright and Reifenstein, 1948). It is, therefore, probable that oestrogens influence bone in Man through an action on mineral metabolism. This has been suggested by Ranney (1959) who found that oestrone neutralised the effects of parathyroid extracts on bone turnover in mice. An alternative explanation may be found in the work of Cushman *et al.* (1965) who made the interesting observation that 17 β-oestradiol perfused into the isolated dog adrenal inhibited corticosteroid secretion. This reminds one that the effects of oestrogens on urinary calcium and citrate excretion are the reverse of those of the adrenocortical steroids.

Another little known effect of oestrogens was reported by Nassim *et al.* (1956) who found that administration of stilboestrol to 5 patients lowered the tubular reabsorption of phosphate. They attributed this to depression of the anterior pituitary and thought it might explain the hypophosphataemic action of the oestrogens previously reported by REIFENSTEIN and ALBRIGHT (1947). An alternative explanation would be, however, that the parathyroid glands were stimulated by the stilboestrol which in turn suggest that stilboestrol may lower the plasma calcium. If this were one of the actions of the oestrogenic hormones it would also explain their effect upon urinary calcium and possibly on urinary citrate, which rises with parathyroid activity (HORWITH *et al.*, 1961). We have tested this hypothesis by the administration of ethinyl oestradiol to postmenopausal women and our preliminary data do in fact suggest that this compound depresses plasma calcium (Fig. 5).

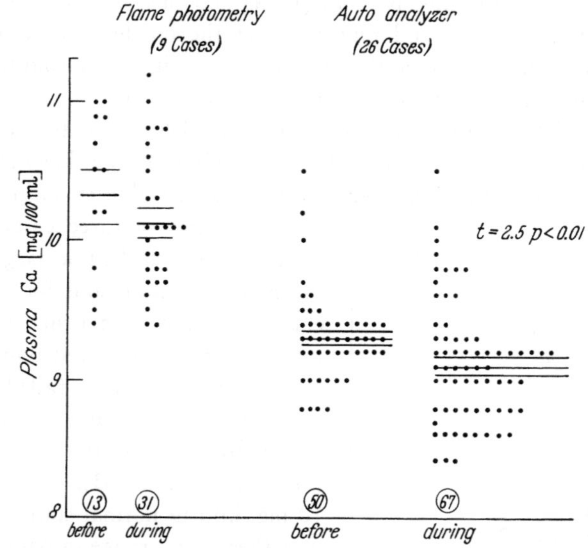

Fig. 5. 50 observations of plasma calcium before and 67 during the administration of ethinyl oestradiol 0.1 mg. daily to 26 patients

To sum up the effects of the gonadal hormones on bone and calcium metabolism, it seems fair to say that the actions of androgenic and anabolic compounds in this field are quite uncertain, though their effect upon nitrogen balance is well established. The oestrogenic hormones, on the other hand, have little effect on nitrogen metabolism but appear to reduce urinary calcium, raise urinary citrate, inhibit bone resorption and depress plasma calcium. The overall effect is an improvement in calcium balance but it is not clear whether this effect is achieved by inhibiting bone resorption or whether bone resorption is inhibited as a result of the improvement in calcium balance. The reverse effects of oestrogens on urinary calcium and citrate are of course reminiscent of a metabolic alkalosis (DEDMON and WRONG, 1962) but there is no convincing evidence that oestrogens have an effect on acid-base balance.

Corticosteroid hormones

Compression fractures and "soft bones" were a feature of the original cases of hyperadrenocorticism described by CUSHING in 1932. ALBRIGHT *et al.* (1941) intuitively attributed this syndrome to an overproduction of the adrenal cortical "sugar" hormone, a prediction which was subsequently confirmed when the hormone was indentified as cortisol. It was also ALBRIGHT (1942—1943) who recognised the bone disease as osteoporosis and who attributed it as well to the antianabolic action of the "S" hormone the existence of which he had himself been the first to postulate. In accordance with this concept, he proposed that the osteoporosis of Cushing's syndrome was due to decreased formation of protein bone matrix, and this hypothesis has remained popular for many years.

That Cushing's syndrome is associated with osteoporosis is beyond doubt, but whether therapy with synthetic corticosteroids has the same effect is a little less certain, although extremely probable. The first cases of osteoporosis from corticosteroid therapy were described by DE MARTINI *et al.* in 1952 and further cases were reported by CURTIS *et al.* (1954) and then by many others. MCCONKEY *et al.* (1962) on the other hand reported that the incidence of osteoporosis was no higher in a series of patients with rheumatoid arthritis on steroid therapy than in a similar group untreated, but they are probably in a minority.

The cause of the osteoporosis in these patients is uncertain. The measurement of bone formation rate with bone-seeking isotopes has not yielded a clear answer. Thus GORDAN and EISENBERG (1963), using stable strontium, found small pool sizes and turnover rates in three cases of Cushing's syndrome. The same authors studied a large number of patients taking synthetic corticoids and found variable pool sizes but generally an *increase* in urinary excretion and bone accretion rates. We have measured bone formation rate by a variety of techniques but have failed to find any consistent difference between the rates in normal and steroid-treated individuals. Using intravenous radiocalcium or radiostrontium (NORDIN *et al.*, 1963), our values ranged from about 2 to 10 mg./kilo in normal subjects and extended over a similar or rather larger range in patients on steroid therapy (Fig. 6). Measurement of retention in a whole body counter yielded lower values but again there was no difference between the controls and the patients on corticosteroids (Fig. 6). Even with continuous feeding of radiocalcium (NORDIN *et al.*, 1964) the bone mineralisation rate appeared to be normal in patients on steroid therapy.

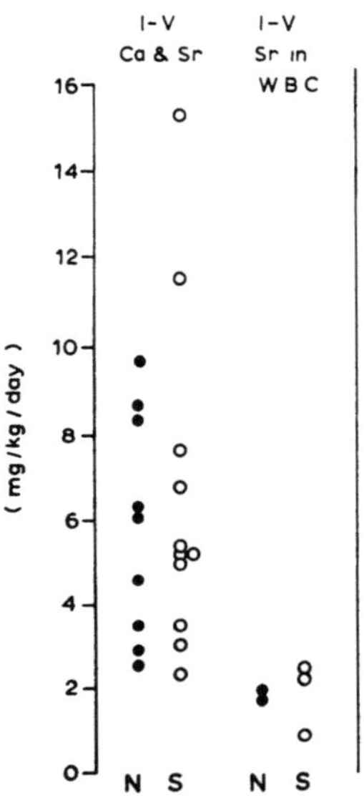

Fig. 6. Bone mineralisation rate values in 9 normal subjects and 11 patients on corticosteroids as determined from conventional excretional collection (left) and 2 measurements in normal subjects and 3 in patients on steroid therapy calculated from measurements in a whole body counter (right)

Balance studies in patients on steroid therapy have also been somewhat inconclusive. SLATER *et al.* (1959) observed malabsorption of calcium in patients on dexamethasone. We have observed the same thing occasionally but not consistently. There is a tendency for both faecal and urinary calcium to be higher than normal in patients on steroid therapy and the theoretical mean calcium requirement (i.e. the level at which calcium intake and output are equal) is therefore somewhat increased but the significance of this is uncertain. Radiocalcium absorption studies have also been rather inconclusive although the results tend to be low particularly in patients on cortisone (NORDIN, 1964). In animals, STOERK *et al.* (1963) implied that hydrocortisone interfered with calcium absorption but suggested that it also interfered with the action of parathyroid hormone on bone whereas CLARK and SMITH (1964) were unable to demonstrate any effect of corticosteroids upon calcium absorption.

STOERK *et al.* (1963) showed that hydrocortisone could lower the plasma calcium and plasma citrate of parathyroidectomised rats and suggested that failure to observe the same effect in normal animals was due to secondary hyperparathyroidism. They found that hypocalcaemia following parathyroidectomy was aggravated by hydrocortisone and that the amount of parathyroid extract required to maintain serum calcium concentration was increased in the presence of hydrocortisone.

In man hypophosphataemia with a raised phosphate clearance is sometimes seen in Cushing's syndrome and could be due to secondary hyperparathyroidism (NORDIN and FRASER, 1960). The hypocalcaemic effect of cortisone is well established in sarcoidosis and it has also been reported in vitamin D intoxication (VERNER *et al.*, 1958) in thyrotoxicosis (SATALINE *et al.*, 1962) and in multiple myeloma (MERIGAN and HAYES, 1961). Cortisone responsive hypercalcaemia has also been reported occasionally in proven hyperparathyroidism (GWINUP and SAYLE, 1961). This hypocalcaemic action is not confined to cortisone itself since it has frequently been reported with prednisone as well (BENTZEL *et al.*, 1964).

The mode of action of the corticosteroids on plasma calcium is quite uncertain but they have at times been thought to be antagonistic to parathyroid hormone (LARON *et al.*, 1958; MYERS, 1962) and at other times to antagonise the action of vitamin D (ANDERSON *et al.*, 1954; SCHOLZ, 1959). As far as the former concept is concerned, the apparently hypocalcaemic action of corticosteroids in parathyroidectomised animals (STOERK *et al.*, 1963) tends to rule it out. As far as the second concept — antagonism to vitamin D — is concerned, the circumstances in which this antagonism operates appear to be quite limited. Thus HARRISON and HARRISON (1958) found that cortisol did not prevent the healing of rickets in rachitic rats given vitamin D, and THOMAS and MORGAN (1958) found that it did not prevent the development of hypercalcaemia in rats given large doses of vitamin D.

JACKSON and DANCASTER (1963) investigated this subject in four male adult volunteers in whom they failed to prevent the development of vitamin D poisoning by the simultaneous administration of large doses of cortisone and vitamin D. Moreover, patients with adrenal insufficiency were no more sensitive to calciferol than those with hyperadrenocortisism.

A hypocalcaemic effect of corticosteroids is again apparent in the hypercalcaemia of adrenal insufficiency (SPRAGUE *et al.*, 1956; LEEKSMA *et al.*, 1957). The nature of this hypercalcaemia has been carefully investigated by ROBINSON and WALSER (1964) and MYERS *et al.* (1964). Both these groups measured calcium fractions in the plasma of normal and adrenalectomised dogs and found that the hypercalcaemia following cortisol withdrawal could be explained by the following processes:

1. Dehydration and consequent increased protein concentration.
2. Increased calcium-binding by the proteins.
3. Increased ultrafiltrable calcium due both to increased calcium citrate and increase in other complexes.

Both groups agreed that the ionic calcium remains normal. These observations are difficult to reconcile with the clinical picture of nausea and vomiting following adrenalectomy described by SPRAGUE *et al.* (1956) which suggests a raised ionic calcium in the blood. The implication that the corticosteroids do not affect ionic calcium concentrations is also difficult to reconcile with their hypocalcaemic action in vitamin D poisoning, hypercalcaemia of malignant disease and other conditions. It is hard to believe that cortisone reduces plasma calcium in these diseases without modifying the ionic fraction.

If there is some doubt about the effects of the corticosteroids on plasma calcium, there is no doubt about their effect on plasma and urinary citric acid, which are depressed by steroid therapy. This was reported in 1958 by HENNEMAN and HENNEMAN who stated that adrenocorticotrophic hormone and operative trauma both lowered the serum concentration and urinary excretion of citric acid in man, and confirmed by AGRELL *et al.* (1961).

HARRISON (1959) found that administration of cortisol to rats produced much lower levels of citric acid in plasma than were found in rachitic or control animals. HARRISON and HARRISON (1958) reported that this effect of cortisol was attributable to its inhibitory action on the efflux of citrate from cells to extracellular fluid rather than to the intracellular accumulation of citrate.

There is little doubt that corticosteroids tend to increase urinary calcium though whether this action is direct or indirect it is impossible to say. According to PECHET *et al.* (1959) the dose required to produce this effect is large but LAAKE (1960) determined calcium clearance in 16 patients on corticosteroid therapy and found the tubular reabsorption of calcium to be decreased in 7 of them.

The effect of corticosteroids upon bone structure varies with the species studied. Thus in Man the bone changes in Cushing's syndrome are essentially those of osteoporosis (SISSONS, 1956) but the presence of normal osteoid seams and the occasional slight increase in osteoclastic activity is perhaps slightly more in favour of increased bone destruction than decreased new bone formation. This is also true in the rabbit in which species STOREY (1961) produced spontaneous fractures after 12 days of cortisone administration. This rapid rarefaction of bone was mainly due to an increased rate of resorption associated with large numbers of osteoclasts at trabecular margins. Old rabbits responded in the same way though rather more slowly. URIST and DEUTSCH (1960) also demonstrated increased bone resorption by cortisone in birds. The effects of corticosteroids on rat bone are more variable and are complicated by the almost invariable interference with growth which this regime produces. Metaphyseal sclerosis has been reported on cortisone treatment but this gave way to osteoporosis when the Ca/P ratio of the diet was adjusted (STOREY, 1961).

To summarise the effects of corticosteroids on calcium and bone metabolism, it would appear that they tend to inhibit calcium absorption, to inhibit renal tubular reabsorption, to depress plasma calcium, and to depress plasma and urinary citrate. Associated with these effects there is a tendency to negative calcium balance and the development of osteoporosis which some workers attribute to reduced bone formation but which experimentally seems more likely to be due to increased bone resorption. In many ways their action is antagonistic to that of vitamin D and the parathyroid hormone and it is possible that the interpretation of steroid action on bone may be complicated by the frequent presence of secondary hyperparathyroidism.

Growth hormone

The effects of growth hormone on bone growth are too well known to require detailed recapitulation. There occurs in acromegaly a "generalised overgrowth of bone characterised by cortical thickening with circumferential increase and coarsening of structure" (FINLAY and MACDONALD, 1954). These effects are understandable in terms of the action of the hormone on growth processes in general. What is less easy to understand is the occurrence of osteoporosis in acromegaly and attributed by ALBRIGHT and REIFENSTEIN (1948) to the effects of secondary adrenocortical overactivity on the synthesis of bone matrix. The hyperphosphataemia is also unexplained.

The frequency of osteoporosis in acromegaly is uncertain but most workers are agreed that a characteristic feature is hypercalciuria (BAUER and AUB, 1941; HARRISON *et al.*, 1960; HAYMOVITZ and HORWITH, 1964). According to ALBRIGHT and REIFENSTEIN (1948) this hypercalciuria is the result of the disease whereas KARAM *et al.* (1961) and HAYMOVITZ and HORWITH (1964) both suggest that the high urinary calcium contribute to the development of bone disease by causing a negative calcium balance.

With the advent of purified human growth hormone it has become possible to observe the effects of this hormone in Man and a striking and consistent observation has been the rise in urinary calcium which follows administration of the hormone to cases of hypopituitarism (IKKOS *et al.*, 1959; HENNEMAN *et al.*, 1960; FRASER and HARRISON, 1960). This rise in urinary calcium is associated with a fall in urinary nitrogen and phosphorus. Various workers have tried to establish whether the hypercalciuria is the result of increased calcium absorption but their results are conflicting. In three of the four cases reported by IKKOS *et al.* (1959) the faecal calcium rose whereas in the hypopituitary cases of HENNEMAN *et al.* (1960) faecal calcium fell, as it did in most of the cases studied by BECK *et al.* (1960). Moreover, FINKELSTEIN and SCHACHTER (1962) found that growth hormone promoted active calcium transport by the rat duodenum. FRASER and HARRISON (1960) confirmed the hypercalciuric effect of growth hormone in hypophysectomised rats but not in normal rats and showed that the rise in urinary calcium was associated with a corresponding rise in the excretion of Sr^{89} with which the skeletons had been labelled. This indicated that the calcium was being withdrawn from the skeleton but since the animals were on a low calcium diet it is difficult to see where else it could have come from. They repeated the observations on rats which had also been parathyroidectomised and found no rise in urinary calcium or strontium. They inferred that the effect of growth hormone on calcium excretion was due to parathyroid stimulation by an overdosage of the hormone. In another paper, HARRISON *et al.* (1960) described a case of acromegaly with hypercalcaemia in which plasma calcium returned to normal after pituitary irradiation.

KARAM *et al.* (1961) pursued this subject further by postulating that the hypercalciuria produced by growth hormone might be the result of a fall in the intracellular concentration of citrate in the renal tubules. They showed that fluoroacetate given to normal rats raised the urinary and kidney citrate and lowered calcium whereas growth hormone given to hypophysectomised rats lowered renal citrate and raised urinary calcium. The idea that urinary calcium is controlled by renal citrate is a good one but the data are not entirely convincing nor is this concept really compatible with the idea of parathyroid stimulation by the pituitary put forward by the same authors.

The hyperphosphataemia of acromegaly (WILLIAMS, 1964) is well recognised and used by many workers as an indicator of pituitary activity and is reminiscent of the hyperphosphataemia of children. It is associated with an increased Tm phosphate which is said by some, however, only to be increased in proportion to the glomerular filtration rate (CATTANEO *et al.*, 1964). Since the urinary phosphate is reduced by the growth hormone as described above, and the plasma phosphate is increased (HENNEMAN *et al.*, 1960) the implication is that tubular reabsorption of phosphate has increased as CORVILAIN *et al.* (1962, 1964) have shown. This could be the result of diminished parathyroid activity such as would be produced if growth hormone tended to raise plasma calcium, as it did in one of Henneman's two cases. The early literature (reviewed by BAUER and AUB, 1941) suggested in fact that pituitary extract raised plasma calcium but it is hard to know how much credence to place in those data now.

If the effect of growth hormone in raising plasma phosphorus were a primary one, it would be expected to depress plasma calcium and stimulate the parathyroids in the manner suggested by TORNBLOM (1949). This would lead to a fall in urinary calcium, SMITH and NORDIN (1964). Since the hormone raises urinary calcium, however, another explanation must be sought — either a rise in plasma calcium or a diminution in parathyroid activity or both. Since a primary action of the hormone is to stimulate new bone growth it presumably increases the proportion of young to old mineral in the skeleton so producing the increased miscible pool and decreased 24-hr. plasma specific activity reported by HAYMOVITZ and HORWITH (1964). MACGREGOR (1962) has suggested that the increased "solubility" of child bone might explain the higher plasma phosphates in children. A similar explanation might be applied to acromegaly. Young bone (probably octocalcium phosphate as suggested by BROWN and MACGREGOR [1965]) being more soluble than old allows the plasma calcium to rise, thus diminishing parathyroid activity and allowing the plasma phosphate to rise. Urinary calcium increases both because of the rise in plasma calcium, however small (MACFADYEN *et al.*, 1965) and because of the fall in parathyroid activity (KLEEMAN *et al.*, 1961).

Thus to summarise the action of growth hormone on calcium metabolism it appears that the hormone stimulates bone growth, raises plasma phosphate and raises urinary calcium and increases tubular phosphate reabsorption. It may tend to elevate plasma calcium but this is speculative. The evidence that it stimulates the parathyroids and/or reduces kidney citrate is still inconclusive, and its effect on calcium absorption is uncertain.

Other hormones

The association between Diabetes and Osteoporosis reported by HERNBERG (1952) is unexplained. NIELSEN (1964) has shown that antidiuretic hormone increases the excretion of calcium and suggests that it inhibits renal tubular reabsorption of calcium. PITIS *et al.* (1964) have reported that noradrenaline may precipitate tetany in Man. Space and time do not permit me to pursue any of these trains of thought, inviting though they seem to be.

Conclusions

It seems that it might be possible to integrate our knowledge of the action of the hormones on calcium metabolism by relating them all to the plasma calcium level. The plasma and extracellular calcium form a pool through which all calcium traffic as it were must pass. The calcium concentration in this pool is governed by the relation of blood to bone. Taking this as the starting point, it appears that the following effects may just be discernible:

1. The thyroid hormone raises plasma calcium, depresses parathyroid activity and increases tubular reabsorption of phosphate. Urinary calcium is increased both because of an increase in filtered load and reduced parathyroid activity. Calcium absorption is reduced (? due to reduced parathyroid activity). Hypercalciuria and malabsorption of calcium lead to negative calcium balance and osteoporosis or osteitis fibrosa according to severity.

2. The corticosteroids depress plasma calcium, reduce calcium absorption, increase calcium excretion and depress plasma and urinary citrate. If citrate were an intracellular calcium carrier it might be suggested that these steroids reduce calcium transport. Malabsorption and hypercalciuria would suffice to explain the osteoporosis but a primary effect on bone protein cannot be excluded.

3. The oestrogens depress plasma calcium, reduce urinary calcium, raise urinary citrate, probably increase calcium absorption. They may promote calcium transport, possibly through the citrate ion. They tend to stimulate the parathyroids and so cause phosphaturia and hypophosphataemia and this contributes to (or may explain) their hypocalciuric action. Loss of oestrogens allows plasma and urinary calcium to rise and so reduces parathyroid activity and increases urinary calcium. Calcium absorption may fall. These effects result in negative calcium balance and osteoporosis but a primary effect on bone resorption cannot be excluded.

4. Growth hormone raises plasma calcium, reduces parathyroid activity, raises plasma phosphate, increases urinary calcium. The effects on plasma and urinary citrate and on calcium absorption are uncertain, but hypercalciuria causes negative calcium balance and osteoporosis despite the stimulating effect of the hormone on new bone formation.

When these actions (which are summarised in Fig. 7) are considered in relation to those of the parathyroid hormone (hypercalcaemic) and calcitonin (hypocalcaemic)

Hormone	*Plasma*		*Urine*		*Absorption*	*Urine*	*Bone*
	Ca	P	Ca	PEI	Ca	CIT	*Resorption*
Thyroid	↑	N	↑	↓	↓	N	↑
Corticoid	↓	↓	↑	↑	↓	↓	↑
Oestrogen	↓	↓	↓	↑	↑	↑	↓
Growth	↑	↑	↑	↓	?	N	↑

Fig. 7. Tentative scheme indicating possible actions of hormones on various aspects of calcium metabolism

a pattern emerges in which the plasma calcium is the resultant of the opposing effects of at least six hormones on bone, 3 tending to raise it and three to lower it. However, although all these six hormones (and possibly others) may influence plasma calcium, only the parathyroid hormone (and possibly calcitonin) is in all probability secreted in direct response to variations in plasma calcium concentration. The intervention of these other hormones presumably makes the work of the parathyroid glands even more critical than it would otherwise be.

References

ACKERMAN, P. G., D. G. TORO, W. B. KOUNTZ, and T. KHEIM: The effect of sex hormone administration on the calcium and nitrogen balance in elderly women. J. Geront. **9**, 450 (1954).

AGRELL, I. G., S. E. LINDELL, and H. WESTLING: Observations on the influence of adrenocortical steroids on the serum critic acid content. Acta. med. scand. **169**, 127 (1961).

ALBRIGHT, F.: Cushing's syndrome. Harvey Lect. **38**, 123 (1942—1943).

—, W. PARSONS, and E. BLOOMBERG: Cushing's syndrome interpreted as hyperadrenocorticism leading to hypergluconeogenesis. J. clin. Endocr. **I**, 375 (1941).

—, and E. C. REIFENSTEIN: The Parathyroid Glands and Metabolic Bone Disease. Baltimore 1948.

—, P. H. SMITH, and A. M. RICHARDSON: Postmenopausal osteoporosis. J. Amer. med. Ass. **116**, 2465 (1941).

ANDERSON, I. A.: Postmenopausal osteoporosis, clinical manifestations and treatment with oestrogens. Quart. J. Med. **19**, 67 (1950).

ANDERSON, J., C. E. DENT, C. HARPER, and G. R. PHILPOT: Effect of cortisone on calcium metabolism in sarcoidosis with hypercalcaemia. Lancet **II**, 720 (1954).

ASKANAZY, M., und E. RUTISHAUSER: Die Knochen der Basedowkranken. Virchows Arch. path. Anat. **291**, 635 (1933).

AUB, J. C., W. BAUER, C. HEATH, and M. ROPES: Studies of calcium phosphorus metabolism; effects of thyroid hormone and thyroid disease. J. clin. Invest. **7**, 97 (1929).

BARTTER, F. C.: Osteoporosis. Amer. J. Med. **22**, 797 (1957).

BAUER, W., and J. C. AUB: Studies of calcium and phosphorus metabolism. J. clin. Invest. **20**, 295 (1941).

BECK, J. C., E. C. MCGARRY, I. DYRENFURTH, R. O. MORGAN, E. BIRD, and E. H. VENNING: The variability in physiological response to growth hormone. Ciba Coll. Endocr. **13**, 156 (1960).

BECK, J. S., and B. E. C. NORDIN: The histological assessment of osteoporosis by iliac crest biopsy. J. Path. Bact. **80**, 391 (1960).

BENOIT, F. L., G. B. THEIL, and R. H. WATTEN: Hydroxyproline excretion in endocrine disease. Metabolism **12**, 1072 (1963).

BENTZEL, C. J., P. P. CARBONE, L. ROSENBERG, and M. BEAN: The effect of prednisone on calcium metabolism and Ca^{47} kinetics in patients with multiple myeloma and hypercalcemia. J. clin. Invest. **43**, 2132 (1964).

BORTZ, W., E. EISENBERG, C. Y. BOWERS, and M. PONT: Differentiation between thyroid and parathyroid causes of hypercalcaemia. Ann. intern. Med. **54**, 611 (1961).

BROWN, W. E., and J. MACGREGOR: Blood bone equilibrium in calcium homeostasis. Nature (Lond.) **205**, 359 (1965).

CATTANEO, C., P. F. MARTINI, and A. MODICA: The maximal tubular reabsorption of phosphate in acromegaly. Acta endocr. **45**, 203 (1964).

CLARK, I., and M. R. SMITH: Effects of parathyroidectomy and hydrocortisone on the intestinal absorption of calcium and phosphate. Endocrinology **74**, 421 (1964).

COOK, P. B., J. R. NASSIM, and J. COLLINS: The effects of thyrotoxicosis upon the metabolism of calcium, phosphorus and nitrogen. Quart. J. Med. **XXVIII**, 505 (1959).

CORVILAIN, J., M. ABRAMOW, and A. BERGANS: Effect of human growth hormone on some renal hemodynamics and on tubular phosphate transport in man. J. clin. Invest. **41**, 1230 (1962).

— — — Effect of growth hormone on tubular transport of phosphate in normal and parathyroidectomised dogs. J. clin. Invest. **43**, 1608 (1964).

CURTISS, P. H., JR., W. S. CLARK, and C. H. HERNDON: Vertebral fractures resulting from prolonged cortisone and corticotrophin therapy. J. Amer. med. Ass. **156**, 467 (1954).

CUSHING, H.: The basophil adenomas of the pituitary body and their clinical manifestations. Bull. Johns Hopk. Hosp. **50**, 137 (1932).

CUSHMAN, P., JR., M. A. PULIDO, and J. G HILTON: The effects of oestradiol on cortisol secretion by the isolated dog adrenal. Acta endocr. **48**, 225 (1965).

DAVID, N. J., J. V. VERNER, and F. L. ENGEL: Diagnostic spectrum of hypercalcemia; case reports and discussion. Amer. J. Med. **33,** 88 (1962).

DEDMON, R. E., and O. WRONG: The excretion of organic anion in renal tubular acidosis with particular reference to citrate. Clin. Sci. **22,** 19 (1962).

DONALDSON, I. A., and J. R. NASSIM: The artificial menopause with particular reference to the occurrence of spinal porosis. Brit. med. J. **1,** 1228 (1954).

DYMLING, J. F., B. ISAKSSON, and B. SJOGREN: Anabolic steroids in the treatment of osteopenia. In Protein Metabolism. GROSS, F. (ed.). Berlin: Springer Verlag, 1962, p. 412.

EVERSE, J. W. R., and P. A. VAN KEEP: Symposium on anabolic steroids. Acta endocr. **39,** suppl. 63 (1961).

FINKELSTEIN, J. D., and D. SCHACHTER: Active transport of calcium by intestine: effects of hypophysectomy and growth hormone. Amer. J. Physiol. **203,** 873 (1962).

FINLAY, J. M., and R. I. MACDONALD: Acromegaly. Canad. med. Ass. J. **71,** 345 (1954).

FOLLIS, R. H.: Skeletal changes associated with hyperparathyroidism. Bull. Johns Hopkins Hosp. **92,** 405 (1953).

FRASER, R., and M. T. HARRISON: Effect of growth hormone on urinary calcium excretion. Ciba Coll. Endocr. **13,** 135 (1960).

— —, and K. IBBERTSON: The rate of calcium turnover in bone. Quart. J. Med. **XXIX,** 85 (1960).

GARDNER, W. U., and PFEIFFER, C. A.: Skeletal changes in mice receiving estrogens. Proc. Soc. exp. Biol. **27,** 678 (1938).

GORDAN, G. S., and E. EISENBERG: The effect of oestrogens, androgens and corticoids on skeletal kinetics in man. Proc. roy. Soc. Med. **56,** 1027 (1963).

GREEN, J., and A. LYALL: Calcium metabolism in hyperthyroidism. Lancet **1,** 828 (1951).

GUYER, P. B.: Hypercalcaemia in thyrotoxicosis. Brit. med. J. **1,** 169 (1965).

GWINUP, G., and B. SAYLE: Cortisone responsive hypercalcemia in proved hyperparathyroidism. Ann. intern. Med. **55,** 1001 (1961).

HARDEN, R. McG., M. T. HARRISON, W. D. ALEXANDER, and B. E. C. NORDIN: Phosphate excretion and parathyroid function in thyrotoxicosis. J. Endocr. **28,** 281 (1964).

HARRISON, H. C., and H. E. HARRISON: Vit. D and citrate metabolism inhibition of vit. D effect by cortisol. Proc. Soc. exp. Biol. **96,** 768 (1958).

HARRISON, H. E.: Factors influencing calcium absorption. Fed. Proc. **18,** 1085 (1959).

HARRISON, M. T., R. McG. HARDEN, and W. D. ALEXANDER: Some effects of parathyroid hormone in thyrotoxicosis. J. clin. Endocr. **24,** 214 (1964).

—, G. F. JOPLIN, M. HARTOG, and R. FRASER: Acromegaly treated by needle — implantation of Au^{198} seeds into the pituitary gland, showing changes in growth, carbohydrate and calcium metabolism. Proc. roy. Soc. Med. **53,** 869 (1960).

HAYMOVITZ, A., and M. HORWITH: The miscible calcium pool in metabolic bone disease — in particular, acromegaly. J. clin. Endocr. **24,** 4 (1964).

HEANEY, R. P., and G. D. WHEDON: Radiocalcium studies and bone formation rate in human metabolic disease. J. clin. Endocr. **18,** 1246 (1958).

HENNEMAN, D. H., and P. H. HENNEMAN: Depression of serum and urinary citric acid levels by 17 hydroxy-corticosteroids. J. clin. Endocr. **18,** 1093 (1958).

HENNEMAN, P. H., A. P. FORBES, M. MOLDAWER, E. F. DEMPSEY, and E. L. CARROLL: Effects of human growth hormone in man. J. clin. Invest. **39,** 1223 (1960).

—, and S. WALLACH: A review of the prolonged use of estrogens and androgens in postmenopausal and senile osteoporosis. Arch. intern. Med. **100,** 715 (1957).

HERNBERG, C. A.: Skelettveränderungen bei Diabetes mellitus der Erwachsenen. Acta med. scand. **136,** 26 (1952).

— Bone phosphorus metabolism in vitro in thyrotoxicosis. Acta endocr. **33,** 577 (1960).

—, and T. JAKOBSEN: Urinary excretion of calcium and 17-nitrogenic steroids in hyperthyroidism. Acta med. scand. suppl. **412,** 151 (1964).

HORWITH, M., C. RICH, D. D. THOMPSON, and H. RASMUSSEN: Renal effects of purified bovine parathyroid extract. In The Parathyroids. GREEP, R. O., and R. V. TALMAGE (eds.). Springfield: Charles C. Thomas 1961, p. 415.

Ikkos, D., R. Luft, and C. A. Gemzell: The effect of human growth hormone in man. Acta endocr. **32**, 341 (1959).

Jackson, W. P. U., and C. P. Dancaster: A clinical study of the postulated antagonism between gluco corticoids and vitamin D. Acta endocr. **44**, 443 (1963).

Karam, J., M. T. Harrison, M. Hartog, and R. Fraser: Renal citrate and urinary calcium excretion — the effects of growth hormone contrasted with those of sodium fluoroacetate. Clin. Sci. **21**, 265 (1961).

Kivirikko, K. K., M. Koivusalo, O. Laitinen, and B. A. Lamberg: Hydroxyproline in the serum and urine of patients with hyperthyroidism. J. clin. Endocr. **24**, 222 (1964).

Kleeman, C. R., D. Bernstein, R. Rockney, J. T. Dowling, and M. H. Maxwell: Studies on the renal clearance of diffusible calcium and the role of the parathyroid glands on its regulation. In The Parathyroids. Greep, R. O., and R. V. Talmage (eds.). Springfield: Charles C. Thomas 1961, p. 353.

—, S. I. Tuttle, and S. M. Bassett: Metabolic observations in thyrotoxicosis with hypercalcemia. J. clin. Endocr. **18**, 477 (1958).

Krane, S. M., G. L. Gordon, J. B. Stanbury, and H. Corrigan: The effect of thyroid disease on calcium metabolism in man. J. clin. Invest. **XXXV**, 874 (1956).

Laake, H.: The action of corticosteroids on the renal reabsorption of calcium. Acta endocr. **34**, 60 (1960).

Labhart, A., und B. Courvoisier: Osteoporose bei Eunuchismus. Helv. med. Acta **17**, 475 (1950).

Lafferty, F. W., G. E. Spencer, Jr., and O. H. Pearson: Effects of androgens, oestrogens and high calcium intakes on bone formation and resorption in osteoporosis. Amer. J. Med. **36**, 514 (1964).

Laron, Z., J. P. Muhlethaler, and R. Klein: The interrelationship between cortisone and parathyroid extract in rats. Arch. Path. **65**, 125 (1958).

Leeksma, J., J. De Graeff, and J. De Cook: Hypercalcaemia in adrenal insufficiency. Acta med. scand. **CLVI**, 455 (1957).

Lindquist, B., A. M. Budy, F. C. McLean, and J. L. Howard: Skeletal metabolism in estrogen treated rats studied by means of Ca 45. Endocrinology **66**, 100 (1960).

Lowe, C. E., E. D. Bird, and W. C. Thomas: Hypercalcaemia in myxoedema. J. clin. Endocr. **XXII**, 261 (1962).

Lund, H.: Corticosteroid osteoporosis and treatment with anabolic hormone. Acta med. scand. **174**, 735 (1963).

MacFadyen, I. J., B. E. C. Nordin, D. A. Smith, D. J. Wayne, and S. L. Rae: Effect of variation in dietary calcium on plasma concentration and urinary excretion of calcium. Brit. med. J. **1**, 161 (1965).

MacGregor, J.: Studies in Bone Solubility. Thesis. Glasgow 1962.

Martini, F. de, A. W. Grokoest, and C. Ragan: Pathological fractures in patients with rheumatoid arthritis treated with cortisone. J. Amer. med. Ass. **149**, 750 (1952).

McConkey, B., G. M. Fraser, and A. S. Bligh: Osteoporosis and purpura in rheumatoid disease; prevalence and relation to treatment with corticosteroids. Quart. J. Med. **XXXI**, 419 (1962).

Merigan, T. C., and R. E. Hayes: Treatment of hypercalcemia in multiple myeloma. Arch. intern. Med. **107**, 133 (1961).

Myers, W. P. L.: Studies of serum calcium regulation. Advanc. intern. Med. **XI**, 163 (1962).

—, E. O. Rothschild, and W. Lawrence, Jr.: Adrenal factors in plasma calcium regulation. In Bone and Tooth. Blackwood, H. J. J. (ed.) Oxford: Pergamon Press 1964, p. 193.

Nassim, J. R., P. D. Saville, and L. Mulligan: The effect of stilboestrol on urinary phosphate excretion. Clin. Sci. **15**, 367 (1956).

Nielsen, B.: Correlation between antidiuretic hormone effect and the renal excretion of magnesium and calcium in man. Acta endocr. **45**, 151 (1964).

Nordin, B. E. C.: Osteoporosis. Advanc. metab. Dis. **1**, 125 (1964).

—, and R. Fraser: Assessment of urinary phosphate excretion. Lancet **1**, 947 (1960).

—, J. MacGregor, and M. M. Bluhm: Determination of bone formation rate with radioactive strontium. Clin. Sci. **24**, 301 (1963).

NORDIN, B. E. C., D. A. SMITH, and J. MACGREGOR: The incidence of osteoporosis among normal women. Quart. J. Med. (in press).

— —, and J. NISBET: Bone mineralisation and destruction rates determined by continuous feeding of radiocalcium. Clin. Sci. **27,** 111 (1964).

PARSONS, V., and J. ANDERSON: The maximal renal tubular reabsorptive rate for inorganic phosphate in thyrotoxicosis. Clin. Sci. **27,** 313 (1964).

PECHET, M. M., B. BOWERS, and F. C. BARTTER: Metabolic studies with a new series of 1,4-diene steroids. Effects on normal subjects of prednisone, prednisolone and 9α-fluoro prednisolone. J. clin. Invest. **38,** 691 (1959).

PFEIFFER, C. A., and W. U. GARDNER: Skeletal changes and blood serum calcium level in pigeons receiving estrogens. Endocrinology **23,** 485 (1938).

PITIS, M., A. I. NICOLESCO-CATARGI, S. PETRESCO, V. CHIVU, et A. GALU: Recherches concernant les facteurs extraparathyroïdiens dans la tétanie. Acta endocr. **47,** 529 (1964).

PRIBEK, R. A., and R. C. MEADE: Thyrotoxicosis simulating hyperparathyroidism. Arch. intern. Med. **100,** 994 (1957).

PUPPEL, I. D., H. T. GROSS, E. K. MCCORMICK, and E. HERDLE: Rationale of calcium phosphorus and vitamin D therapy in clinical hyperthyroidism. Surg. Gynec. Obstet. **81,** 243 (1945).

RANNEY, R. E.: Antagonism between estrone and parathyroid extract in their effects upon bone accretion. Endocrinology **65,** 594 (1959).

REIFENSTEIN, E. C., JR., and F. ALBRIGHT: The metabolic effects of steroid hormones in osteoporosis. J. clin. Invest. **26,** 24 (1947).

ROBINSON, B. H. B., and M. WALSER: Plasma calcium concentration. In Bone and Tooth. BLACKWOOD, H. J. J. (ed.). Oxford: Pergamon Press 1964, p. 185.

ROSE, E., and R. S. BOLES, JR.: Hypercalcemia in thyrotoxicosis. Med. Clin. N. Amer. **37,** 1715 (1953).

SATALINE, L. R., C. POWELL, and G. J. HAMWI: Suppression of the hypercalcemia of thyrotoxicosis by corticosteroids. New Engl. J. Med. **267,** 646 (1962).

SAVILLE, P. D.: Quoted by BRONNER, F. In Radioisotopes and Bone. LACROIX, P., and A. M. BUDY (eds.). Oxford: Blackwell Scientific Publications 1962, p. 462.

SCHOLZ, D. A.: Effects of steroid therapy on hypercalcaemia and renal insufficiency in sarcoidosis. J. Amer. med. Ass. **169,** 682 (1959).

SHORR, E.: The possible usefulness of estrogens and aluminium hydroxide gels in the management of renal stone. J. Urol. **53,** 507 (1945).

SISSONS, H. A.: The osteoporosis of Cushing's syndrome. J. Bone Jt Surg. **38 B,** 418 (1956).

SLATER, J. D. H., E. F. HEFFRON, A. VERNET, and J. D. N. NABARRO: Clinical and metabolic effects of dexamethasone. Lancet **1,** 173 (1959).

SMITH, D. A., and B. E. C. NORDIN: The effect of a high phosphorus intake on total and ultrafilterable plasma and on phosphate clearance. Clin. Sci. **26,** 479 (1964).

SPRAGUE, R. G., R. V. RANDALL, R. M. SALASSA, D. A. SCHOLZ, J. T. PRIESTLEY, W. WALTERS, and A. H. BULBULAN: Cushing's syndrome. Arch. intern. Med. **98,** 389 (1956).

STOERK, H. C., A. C. PETERSON, and V. C. JELINEK: The blood calcium lowering effect of hydrocortisone in parathyroidectomised rats. Proc. Soc. exp. Biol. **114,** 690 (1963).

STOREY, E.: Cortisone induced bone resorption in the rabbit. Endocrinology **68,** 553 (1961).

THOMAS, W. C., and H. G. MORGAN: The effect of cortisone in experimental investigations. Endocrinology **63,** 57 (1958).

TORNBLOM, N.: On the functional relationship between the pituitary gland and the parathyroids. Acta endocr. Suppl. **4,** 178 (1949).

TURNER, H. H.: Syndrome of infantilism, congenital webbed neck, and cubitus valgus. Endocrinology **23,** 566 (1938).

URIST, M. R., and N. M. DEUTSCH: Effects of cortisone upon blood, adrenal cortex, gonads and the development of osteoporosis in birds. Endocrinology **66,** 805 (1960).

VERNER, J. V., F. L. ENGEL, and H. T. MCPHERSON: Vitamin D intoxication: report of two cases treated with cortisone. Ann. intern. Med. **48,** 765 (1958).

WHEDON, G. D.: The combined use of balance and isotopic studies in the study of calcium metabolism. In Nutrition. MILLS, C. F., and R. PASSMORE (eds.). Edinburgh: Livingstone 1964 p. 425.

WILLIAMS, P. H.: Textbook of Endocrinology. London: Saunders 1964, p. 73.

Mode of Action of Calcitonin

H. A. SOLIMAN *, C. J. ROBINSON, G. V. FOSTER, I. MACINTYRE

Department of Chemical Pathology, Postgraduate Medical School, Ducane Road, London, England

In our laboratory perfusion studies in the dog and goat have demonstrated the secretion of calcitonin by the thyroid gland. Our findings in the dog have been confirmed by BERNSTEIN *et al.* (1965). We present here studies of the mode of action of the new hormone.

Acetone-dried pig thyroid was extracted with hot hydrochloric acid, dialysed, fractionated with NaCl and the active precipitate dissolved in acetate buffer. This salt precipitated fraction was used in these studies. A single intravenous dose of calcitonin in the rat produced a prompt fall in plasma calcium and phosphate. The possibility of the existence of plasma calcium lowering principles in other tissue extracts was examined. Beef parathyroid, pig liver and ox kidney were dealt with in a similar manner to the thyroid tissue. Equal doses, on the basis of protein nitrogen content of these extracts, and one-tenth of this dose of thyroid extract were tested in the rat. Extracts from the other tissues produced a small, non-specific fall in plasma calcium, compared to the marked drop produced by the thyroid extract.

In vitamin D-induced hypercalcemia and hyperphosphataemia in the rat, the hormone was found to be still potent in lowering both plasma calcium and phosphate. Calcitonin was also active in calcium deficient and in magnesium deficient rats. The hormone lowered the plasma calcium in vitamin D deficient rats, and therefore its activity is not dependent on vitamin D.

Removal of the kidneys did not alter the plasma calcium-lowering response to the calcitonin injection and, therefore, this effect is not mediated via a renal mechanism. The plasma calcium lowering effect was not accompanied by an increase in soft tissue calcium.

These two facts, that the calcium lowering activity is not mediated through a renal mechanism and is not accompanied by an increase in soft tissue calcium, point strongly to the bone as the site of action of calcitonin.

A new concept of the mode of action of hormones is that they may act by control of gene activity. The possibility of a genotropic action for calcitonin was investigated. The antibiotic, actinomycin D is a specific inhibitor of DNA-dependent synthesis of RNA. Actinomycin injected three hours prior to calcitonin did not block its action.

The conclusion is that concurrent synthesis of RNA is not necessary for calcitonin to exert its two cardinal acute actions on plasma calcium and phosphate. This is analogous to the rapid glucose lowering action of insulin, which cannot be blocked by actinomycin D.

In parathyroidectomised rats calcitonin produced a marked drop in the plasma phosphate, without an appreciable effect on plasma calcium. However, in parathyroidectomised rats fed a high calcium, low phosphate diet, the hormone lowered both plasma calcium and phosphate.

---

* United Arab Republic Scholar.

From these two experiments we gather that:

1. Calcitonin does not act by inhibition of the parathyroid hormone.
2. Its action on plasma phosphate can occur without an effect on calcium.
3. It cannot lower plasma calcium below a certain level.

Summary

1. Calcitonin is a thyroid hormone which lowers plasma calcium and phosphate.
2. It is extremely potent.
3. Its site of action seems to be the bone.
4. It does not act by inhibition of the parathyroid hormone; concurrent synthesis of RNA is not necessary for its acute actions.
5. It appears to have therapeutic potentialities.
6. Calcitonin will change our views on calcium homeostasis and bone physiology.

Reference

BERNSTEIN, D., C. R. KLEEMAN, and S. PINE: The effect of thyro-parathyroid perfusion with hyper- and hypocalcaemic blood on calcium, phosphorus and magnesium metabolism. Clin. Res. **13**, 105 (1965).

On the Influence of Thyroxine, Thiouracil, Cortisone, Estrogen and Testosterone on Endochondral Ossification Utilizing Autoradiography

E. UEHLINGER

Pathologisches Institut, Universität Zürich, Schweiz

The experiments which will be dealt with in my report have as their goal a further clarification of the influence exerted by hormones on endochondral ossification. Tritiated thymidine was employed in separate studies in conjunction with the various individual hormones and my report will deal primarily with the results obtained with *thyroxine* and *thiouracil*. Tritiated thymidine, a precursor of DNA, is presently being utilized to label the mitotic activity of various tissues. During a 40 minute period after intravenous or intraperitoneal application, tritiated thymidine is incorporated by all those cells which are actively synthesizing DNA so that they may double their chromosomes during mitosis. The number of labelled cells is therefore proportional to the proliferation of a specific tissue or a group of cells. This allows the calculation of the *proliferation index* (H_3-Index), which is the ratio of the labelled cells to the total number of identical cells in percent (ROHR, 1963).

Two month old, 250—300 gram, male Wistar rats received daily during the entire experiment 0.05 mg (50 γ) thyroxine subcutaneously, or 50 mg thiouracil enterally. The animals were then killed at regular intervals of 7, 14, 21 and 28 days. 40 min. prior to death each rat also received a single intraperitoneal injection of 25 μC of tritiated thymidine.

The experiments with *thyroxine* yielded the following results: A comparison of the cartilaginous proliferation of the epiphyseal plate with control animals showed no marked differences. A certain degree of unrest is observed in the proliferating zone, which may, however, be ascribed to chance. A distinct impression is obtained that a slightly increased ossification has taken place in the primary ossification zone, but this is in no case certain. However, the labelling process with tritiated thymidine reveals a significant increase of labelling of the preosteoblasts. The proliferation index of preosteoblasts in the normal rat is 7.5%, (Table 1). In these experiments, in which

Table 1

^{3}H-Index of the Pre-Osteoblast in %						
	Control	1. W.	2. W.	3. W.	4. W.	
Thyroxine	7—8	16	18	24	18	%
Thiouracil	7—8	12	26	17	15	%

more than 2000 cells were counted per animal, the preosteoblast proliferation-index more than doubled itself with values over 14% being obtained. In other words, thyroxine practically selectively stimulated the preosteoblasts and thus furthered the endochondral ossification, (Uehlinger *et al.*, in press).

The experiments utilizing the thyroid inhibitor, *thiouracil,* were more impressive and significant. These experiments clearly exhibited a remarkably intensive shortening of the epiphyseal cartilage plate, especially in the zone of proliferation and vesicular cartilage. This shortening occurs simultaneously with a certain repositioning of the cartilage columns. In contrast to the inhibitory effect upon the chondrocytes, which is also clinically observed in thyrogenic growth retardation, the effect on the osteoblasts is little different to that of thyroxine. The zone of vesicular cartilage is, as in normal tissue, invaded by capillaries, its cells are loosened, and the cartilaginous ground substance is covered by bone. Remarkably broad primary spongiosa trabeculae result. The preosteoblast counts support this histological observation. The proliferation-index is again increased from a norm of 7% to values over 14%. Why thyroxine and thiouracil both induce the same degree of preosteoblastic stimulation is as yet not clear.

Table 2

^{3}H-Index of the Pre-Osteoblast in %						
	Control	1. W.	2. W.	3. W.	4. W.	
Oestradiol (mice)	7	16	33	33	33	%
Testosterone (mice)	7	7	7	7	7	%
Cortisone (rats)	7	1,5—0,7				%

By the same technique we investigated the influence of cortisone, estrogen and testosterone (Rohr, 1964; Holzer, 1965). Wistar rats after 10 days of *cortisone* treatment showed a reduction of the proliferation-index of the preosteoblasts to

0.7—1.5%. The suppression of mitosis in the preosteoblasts results in a delayed chondrocytolysis and therefore in a delay of the longitudinal growth (Table 2).

Finally we treated 5—6 month old male Swiss mice, weighing approximately 25 g, daily by intraperitoneal injections of 2 mg estrogen or testosterone. The mice were killed 7, 13, 20 and 27 days after the beginning of the experiment.

In *testosterone* treated mice the proliferation-index of the preosteoblasts remains unchanged at the normal value of 7%. In contrast, *estrogen* increases the proliferation-index of the preosteoblasts from 7% to 16% after the first week of treatment, which then stabilizes at 33% (Table 2). The increase of preosteoblasts causes an exceptional increase of endochondral, endosteal and periosteal new bone formation. A weight comparison of bone tissue to the total metaphysis yields a percentage of 28.6 for the control mice, 24.6 for the testosterone treated mice, and 39.6 for the estrogen treated mice.

In conclusion: The combined method of light microscopic and autoradiographic investigation offers a clearer and finer understanding as to the exact influence of hormones on the endochondral ossification. The transposition of these experimental results from animal to man is not within the scope of this work.

References

Holzer, F.: Autoradiographische Untersuchungen über die Zellkinetik der enchondralen Ossifikation der Maus nach Oestrogen- und Testosteronverabreichung. Z. ges. exp. Med. **139**, 213 (1965).

Rohr, H. P.: Reifung der Knorpelzellen der Epiphysenfuge bei der experimentellen Rattenrachitis. Z. ges. exp. Med. **137**, 532 (1963).

— Autoradiographische Untersuchungen über den Wirkungsmechanismus des Cortisons (17-oxy-dehydrocorticosteron) auf das enchondrale Knochenlängenwachstum der Ratte. Z. ges. exp. Med. **138**, 150 (1964).

Uehlinger, E., H. P. Rohr und F. Holzer: Über den Wirkungsmechanismus von Thyroxin und Thiouracil auf das enchondrale Knochenlängenwachstum der Ratte. Z. ges. exp. Med. (in press).

The Effect of Cortisone and Anabolic Agents on Bone

J. A. Fernandez de Valderrama, L. M. Munuera

Nuffield Orthopaedic Centre, Oxford, England
Now: Madrid, España

An excess of cortisone causes an osteoporosis which resembles that of Cushing's syndrome (Sissons, 1956) and also the osteoporosis of the elderly (Valderrama and Little, 1965). Although the detailed mechanism has been only partially elucidated, anabolic agents have been used clinically to provide symtomatic relief, but practically nothing has been reported which might suggest a mechanism of action. In the present investigation rabbits were used as the experimental animal, and given cortisone alone, or an anabolic agent alone, or various combinations of the two. "Stromba" (17β-hydroxy-17α-methylandrosteno(3.2-C)pyrazole) was the anabolic agent of choice as it is reported to give a typical anabolic action with minimal side effects.

1. Cortisone alone

Using high doses of cortisone acetate (15 to 25 mg/kg), our observations, although inter-related, fall into four main categories.

1. In the first place, cell division is diminished or ceases. No new bone is laid down in the cortex, and in growing animals the production of metaphyseal bone is almost stopped when doses of 25 mg/kg are used. In the growth cartilage the proliferative zone is smaller than normal, and the enlarging zone wider. The cells in the enlarging zone do not reach the stage of complete hypertrophy, and at the base of this area a horizontal layer of bone is formed. In the metaphysis the number and calibre of the vessels is greatly decreased.

2. In the early stages there is resorption of bone, particularly in those regions where turnover is normally the most rapid. Osteoclasts may be seen on almost every bone surface (Fig. 1), and in the cortex some sinusoids appear to be irregularly

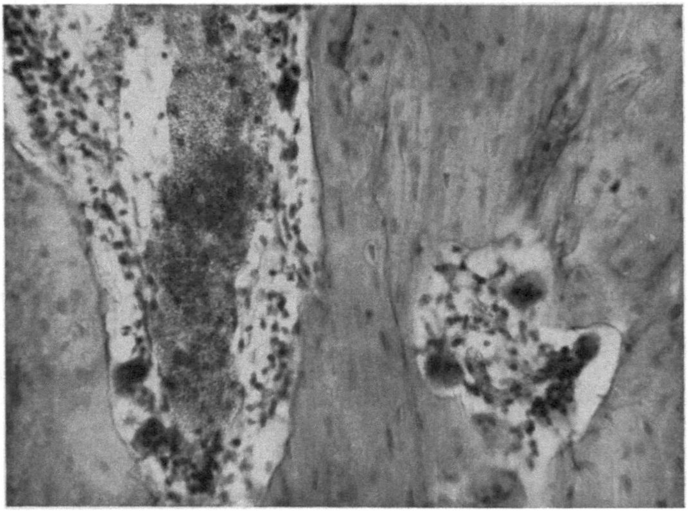

Fig. 1. One week after the administration of cortisone some sinusoids are dilated, and on the resorbing bone surfaces numerous osteoclasts are seen

enlarged. With high doses osteoclast formation and consequent bone resorption continue until no more osteoblasts and osteoblast precursors are left to coalesce into osteoclasts. In electron microscope photographs of the resorbing bone, all the matrix components appeared to be degraded simultaneously. This is in contrast to the resorption seen in disuse osteoporosis (Valderrama and Little, 1965) where the non-collagenous matrix components dissapear first, and the collagen later. Even at some distance from the bone there is a tendency for osteoclast-like cells to form around sinusoids.

3. As bone resorption takes place and proliferation ceases the tissue is replaced by an irregular fatty marrow network, even in the Volkman's canals. By 21 days very few osteoclasts could be seen (their half-life is rather less than 48 hours — Trueta and Rigal, in press), and the remaining osteoblasts on the bone surfaces had

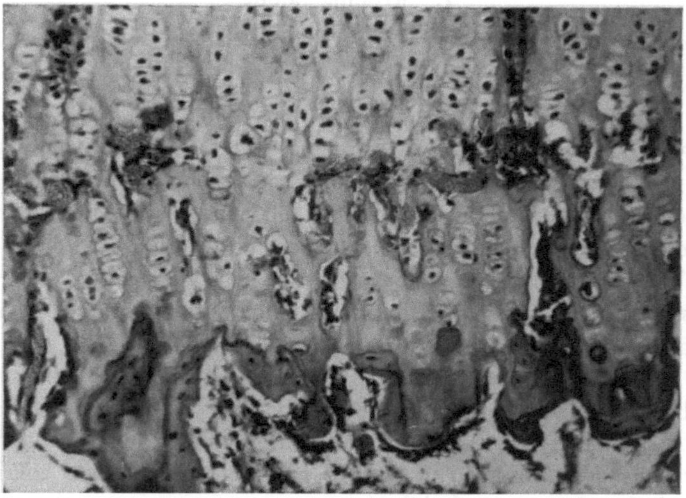

Fig. 2. 16 days of cortisone administration followed by 5 days of cortisone plus "Stromba". The metaphyseal capillaries penetrate to the normal level of the growth plate leaving behind an area of arrested cartilage cells. Sealing of the cartilage by a horizontal plate of bone as produced by the cortisone alone is clearly demonstrated

an abnormal appearance, small and heavily stained. Resorption seemed to have come to a halt, and the appearance of the bone showed very little alteration with continuous cortisone administration for up to 6 weeks.

4. The sinusoid walls and surfaces of the cells in the bone and marrow had an irregular appearance, in contrast to the sharp outlines observed in control sections prepared under the same conditions. That these cells have their surface structure disturbed provides a probable explanation for the changed sinusoids and the relaxation of the cell walls which may initiate the first stages of osteoclast formation. In connective tissue cells the channels along which chromatin precursors travel to the nucleus appear to be continuous with the surface membranes of the cells, as described by Rigal and Little (1962). A disturbance of the walls of such channels leading to the nucleus could prevent adequate surface transport of materials needed for cell division.

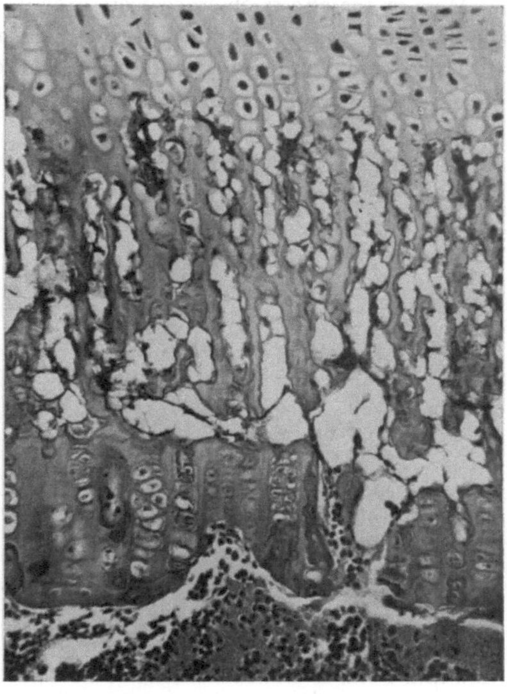

Fig. 3. 7 days cortisone alone followed by 14 days cortisone plus "Stromba". Further penetration of the vessels and resumption of endochondral ossification

2. "Stromba" alone

No definite changes from the normal were observed.

3. Cortisone followed by "Stromba"

5 days after the administration of "Stromba" had begun there were many plump osteocytes, together with evidence of new bone formation in the cortex. There was also new bone formation in the metaphysis, and many new vessels. On the metaphyseal side of the growth cartilage the number and calibre of vessels had returned to normal. The greatly enlarged cartilage cells did not take part in subsequent endochondral ossification but the vessels reached to the normal distance from the proliferative zone, which had also regained its normal activity.

STOREY (1958) has shown that after cessation of cortisone administration in growing rabbits there is a surge of new bone formation. To establish that the anabolic agent has a direct effect, and that we were not merely observing a "rebound" phenomenon, cortisone administration in a third group of animals was continued concurrently with the "Stromba" administration.

4. Cortisone followed by Cortisone plus "Stromba"

Most of the effects observed were exactly the same as those seen when cortisone administration was discontinued before the anabolic agent was given (5 mg/kg).

There were plump matrix forming cells. Proper vessel formation was seen and the vessels reached to the normal distance from the proliferative zone (Fig. 2). Normal

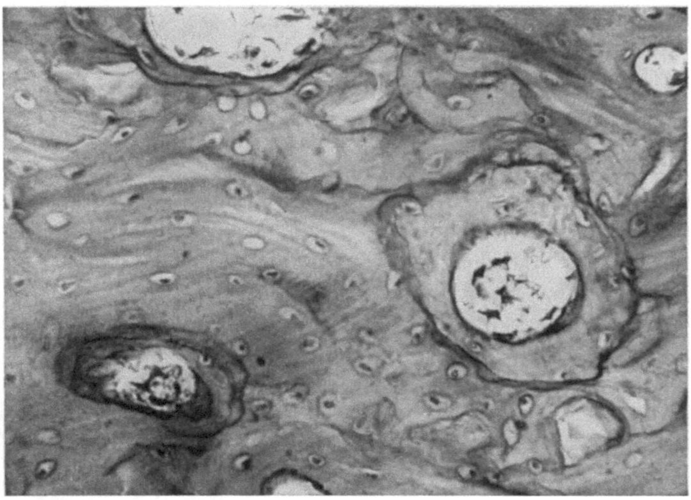

Fig. 4. After 1 week administration of cortisone and cortisone and "Stromba" during a further 2 weeks, there is obvious new bone formation with partially filled cavities in the cortex

enchondral ossification was also in progress (Fig. 3). The abnormal cartilage remained unresorbed, and in many areas was covered by a surface layer of bone. In the cortex some of the enlarged osteocyte lacunae filled in again; and resorption cavities became filled with new bone (Fig. 4).

Conclusions

We deduce from these observations that the osteoporosis caused by the administration of cortisone results not only from a cessation of bone formation, but primarily from a direct degrading effect which causes a massive resorption of bone. In the experiments described this took place during the first two weeks of cortisone administration. With continuous administration of cortisone (up to 6 weeks) the total amount of bone resorption observed, however, was rather less than that caused by experimentally induced disuse osteoporosis in equivalent bones. This was confirmed both by radiographs and in histological section.

The increase in fatty marrow, the disturbance of cell surfaces which are commonly believed to contain phospholipids, and the deposition of fat in the liver and other organs, all point to a general disturbance of lipid metabolism, though we are not sure whether the production of abnormal fat is a direct or indirect effect of the cortisone.

The action of the anabolic agent is very striking in that it reversed in almost every detail the abnormalities caused by cortisone in the bone and growth cartilage.

Summary

In rabbit bone cortisone inhibits osteoblast action and causes massive bone resorption until the osteoclast precursors are exhausted, and abnormal fatty marrow is produced. In growth cartilage the enlarged cells fail to hypertrophy and endochondral ossification ceases.

When the anabolic agent ("Stromba") was given the changes in the bone and marrow were reversed in almost every detail, and in the growth cartilage metaphyseal vessels reached to the normal distance from the proliferative zone. Normal endochondral ossification was resumed.

We are grateful to Dr. K. Little for her help throughout this work; to Professor Trueta for encouragement and helpful discussion; to the Roussel Laboratories Ltd. for the gift of cortisone; and to Bayer Pharmaceutical Products for the gift of "Stromba".

This work was carried out at the Nuffield Orthopaedic Centre, Oxford, while J. A. F. de Valderrama was holding the Nuffield Scholarship in orthopaedic surgery and L. Munuera a British Council Scholarship.

References

Rigal, W. M., and K. Little: Some observations on nuclear structure. J. roy. micr. Soc. **80**, 279 (1962).

Sissons, H. A.: The osteoporosis of Cushing's syndrome. J. Bone Jt Surg. **38 B**, 418 (1956).

Storey, E.: The effect of intermittent cortisone administration in the rabbit. J. Bone Jt Surg. **40 B**, 103 (1958).

Trueta, J., and W. M. Rigal: The use of tritiated thymidine in the study of the mechanism of formation of osteoclasts. (in press).

Valderrama, J. A. F. de, and K. Little: Mechanisms involved in the osteoporotic process. J. Bone Jt Surg. **47 B**, 193 (1965).

Sites and Mode of Action of Growth Hormone

W. M. Rigal, W. M. Hunter

Department of Orthopaedic Surgery, University of Edinburgh, Edinburgh, Scotland; Medical Research Council, Clinical Endocrinology Research Unit, University of Edinburgh, Edinburgh, Scotland

Towards the end of puberty a profound change occurs in bone. This is so striking that it might, for want of a better term, be called "bone puberty". There is as yet no clear correlation between this event and chronological age, cessation of growth, sexual maturation or bone age. Before bone puberty, bone has great reparative power and is in some respects plastic. For example, fracture union is rapid and non-union is rare; a tibia or femur can be lengthened four inches (10 cm.) or more following a simple transverse osteotomy and reconstitution of the defect occurs rapidly; the curve in idiopathic (spinal) scoliosis continues to progress; and imbalanced muscle pull produces bone malalignment.

After bone puberty the reparative power of the tissue is much reduced and its apparent plasticity disappears. Anterior pituitary growth hormone (G. H.) presumably plays some part in this alteration that occurs in bone tissues (Koskinen, 1965). This assumption has prompted an investigation into the sites of action of the hormone and its activity during puberty.

Sites of action

In young growing rabbits 5% of the cells of the germinal zone (zone one) of the epiphyseal growth cartilage are generatively active. Within the articular cartilage, and also in the anlage cartilage while it still persists, a single line of cells exhibits reproductive activity (Rigal, 1962). Growth hormone, in the intact animal, exerts its greatest influence on growth by stimulating these stem cell zones (Rigal, 1964). Injection of excess growth hormone results in 25% to 50% of the germinal zone cells becoming generatively active, and, in the articular and anlage cartilage the two narrow lines of widely spaced active cells become continuous and several cells wide. A similar effect could not be demonstrated *in vitro*.

Mode of action

Methods

The radio-immuno-electrophoretic assay of Hunter and Greenwood (1964) has been used to measure plasma human growth hormone under varying conditions in children between the ages of 9 years and 15 years who were normal from the endocrine point of view.

1. Diurnal studies: the children were confined to bed and plasma samples taken at hourly intervals during day-light hours and at two hour intervals during sleep at night.

2. Nocturnal studies: samples were taken at half-hourly intervals during a 14 hour period which included the whole night.

* These investigations are supported by British Medical Research Council Grant No. G. 963/134.

3. Test meal studies: growth hormone was measured for six hours following the ingestion of 0.71 g. of glucose per kilogram body weight. Here plasma nonesterified fatty acids (N.E.F.A.) were also monitored.

4. Surgery: the hormone levels were determined at short intervals throughout various surgical procedures.

Blood sugar was measured in all samples. Bone age was assessed using the GREULICH and PYLE atlas (1959) and sexual maturation scores (S.M.S.) were made using TANNER's method (1962). Estimations of the urinary 17-Hydroxycortico-steroids during diurnal studies showed that these investigations did not produce a stress response.

Results

The graphs, which are representative of our findings in the whole series, show plasma human growth hormone levels in μ mg. per millilitre of plasma. Arrows

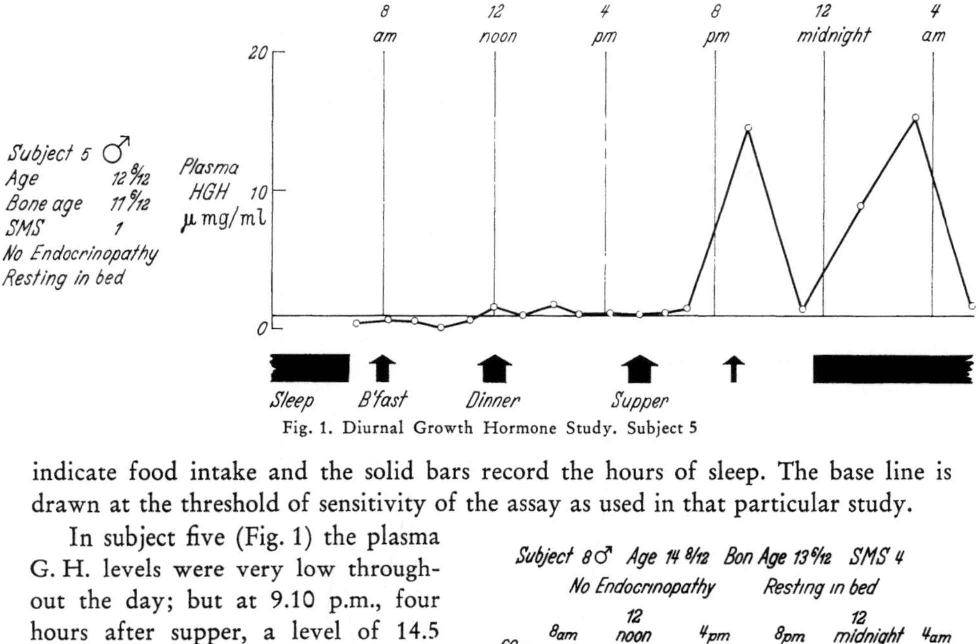

Fig. 1. Diurnal Growth Hormone Study. Subject 5

indicate food intake and the solid bars record the hours of sleep. The base line is drawn at the threshold of sensitivity of the assay as used in that particular study.

In subject five (Fig. 1) the plasma G. H. levels were very low throughout the day; but at 9.10 p.m., four hours after supper, a level of 14.5 μmg./ml. was recorded.

Subject eight (Fig. 2) was a 14 years and 8 months old boy, bone age $13^1/_2$ years and S.M.S. four. During the daytime he produced two high levels, viz. before lunch (> 30 μmg./ml.) and before supper (4.3 μmg./ml.). In each case it fell rapidly to the base line following the respective meals. During sleep the highest level (53 μmg./ml.) was recorded.

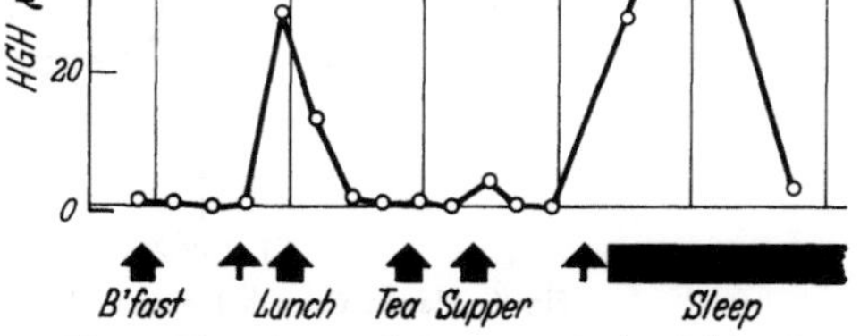

Fig. 2. Diurnal Growth Hormone Study. Subject 8

During the night the total secretion of growth hormone (Fig. 3) was many times greater than that for the same subjects during the daytime. Immediately following the evening meal the hormone level fell to base line. During the second three hours after the meal the levels rose (secondary rise) and fell spontaneously to base line

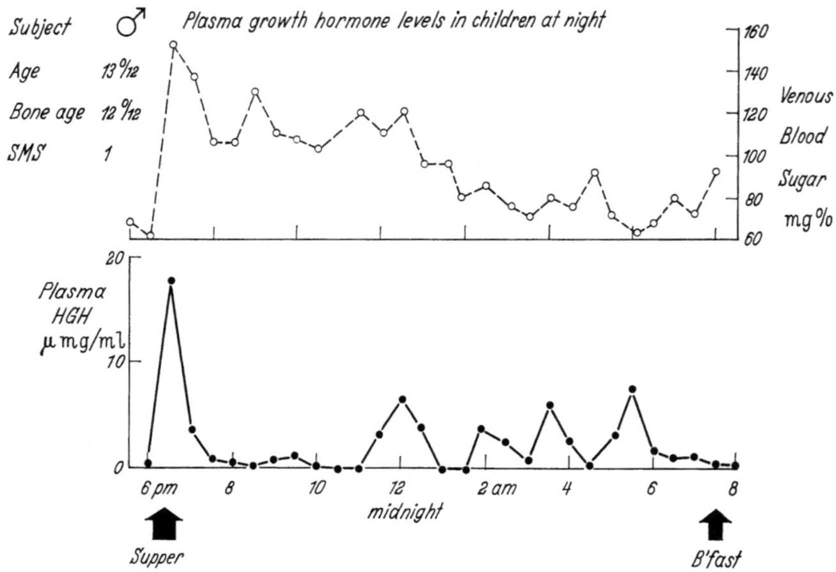

Fig. 3. Nocturnal Growth Hormone Study. Subject 5

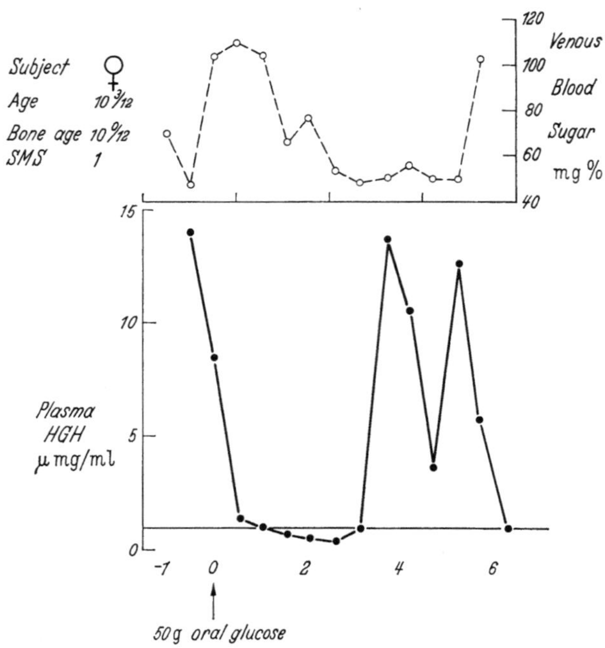

Fig. 4. Plasma Growth Hormone Levels Following a Glucose Test Meal

again. For the remainder of the night the plasma hormone levels fluctuated between the base line and a maximum which was remarkably constant for a particular individual.

Three children given 0.71 g./kg. glucose at 6.0 o' clock in the evening showed an immediate abolition of hormone secretion. Four children given the same dose of glucose at 7.0 o' clock in the morning (Fig. 4) showed no measurable growth hormone during the following three hours. After this period a secondary rise occurred. Plasma N.E.F.A. was low during the first three hours, then rose steadily till the end of the six hour study period.

Lastly, during elective surgical operations, irrespective of the time of day, plasma growth hormone levels rose rapidly to heights comparable to, or higher than, the peaks found at rest.

Discussion

Growth hormone ultimately influences growth by an effect on the stem cells in the cartilages of the epiphysis. How this action occurs is not clear.

In nine of the children submitted to diurnal studies G. H. was detected in 72 of 142 plasma samples [compared to only 8 of 41 samples from a comparable adult series (Hunter *et al.*, in press)]. The mean level in the children was 4.28 ± 7.14 S. D. μmg./ml. and the range was 0 to 53 μmg./ml. (compared to a mean of 0.52 ± 0.46 S.D. μmg./ml. and a range of 0—2.7 μmg./ml. in the adults). This study reveals that the difference between adults and children is due to much higher and more frequent peaks, but *not* due to a continuously elevated secretion, in the children. This finding emphasises the futility of attempting to estimate growth hormone status from a single randon sample.

Before 11 of 30 meals high levels of hormone were recorded. After the meal the levels fell to base line in all cases except one where the child vomited soon after his supper. A complex situation was simplified by the glucose test meal studies. For three hours following the intake of glucose (whether during the morning or the evening) the G. H. levels remained at the base line. A secondary rise occurred during the second three hour period (which tends to correspond to the time preceding the next meal). At the time the hormone level rises plasma N.E.F.A. levels also rise. This is a reflexion of the hormone's known fat mobilisation action.

At least during the daytime the pattern of secretion is similar in children and adults and appears to be related to energy requirements. (G. H. providing N.E.F.A. as energy substrate.)

High night-time secretion was a consistent finding in adequately tested cases. But even during this period a consistent measurable level of G. H. does not occur. Total night secretion is much higher than that which occurs during the day.

Anaesthesia and surgery regularly evoked G. H. secretion. Many factors are at play under these conditions but the demands of growth are presumably not involved.

It would now be desirable to relate these actions of the hormone to its growth promoting function. So far it has not been possible to relate plasma levels directly to skeletal growth. Acute administration of the hormone, as has now been well confirmed, is followed by (i) increase in plasma N.E.F.A. due to lipolysis of depot fat (Raben and Hollenberg, 1959) and by (ii) increased amino acid uptake by tissues (Kostyo and Engel, 1960; Peckham and Knobil, 1960). Utilisation of fatty acid for energy demands can spare carbohydrate and proteins. These factors would produce conditions conducive to tissue growth.

These interpretations still do not fully explain how this substance, which fluctuates in level over very short periods (half life in plasma being 20—30 minutes) and is influenced by food intake and starvation, controls growth rate.

Mitotic rates, as is well known, are higher at night than during the day. The high night-time secretion may, therefore, be more intimately related to growth than to the stabilization of the supply of energy substrate.

Two final points require emphasis. As the plasma levels of growth hormone fluctuate widely and rapidly a single or even a limited number of samples cannot give an adequate picture of the "growth hormone status" of an individual. Secondly the hormone influences several functions and many tissues in the body; its therapeutic administration to produce a single effect should be undertaken with caution.

References

Greulich, W. W., and S. I. Pyle: Radiographic Atlas of Skeletal Development of the Hand and Wrist. Stanford: Stanford University Press. London: Oxford University Press 1959.

Hunter, W. M., J. A. R. Friend, and J. A. Strong: (in press).

—, and F. C. Greenwood: A radio-immuno-electrophoretic assay for human growth hormone. Biochem. J. **91**, 43 (1964).

Koskinen, E. V. S.: Clinical and metabolic effects of hormonal treatment in bone repair. In Calcified Tissues. Richelle, L. J., and M. J. Dallemagne (eds.). Liège: Université de Liège 1965, p. 157.

Kostyo, J. L., and F. L. Engel: *In vitro* effects of growth hormone and corticotrophin preparations on amino acid transport by isolated rat diaphragma. Endocrinology **67**, 708 (1960).

Peckham, W. D., and E. Knobil: Amino acid concentration by the rat diaphragm in response to injury and some metabolic inhibitors. Biochim. biophys. Acta **63**, 207 (1962).

Raben, M. S., and C. H. Hollenberg: Effect of growth hormone on plasma fatty acids. J. clin. Invest. **38**, 48 (1959).

Rigal, W. M.: The use of tritiated thymidine in studies of chondrogenesis. In Radioisotopes and Bone. McLean, F. C., P. Lacroix, and A. M. Budy (eds.).: Oxford: Blackwell Scientific Publications 1962, p. 197.

— Sites of action of growth hormone in cartilage. Proc. Soc. exp. Biol. **117**, 794 (1964).

Tanner, J. M.: Growth at adolescence. In The Development of Reproductive Systems, II Edition: Oxford: Blackwell Scientific Publications 1962, Chapter 2.

Intestinal Absorption and Skeletal Dynamic of Calcium in Acromegaly

G. F. Mazzuoli, L. Terrenato

Istituto di Patologia Medica dell'Università di Roma, Roma, Italia

Intestinal calcium absorption in acromegaly has been investigated by a combination of balance and isotope techniques and calcium absorption has been correlated with other parameters of calcium metabolism. Moreover, calcium balance data from our own and other studies in acromegalic patients have been statistically evaluated.

Materials and methods

The study was performed on six acromegalic patients, aged 19 to 51 years, maintained on a constant calcium and phosphorus diet. Four patients received approximately 450 mg Ca and 1000 mg P, one 200 mg Ca and 800 mg P, and one 750 mg Ca and 1200 mg P daily. All patients were maintained on the specified diets for 8 to 10 days before the balance and kinetic studies were started. Metabolic periods (lasting

12 to 24 days) included kinetic study periods (lasting 8 to 12 days). Four patients were given ^{45}Ca orally as well as intravenously. Two patients received only ^{45}Ca orally. Urine and stools were collected daily. Stools were separated at intervals of four days with carmine markers. Feces and food were homogenized and converted to ash before analysis. Daily determinations of ^{45}Ca were made on samples of plasma, urine, and stools.

After intravenous ^{45}Ca administration, calcium pool and bone accretion rate were determined according to the equation of BAUER *et al.* (1957): $Bt = E\,St + A\int_0^t S(t)\,dt$ *; endogenous fecal calcium according to the equation of BLAU *et al.* (1954): Endogenous fecal $Ca = \frac{S.A.\ stool}{S.A.\ serum} \times$ total stool calcium; bone resorption by subtracting calcium balance from accretion rate. Calcium intestinal absorption was calculated by the following relationship: Dietary calcium absorbed = dietary calcium — (total fecal calcium — endogenous fecal calcium).

After oral ^{45}Ca administration the percentage of absorption was calculated by subtracting from the total radiocalcium excretion recovered the amount of radiocalcium excreted during the intravenous study. In two patients, who received only the oral dose, it was calculated by extrapolating to zero the S.A. of stool following the excretion of the unabsorbed portion of the dose.

Results and discussion

Fig. 1 shows the results of our balance studies and also data collected from the literature. A high correlation exists between calcium intake and output, calcium balance becoming increasingly positive as calcium intake rises. The figure also shows the regression line of calcium output (y) on calcium intake (x) and the 95 per cent confidence limits. The point at which the mean regression line intercepts the 45 degree line corresponds to the mean calcium requirement, that is, the mean value at which

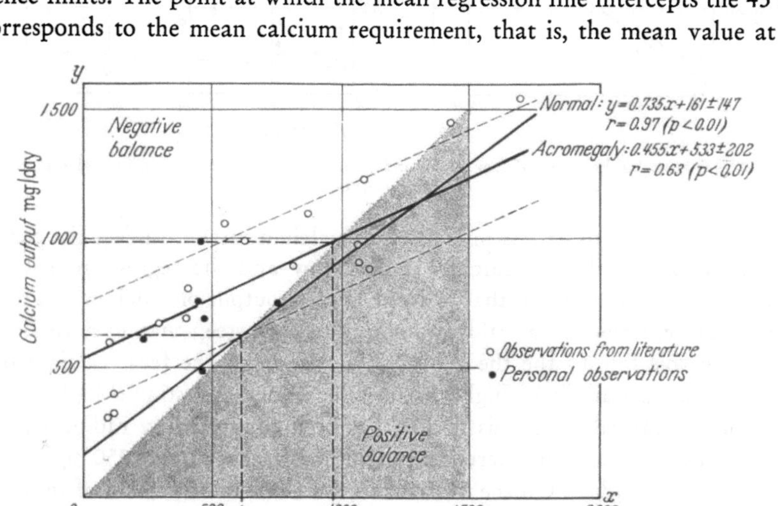

Fig. 1. The regression of calcium output on calcium intake in normal subjects and in acromegaly (6 personal and 21 cases collected from literature)

* Where: Bt = Amount of isotope retained in the body at time t. E = Amount of exchangeable calcium. A = Rate of calcium accretion. St = Serum specific activity at time t. $\int_0^t S(t)\,dt$ = Integrated specific activity.

calcium intake and output are equal and balance reaches the equilibrium. Fig. 1 also shows the mean calcium requirement of normal subjects on the basis of data collected from the literature and analyzed by Nordin (1962). The data indicate that calcium metabolism in acromegaly differs from that of normal subjects in two respects. In the first place, the calculated mean requirement is significantly greater. Secondly, the regression of output on intake is less steep than in normal subjects, so that both the negative balance in patients on low calcium diets, and the positive balance in those on high calcium diets, are greater than normal.

Fig. 2 shows the regression line of fecal calcium on calcium intake found in acromegalic patients and the regression line of the two parameters in normal subjects as reported by Nordin (1962). The figure also shows the values of urinary calcium excretion on calcium intake of acromegalics and the regression line found in normals by Nordin (1962). At all intake levels, urinary calcium of acromegalic patients is higher and this contributes to their higher calcium requirement. On the other hand

	Linear regressions on calcium intake	
Subjects	of fecal calcium	of urinary calcium
Normal	$y=0{,}67x+31\pm224$ / $r=0.94\cdot p<0.01$	$y=0.056x+147$ / $r=0.34$ / $p<0.01$
Acromegaly	$y=0.52x+137\pm202$ / $r=0.91\cdot p<0.01$	— / $r=0.43$ / $p<0.05$

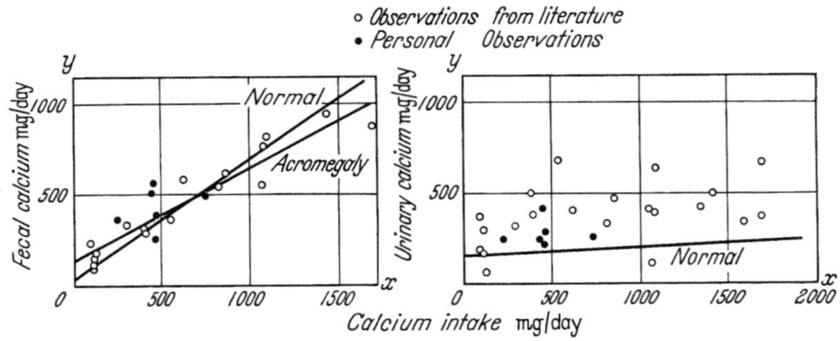

Fig. 2. The relationship between calcium intake and fecal and urinary calcium in normal subjects and in acromegaly

urinary calcium seems to be less influenced by calcium intake. In fact the correlation between urinary and dietary calcium is very low and the regression line of fecal calcium on intake is parallel to that of total calcium output on calcium intake.

The regression line of fecal calcium on intake is less steep than in normal subjects. Extrapolating this line to the theoretical intake of zero, the fecal calcium of acromegalic patients appears to be higher than in normals, suggesting a higher excretion of endogenous fecal calcium. This finding has been confirmed by radiocalcium data, the endogenous fecal calcium excretion ranging between 180 and 250 mg/day in five out of six patients studied. On the other hand, the slope of regression of fecal calcium on intake suggests that the percent absorbed decreases on low calcium diets and increases on high calcium intakes. It seems therefore, that in acromegaly the higher values of both the negative and positive calcium balances, at respectively low or high calcium intakes, are due to both the urinary and fecal calcium excretion.

The percentage of radiocalcium absorbed in acromegalics ranged between 24 to 71% of the administered dose. Wide ranges have also been observed by many authors in normal subjects (BLAU *et al.*, 1954; BRONNER *et al.*, 1956, 1963; DE GRAZIA and RICH, 1964). In view of these results, DE GRAZIA and RICH (1964) maintained that the percentage of absorption may be an individual biological constant. However, the absolute rate of intestinal absorption of calcium may have a greater physiological significance. BRONNER *et al.* (1963) have shown that in normal and osteoporotic subjects, the amount of calcium absorbed and the bone formation rate are linked by a linear relationship. The results of BRONNER indicate also that a linear relation exists between the two bone remodelling processes and that bone formation increases more rapidly than bone resorption. Therefore, the balance appears to be a direct function of the intensity of bone formation, since it represents the difference between the two processes.

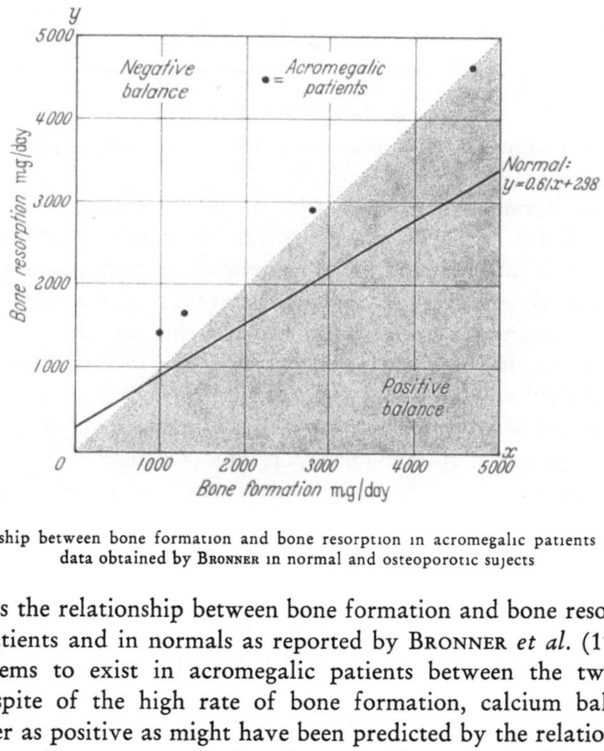

Fig. 3. The relationship between bone formation and bone resorption in acromegalic patients compared with the data obtained by BRONNER in normal and osteoporotic sujects

Fig. 3 shows the relationship between bone formation and bone resorption in four acromegalic patients and in normals as reported by BRONNER *et al.* (1963). A linear relationship seems to exist in acromegalic patients between the two parameters. However, in spite of the high rate of bone formation, calcium balance in these patients is never as positive as might have been predicted by the relationship between bone formation and bone resorption found to prevail in normal subjects.

Also the intestinal absorption of calcium seems to be directly correlated with bone accretion rate as shown in Fig. 4. However calcium absorption, although normal or even increased, never reaches the values which would be expected on the basis of bone formation rate.

If calcium homeostasis implies that the calcium pool is constant, losses and entries of calcium must be equal. Assuming that changes in calcium metabolism in acromegaly are due to the effects of growth hormone on bone metabolism, two different explanations of the data presented may be considered:

1. The growth hormone affects primarily the bone formation rate; the relatively higher rate of bone resorption would be the consequence of the inadequate intestinal calcium absorption and the increased calcium urinary excretion. If so, the high

urinary calcium excretion and its inverse relationship to the amount of calcium absorbed, remain to be explained.

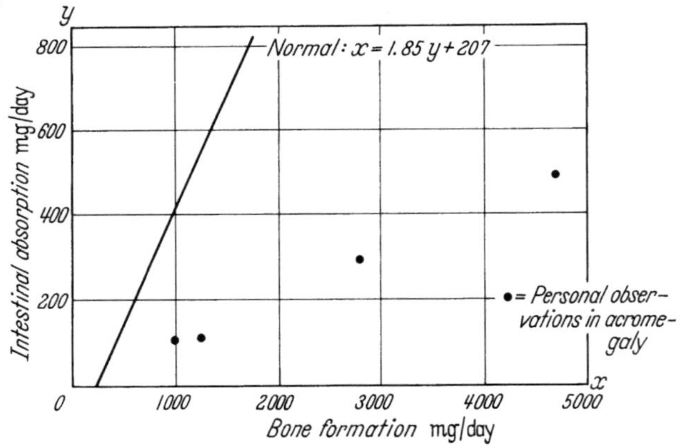

Fig. 4. The relationship between calcium absorption and bone formation in acromegalic patients and in normal and osteoporotic subjects as reported by Bronner *et al.*

2. The growth hormone affects primarily the bone resorption: the equilibrium of the balance would depend on the ability of bone formation to adapt to the rate of bone resorption. This interpretation would provide a more adequate explanation for both metabolic and skeletal dynamic changes observed in acromegaly.

In conclusion our findings in acromegalic patients indicate that:

1. The mean calcium requirement is increased due to both higher urinary and endogenous fecal calcium excretion.

2. Bone turnover is increased but the balance is never as positive as would be expected by the high values of bone formation rate. This suggests that the abnormality of skeletal metabolism may be due to a primary action of growth hormone on bone resorption.

3. The intestinal absorption of calcium may be normal or even high, but it is always inadequate for the bone accretion rate.

Acknowledgement

The authors are indebted to Miss Antonella Scarda for her invaluable technical assistance.

References

Bauer, G. C. H., A. Carlsson, and B. Lindquist: Bone salt metabolism in humans studied by means of radiocalcium. Acta med. scand. **158,** 143 (1957).

Blau, M., H. Spencer, J. Swernov, and D. Laszlo: Utilization and intestinal excretion of calcium in man. Science **120,** 1029 (1954).

Bronner, F., R. S. Harris, C. J. Maletskos, and C. E. Benda: Studies in calcium metabolism. J. Nutr. **59,** 393 (1956).

—, L. J. Richelle, P. D. Saville, J. A. Nicholas, and J. R. Cobb: Quantitation of calcium metabolism in postmenopausal osteoporosis and in scoliosis. J. clin. Invest. **42,** 898 (1963).

Grazia, J. A. de, and C. Rich: Studies of intestinal absorption of Ca45 in man. Metabolism **13,** 650 (1964).

Nordin, B. E. C.: Calcium balance and calcium requirement in spinal osteoporosis. Amer. J. clin. Nutr. **10,** 384 (1962).

The references concerning the metabolic balance data collected from literature have been omitted for space requirement.

Ultrastructure of Human Dentine

R. M. FRANK
Institut Dentaire, Faculté de Médecine, Strasbourg, France

1. Introduction

An extensive literature has been published on the structure and ultrastructure of adult dentine and, through the use of different but convergent techniques, fairly good agreement has been reached concerning the structure and ultrastructure of calcified dentine. One of the main results of recent research, obtained through classical methods of investigation as well as through histochemistry, microradiography, electron microscopy and diffraction has been the recognition of the true nature of the tubular wall. This peritubular zone is more calcified than the intertubular dentine, but both regions possess the same inorganic constituent, namely apatite crystals.

However, a certain number of problems remain unresolved among which the ultrastructure of the adult odontoblast and its process, and the precise contents of the dentinal tubules at different levels within the dentine have yet to be defined. Another important though controversial point is the innervation of dentine and predentine. Whereas, there is a general agreement concerning the presence of myelinated and unmyelinated nerve fibres in the dental pulp as observed with light and electron microscopy, the presence of unmyelinated nerve fibres in the predentine and dentine has alternatively been confirmed and denied by a number of authors using light, or polarizing microscopy. With the electron microscope, no nerve fibres could be located at either of these sites, so that serious doubts have been raised concerning the specificity of the silver impregnation in the identification of nerve fibres in dentine (ANDERSON, 1963).

The purpose of this report is not only to review our present knowledge of the ultrastructure of adult dentine but, through improvements of fixation and embedding techniques, new observations will be presented concerning the ultrastructure of human adult dentine and predentine with special emphasis on the odontoblast and its process. For the first time, unmyelinated nerve fibres will be described under the electron microscope in the predentine and dentine.

2. Technical remarks

Erupted normal premolars from young people 12 to 15 years old, extracted for orthodontic reasons, were immediately cleaved into small pieces. After 5 to 10 minutes fixation in phosphate buffered glutaraldehyde solution (SABATINI *et al.*, 1963), the coronal dentine fragments were postfixed in 1% phosphate buffered osmic acid solution (MILLONIG, 1961). The tissue blocks irrespective of their degree of calcification were embedded in Epon 812 (LUFT, 1961) and cut with a Servall-Porter microtome, equipped with a diamond knife. The ultrathin sections were observed under an electron microscope "Optique et Précision de Levallois", unstained or impregnated with lead citrate (REYNOLDS, 1963). In some cases uranyl acetate in saturated fresh alcoholic solution was used alone or followed by lead citrate staining. Adjacent thick sections of Epon-embedded blocks, stained with toluidine blue, were examined under the light microscope for purposes of orientation and comparison.

3. Ultrastructure of the adult odontoblast

An investigation of the ultrastructure of the adult odontoblast cannot be dissociated from a study of dentine as this should also provide a better understanding of the odontoblastic process. Accurate electron microscopical observations on the adult odontoblast have not been reported and most authors have investigated the characteristics of these cells during dentinogenesis (WATSON and AVERY, 1954; NYLEN and SCOTT, 1958, 1960; LENZ, 1959; NALBANDIAN and FRANK, 1962; NOBLE *et al.*, 1962; FRANK and NALBANDIAN, 1963 a). The similarity of the adult cell cytoplasm to the contents of the odontoblastic process near the pulpo-dentinal border, has been noticed by BERNICK *et al.* (1952) and FRANK (1957).

In the present study, the mature human odontoblast appeared as an elongated cell limited by a cell membrane. Glutaraldehyde fixation gave a typical appearance to the nucleus in which the chromatin was condensed peripherally and in the cytoplasm more of the ultrastructural elements were retained (Fig. 1 and 2).

The nucleus of the odontoblast is normally located near the pulpal end of the cell and in its larger diameter measures 4 to 5 microns. With glutaraldehyde fixation it was difficult to determine accurately the nucleoli but with osmic fixation alone, the nucleolar material appeared as denser chromatin granules arranged in irregular rows surrounding clear areas of pars amorpha. A double membrane surrounded the nucleus (Fig. 1). In the vicinity of the latter, a pair of centrioles are located near a well-developed Golgi apparatus situated between the nucleus and the predentine layer.

In transverse sections, the Golgi apparatus was seen to occupy the core of the odontoblast and consist of a smooth-surfaced system of lamellae, micro-vesicles and granules (Fig. 2). Around the Golgi appartus, rough-surfaced endoplasmic reticulum in close association with mitochondria could be seen. With aldehyde fixation, a finely granular material masked the cristae mitochondrialis (Fig. 1 and 2). In the pulpal cytoplasmic part of the odontoblast and around the nucleus the sacs of the endoplasmic reticulum were scarcer, but numerous mitochondria could be seen in these regions.

Numerous grains of ribonucleoprotein were disseminated throughout the cytoplasm as well as small filaments, 50 to 80 Å in diameter, similar to the intracytoplasmic filaments found in young mesenchymal cells of the dental papilla (FRANK, 1965). Clusters of glycogen granules were dispersed in the cytoplasm (Fig. 2).

Near the pulpo-dentinal border, the odontoblast cytoplasm is filled mainly with these filaments, with ribosomes and some endoplasmic reticulum and mitochondria. In these regions some vacuoles 0.4 to 0.5 μ in diameter, composed of an amorphous transparent material limited by a dense membrane, could be seen beside larger vacuoles, 1.5 μ to 2.5 μ in diameter. These larger vacuoles contained in addition a loose filamentous and granular material. The large vacuoles seemed to arise from fusion of smaller vacuoles.

A continuous cell membrane limits the odontoblast and its small lateral extensions which, in transverse section, appear as small rounded or oval cytoplasmic islands in the intercellular spaces (Fig. 1 and 2). When the plasmalemma is properly sectioned, it appears to be composed of an inner leaflet separated from an outer leaflet by a small clear space. Two types of attachment devices were noticed between adjacent odontoblasts. At the level of the nucleus, desmosome-like structures could be seen

Fig. 1

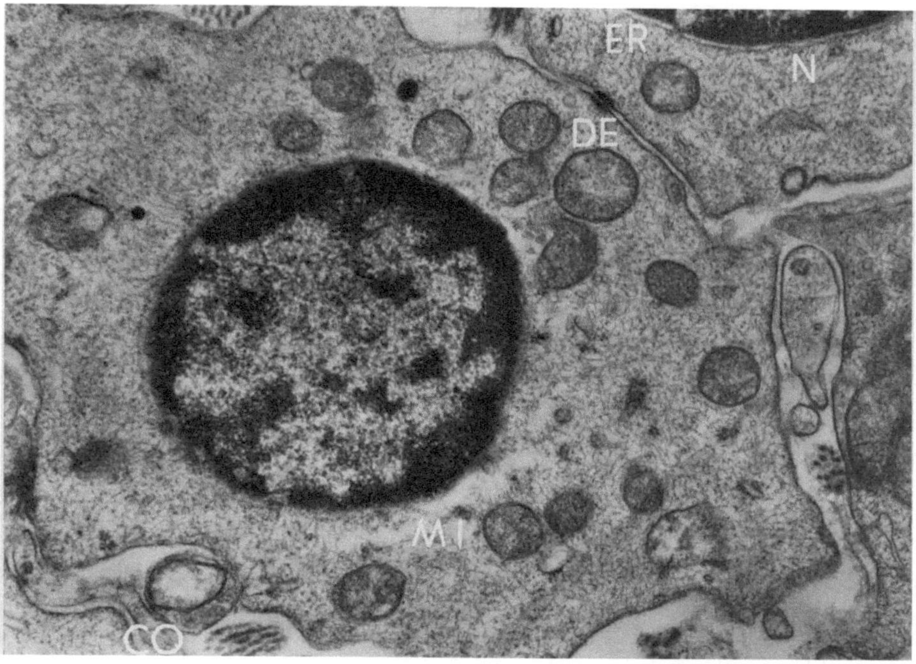

Fig 2

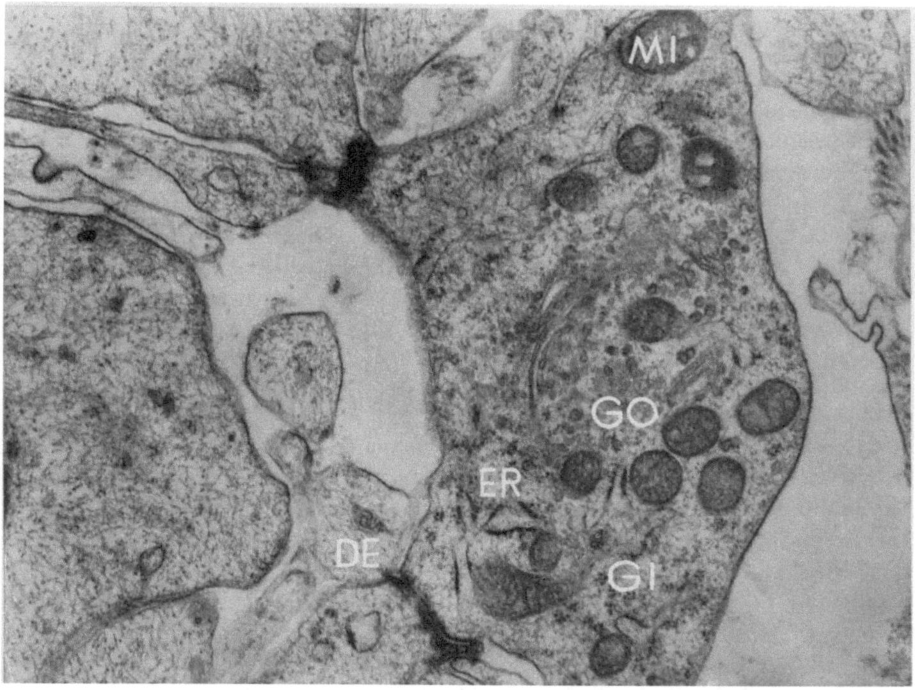

Fig. 1. Transverse section through the nuclear region of human mature odontoblasts. ER = endoplasmic reticulum vesicle continuous with the outer membrane of the nucleus (N) MI = mitochondria. DE = desmosome-like structure. CO = collagen bundle (×21,500)

Fig. 2. Transverse section through human mature odontoblasts. The Golgi apparatus (GO), in the core of the cell is surrounded by endoplasmic reticulum (ER) and mitochondria (MI). Clusters of glycogen granules (GI) are scattered in the cytoplasm. DE = desmosome-like structure (×36,000)

(Fig. 1). Similar structures have been described in the osteoblast by Dudley and Spiro (1961). Around the odontoblasts near the predentine, terminal bar-like structures form a continuous belt-like attachment between adjacent cells. Rounded spaces occupied by bundles of collagen fibrils can be seen at these levels permeating the intercellular regions. These collagen bundles, visible all along the intercellular spaces between lateral walls of the odontoblasts, are embedded in a ground substance denser than the adjacent areas and containing granular and short filamentous structures. These bundles, also noticed by Nylen and Scott (1960), Johansen and Parks (1962) and Frank (1965) correspond to the classical Korff's fibres.

Compared with the fetal odontoblast during dentinogenesis, it would appear that in the adult odontoblast there is a reduction in the importance of the Golgi apparatus and the number of endoplasmic reticulum vesicles and mitochondria. However, all these cytoplasmic organelles are well-developed and the cell exhibits all the ultrastructural characteristics of secretory activity.

4. Ultrastructure of predentine

The predentine is essentially composed of odontoblastic processes separated by a non-calcified collageneous matrix (Fig. 2 and 3). In transverse sections, it appears clearly that the odontoblastic process is a cytoplasmic extension of the odontoblast, limited by a cell membrane and containing dense granules with the same appearance and size as the ribosomes, also numerous filaments 50 to 80 Å in diameter and some scarce endoplasmic reticulum vesicles. Large vacuoles, delineated by a dense membrane, which is sometimes folded, and containing a loosely dispersed granular and filamentous material, are located in the core of the process and have a similar ultrastructure than the large odontoblastic vacuoles.

The non-calcified collagen matrix is made up of numerous collagen fibrils with 640 Å periodicity, interweaving obliquely and transversely around the odontoblastic process. A minority of the collagen fibrils have a longitudinal orientation (Fig. 3). All the collageneous material is located outside the cell membrane of the odontoblastic process, but in close association with it. The collagen fibrils are embedded in a transparent ground substance in which is dispersed a granular and finely filamentous material.

5. Ultrastructure of dentine

One of the main difference of dentine compared to predentine is that in dentine the collageneous matrix embedded in a ground substance is highly calcified and the odontoblastic processes are enclosed in tubules.

In the inner dentine layer situated next to the predentine, these odontoblastic processes have the same ultrastructure as previously described in the predentine. They are limited by a cell membrane and contain a cytoplasmic mass with numerous small filaments, ribosome-like granules and very occasionally some endoplasmic reticulum vesicles (Fig. 5). Similar large vacuoles, previously described in the odontoblast cytoplasm and the predentinal odontoblastic process, are observed in these dentinal processes. Between the calcified wall of the tubule and the cell membrane of the odontoblastic process a small space is visible (Fig. 5). This space contains non-calcified collagen fibrils embedded in a ground substance containing some finely granular and filamentous material (Fig. 5 and 8). Small lateral extensions of the

Fig. 3

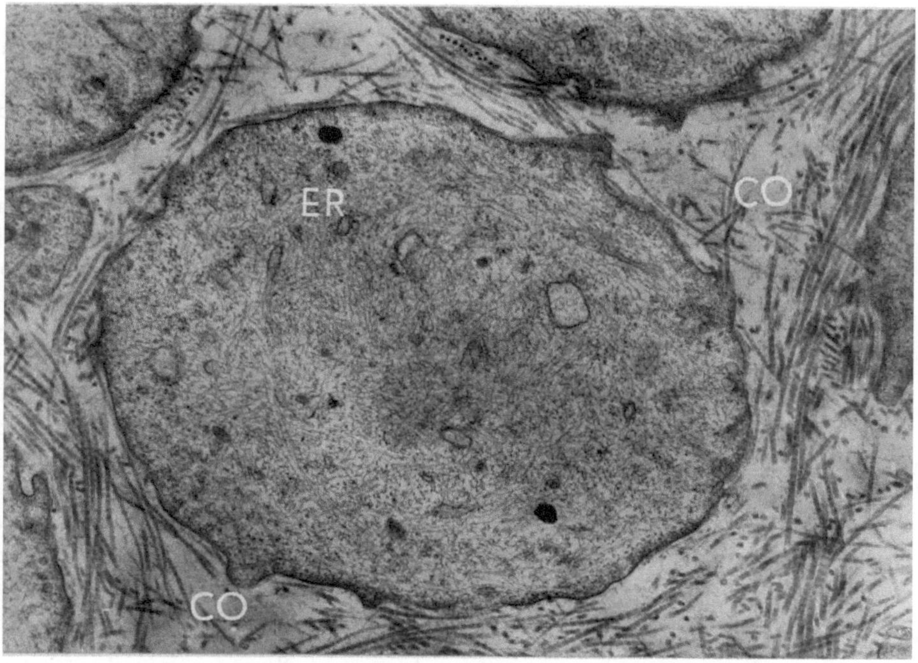

Fig. 4

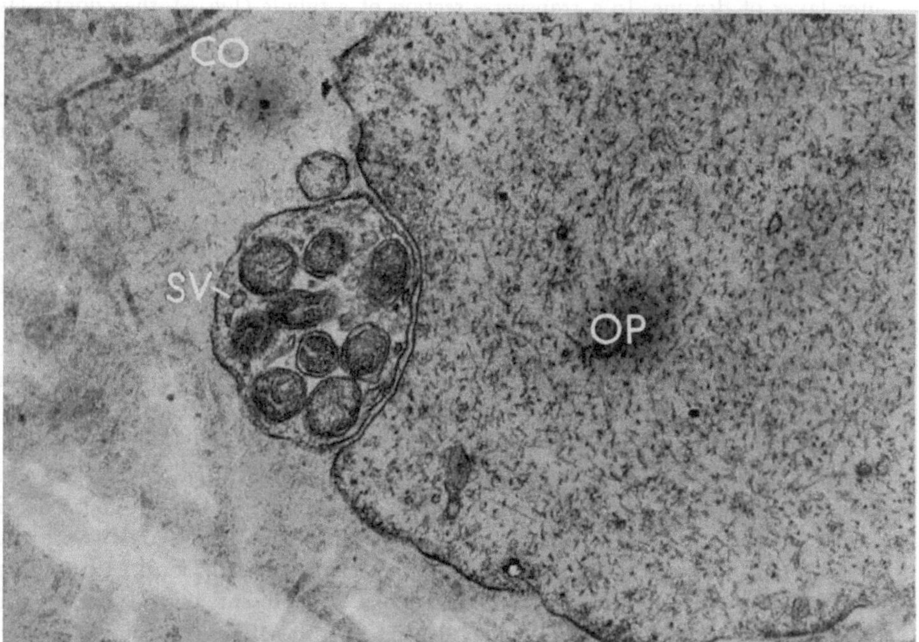

Fig. 3. Transverse section through the predentine layer. Odontoblastic processes, limited by a cell membrane, contain a cytoplasmic mass rich in small filaments, ribosome-like structures and some scarce endoplasmic reticulum vesicles (ER). Numerous collagen fibrils (CO) embedded in a transparent ground substance separate adjacent odontoblastic processes (×28,000)

Fig. 4. Transverse section through an odontoblastic process (OP) in the predentine layer. A transverse section of an unmyelinated nerve fibre can be seen in close association to the process. The axoplasm contains numerous mitochondria and some synaptic vesicle-like structures (SV) CO = non calcified collageneous matrix of predentine (×67,000)

odontoblastic process can be seen in this space (Fig. 5). In fact they cross it and penetrate in the lateral interconnecting micro-tubules.

This small periodontoblastic organic space, limited on the inside by the cell membrane of the odontoblastic process and on the outside by the calcified wall of the tubule, seems to correspond to the "manchon juxta-cytoplasmique immature" of WEILL (1959), confirmed by SYMONS (1961). According to WEILL (1959), this space exhibits metachromasia with methylene blue and stains with alcian blue and with fuchsin paraldehyde after potassium permanganate oxidation. This space is, therefore, rich in acid mucopolysaccharides.

The large vacuoles, located within the odontoblastic process, can approach the cell membrane where their limiting membrane fuses with the plasmalemma. At the point of fusion, there is rupture of the membrane so that the content of the vacuoles is secreted in the periodontoblastic organic space without any discontinuity in the cell membrane. A similar mechanism of secretion has been noticed in the ameloblast (FRANK and NALBANDIAN, 1963 b). Numerous collagen fibrils, with 640 Å bandings, appear in the space where the vacuoles discharge their secretion (Fig. 8). It is interesting to note that WEILL (1959) also mentions the secretion of globules from the odontoblastic process as well as from the odontoblast. These globules stain with alcian blue.

The ultrastructure of the odontoblastic process changes in the more peripheral or outer layer of dentine. In a transverse section of a tubule (Fig. 6), the odontoblastic process contains a large vacuole centrally surrounded by an annular peripheral layer of cytoplasm with a hyaline appearance close to the calcified wall of the tubule (Fig. 6 and 7). That this annular layer is a peripheral cytoplasmic condensation can be deduced from the presence at this level of typical lipo-pigment inclusions and from intermediate stages ranging from typical cytoplasmic contents to the hyaline appearance. This centrally located vacuole containing fine granular material (Fig. 7) has an ovoid or elongated form, as judged from different planes of section. The long axis of the oval type of vacuole occurs parallel to the long axis of the odontoblastic process. This configuration has previously been described as the thin-walled or tube-like odontoblastic process (HELMCKE, 1955; SCOTT, 1955; FRANK, 1957, 1959).

It must be mentioned that in some tubules of the peripheral dentine, no structure could be located except an amorphous epon content. This observation is either related to a fixation defect or to the so-called dead tracts (BRADFORD, 1960).

The calcified parts of the dentine can be divided into peritubular dentine and intertubular dentine. In the inner dentine, near the predentinal layer, the tubule lumen is immediately surrounded by intertubular dentine and no peritubular dentine is present, this has been shown by microradiography (FRANK, 1957; BLAKE, 1958; WYCKOFF and CROISSANT, 1963), and by electron microscopy (FRANK, 1959). In the outer layer of dentine, the peritubular zone is also absent around some tubules (FRANK, 1959) and in the interglobular dentine (BLAKE, 1958). Elsewhere, however, a typical peritubular zone surrounds the lumen of the tubules as a densely calcified wall, whose inner side is in contact with the odontoblastic process or the periodontoblastic organic space and whose outer surface is continuous with the intertubular dentine (Fig. 6 and 7).

This peritubular dentine has been described by BRADFORD (1955) using the optical microscope and by MILLER (1954), BAUD and HELD (1956), BLAKE (1958), DREYFUSS

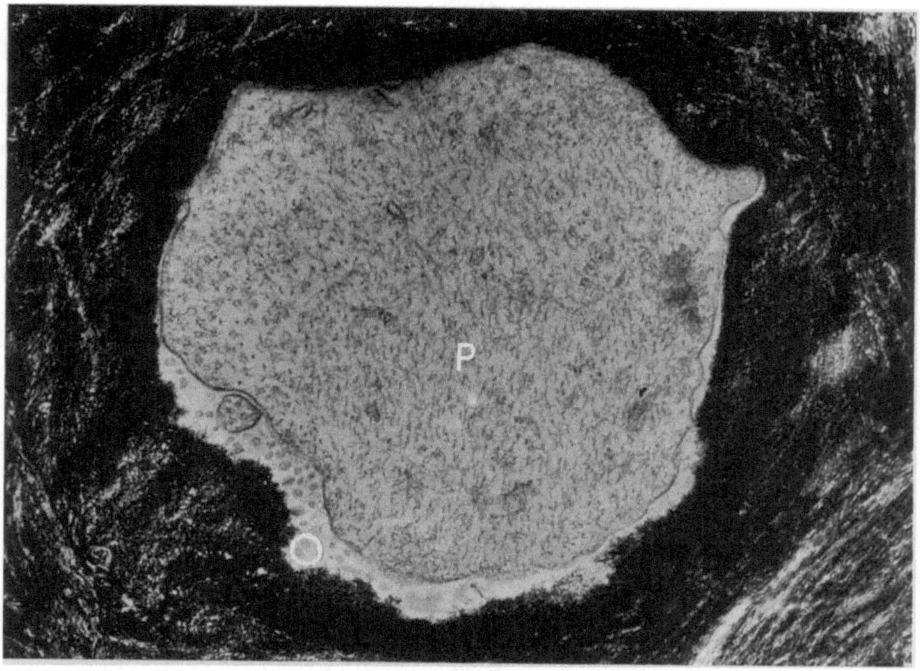

Fig. 5

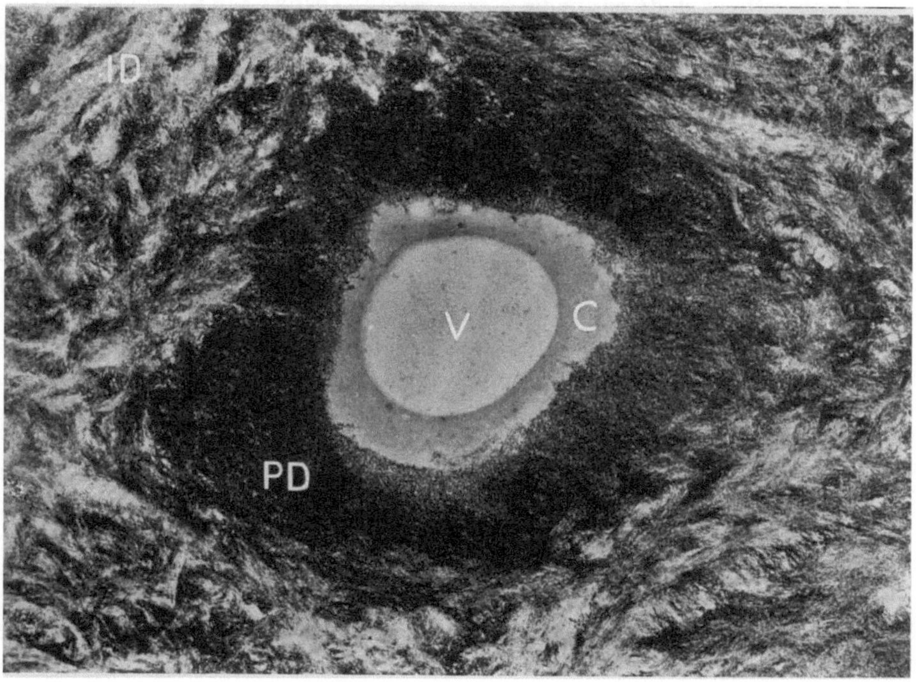

Fig. 6

Fig. 5. Transverse section through a dentinal tubule. Between the cytoplasmic odontoblastic process (P), limited by a cell membrane, and the calcified wall of the tubule (in black), an organic periodontoblastic space (O) can be seen. It contains cross-sectioned collagen fibres embedded in ground substance as well as a cross-sectioned lateral extension of the process (×52,000)

Fig. 6. Transverse section through a dentinal tubule. The odontoblastic process is composed by a centrally located vacuole (V) with peripheral annular condensation of hyaline cytoplasm (C). An electron-dense peritubular zone (PD) surrounds the odontoblastic process. ID = intertubular dentine (×35,000)

et al. (1964), using microradiography and by ROUILLER (1951), FRANK (1959), PLACKOVA and STEPANEK (1960), TAKUMA (1960), AWAZAWA (1962), JOHANSEN and PARKS (1962) with the electron microscope. The presence of peritubular dentine has been noted in fetal dentine (TAKUMA, 1960; FRANK and NALBANDIAN, 1963 a) and in young third molars (FRANK, 1959) so that this zone has to be considered as a normal constituent of developing and adult dentine.

In the present study, the peritubular dentine appeared in non-decalcified sections as a electron dense annular zone (Fig. 6), which at higher magnification was seen to be built up by a grouping of dark dots more apparent on transverse section (Fig. 6) and predominantly as dark long profiles on longitudinal section. Electron diffraction of peritubular dentine shows ring patterns typical of the apatite group and when selective area electron diffraction patterns from this region are made with a small selection diaphragm, the presence of line arcing is noted on the pattern indicating a preferential orientation of the apatite crystals (Fig. 11).

It has been shown that this peritubular dentine has a loose fibrillar matrix, easily destroyed by histological decalcifying methods (FRANK, 1959). According to TAKUMA (1960) and JOHANSEN and PARKS (1962), the fibrils of the peritubular zone are collagen fibrils. However AWAZAWA (1962) did not find any collagen striations and BRADFORD (1963) noticed after ethylene diamine maceration, followed by decalcification in weak buffered formic acid that a larger part of the peritubular matrix still remained.

In the present study our findings agree with PLACKOVA and STEPANEK (1960) who state that the peritubular dentine contains more minerals, less fibrils and more ground substance than the intertubular dentine. The rich content of acid mucopolysaccharides in the peritubular matrix has been confirmed by histochemical methods (WISLOCKI *et al.*, 1948; WISLOCKI and SOGNNAES, 1950; WEILL, 1959; SYMONS, 1961).

In the young premolar teeth examined in the present investigation, we noticed that the peritubular zone is formed and enlarges progressively by calcification of its inner wall at the expense of the tubular lumen. The presence of collagen fibrils in the periodontoblastic organic space (Fig. 8) and their subsequent calcification and embedding in the peritubular zone points to the fact that the loose fibrillar matrix of this zone is collagen. In the peripheral layer of dentine complete obliteration of the tubular content occucrs in some tubules. Therefore, dentinal sclerosis which has been noted in different pathological conditions as well as in old dentine (DREYFUSS *et al.*, 1964), is also present in young coronal dentine under physiological conditions.

The intertubular dentine immediately surrounds the lumen of tubules in areas where no pertitubular dentine is present and also fills the regions between the outer parts of the peritubular zones. Compared with the latter the intertubular dentine contains less apatite crystals and ground substance, but is richer in collagen fibrils with 640 Å periodicity. JOHANSEN (1964) considers the apatite crystals of the intertubular dentine as plates of 1000 Å in length and 20—35 Å in thickness. Like HÖHLING (1963), we have also noticed the absence of preferential orientation of the electron diffraction pattern of large areas of intertubular dentine (Fig. 10). However, with selective area electron diffraction pattern performed with a small selection aperture, preferential orientation of the crystals has been noticed. Electron micrographs of human amelo-dentinal junction (Fig. 9) show that the intertubular dentine is closely interconnected with enamel and it is difficult to follow the exact limit of both tissues.

Fig. 7

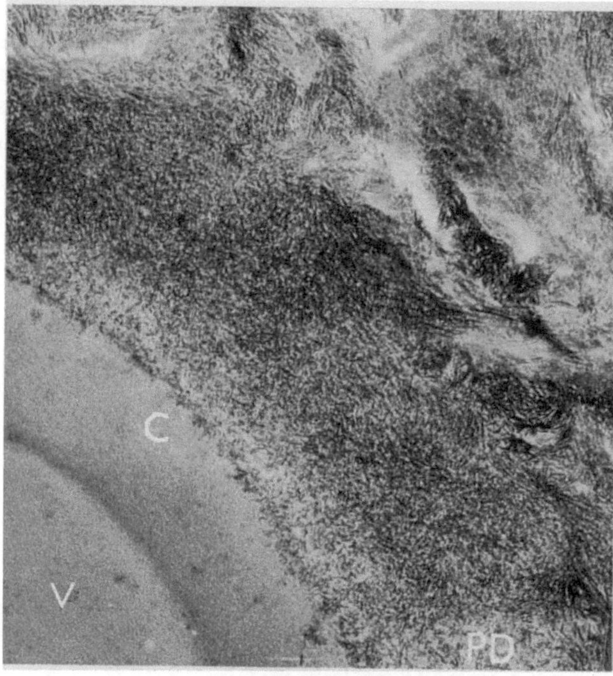

Fig. 8

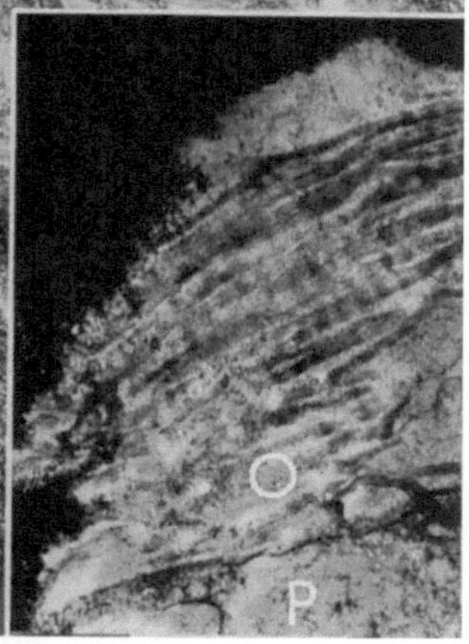

Fig. 9

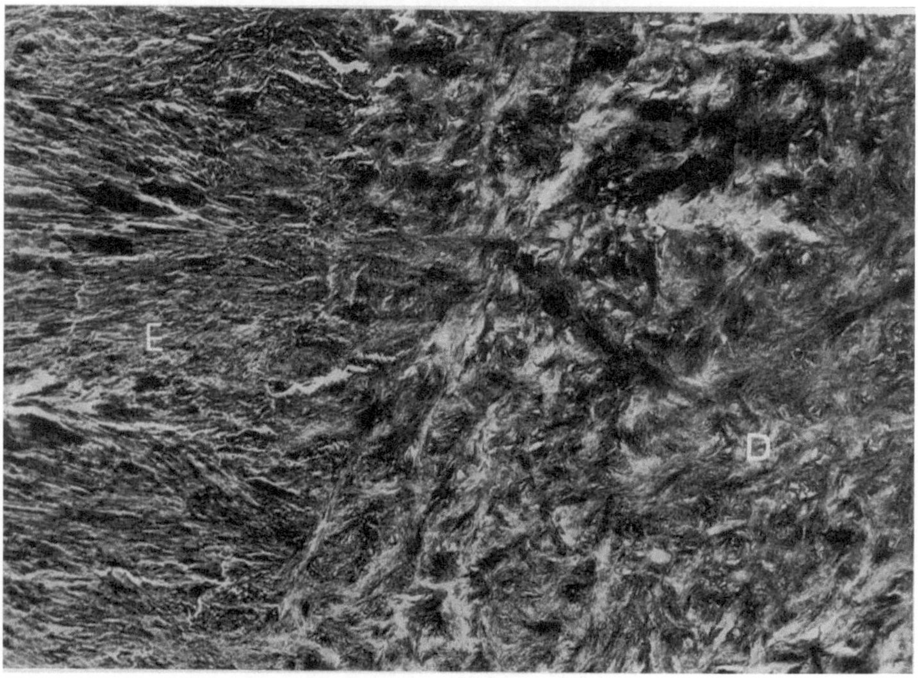

Fig. 7. Higher enlargement of the central vacuole (V), the hyaline cytolasma (C) of an odontoblastic process in cross-section. PD = peritubular dentine. ID = intertubular dentine (×85,000)

Fig. 8. Presence of numerous collagen fibrils in the periodontoblastic space (O). P = odontoblastic process (×61,000)

Fig. 9. The precise outlines of the dentino-enamel junction is difficult to follow. E = enamel. D = dentine (×11,000)

The last ultrastructural problem to be discussed is the innervation of predentine and dentine. It is impossible to review all the very extensive literature on the light microscopical investigations dealing with the presence or absence of nerves in this tissue. It can be mentioned, however, that BAUD and HELD (1953), FEARNHEAD (1957,

Fig. 10

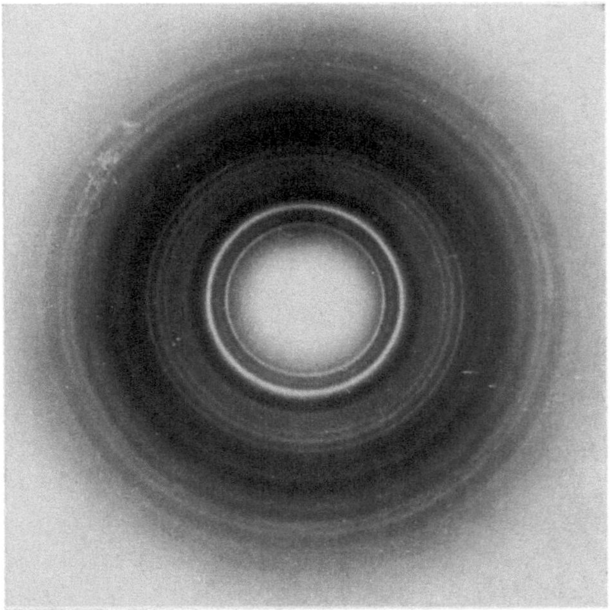

Fig. 11

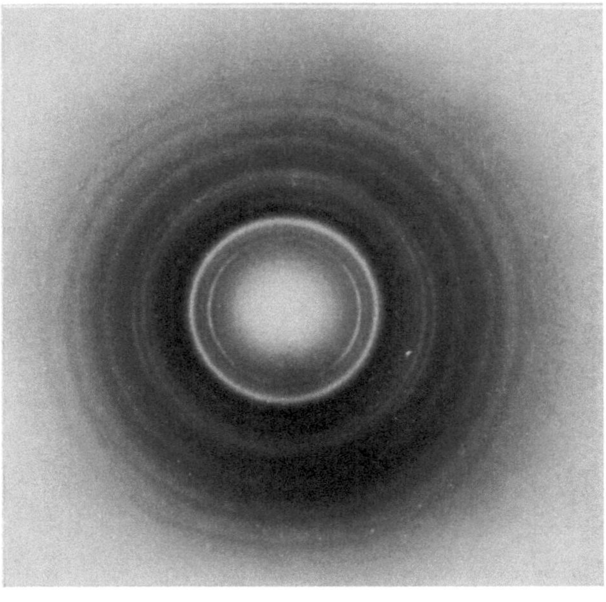

Fig. 10. Electron diffraction pattern of the intertubular substance
Fig. 11. Selective area electron diffraction pattern of peritubular dentine with line arcing indicative of preferential orientation of the apatite crystals

1963), HATTYASY (1961) and STELLA and FUENTES (1963) have described amyelinated beaded intratubular nerve fibres in the calcified dentine of erupted teeth, whereas amyelinated nerve fibres could be located only in the predentine by ARWILL (1958), ZEROSI (1959), KEREBEL (1964) and BERNICK (1964). With the electron microscope, myelinated and unmyelinated nerve fibres have been described in the pulp tissue (ARWILL, 1958; MATHEWS *et al.*, 1959; UCHINOZO and HOMMA, 1959; ÖHMAN and ENGSTRÖM, 1960) but no nerve fibres could be located in the predentine and dentine with the electron microscope (FEARNHEAD, 1957; ARWILL, 1958).

In the present study, typical unmyelinated nerve fibres have been identified for the first time under the electron microscope in the human predentine and dentine of erupted teeth (Fig. 4). These free sensory axons are in close contact with the odontoblastic process. Their limiting cell membranes are parallel to the cell membrane of the odontoblastic process and separated by a small space about 150 Å to 220 Å wide (Fig. 4). No specific relationship of the nerves to odontoblasts could be observed so far. In cross section, at the predentinal level, the axoplasm of the nerve fibre, about 0.5 μ to 0.7 μ in diameter, contains numerous mitochondria and some synaptic vesicle-like structures. Such sensory nerve fibres of a terminal type are also present in transverse sections of calcified dentine, where they present the same ultrastructure and relationship to the odontoblastic process. At the latter level they are, however, smaller, about 0.5 to 0.3 μ in diameter, and contain less mitochondria and synaptic vesicle-like structures.

This ultrastructural demonstration of non-myelinated nerve fibres in the predentine and dentine of erupted teeth confirms the light microscopical investigations performed mainly with silver impregnation methods and with polarizing microscopy. As has been pointed out by FEARNHEAD (1963), the demonstration of nerve fibres in human dentine is indicative of and provides anatomical basis for the sensitivity of this tissue.

6. Conclusion

From this survey on the ultrastructure of dentine, it appears that this tissue is permeated by numerous cytoplasmic extensions of the odontoblasts. In mature erupted teeth, these cells and their processes assume a definite secreting activity. Secretion vacuoles discharge their content through a membrane fusion phenomenon in the periodontoblastic organic space, located between the cell membrane of the odontoblastic process and the calcified wall of the tubule. From electron microscopical evidence and histochemistry it seems that organic matrix precursors of the peritubular dentine are secreted by the odontoblast through this mechanism. The periodontoblastic organic space, surrounding the cell process, contains collagen fibrils embedded in ground substance. Amyelinated nerve fibres are also located in this space in close association with the odontoblastic process. This organic space can undergo calcification and participate to the elaboration of the peritubular dentine. A new periodontoblastic organic space is then elaborated under the control of new odontoblastic secretions.

In peripheral dentine, the odontoblastic process shows structural changes. Large vacuoles collect in the center of the process. These elongated vacuoles are not discharged into the periodontoblastic space, on the contrary, they cause condensation of the cytoplasm peripherally. This cytoplasmic extension of the odontoblast becomes progressively more hyaline in character and is then applied directly along the calcified walls of the tubule. Complete obliteration of the dentinal lumen through apatite crystal growth sometimes occurs in these processes. In young erupted coronal dentine, the presence of dentine sclerosis has, therefore, to be considered as a physiological phenomenon.

The study of the ultrastructure of human mature dentine suggests that this hard tissue, containing in contrast to enamel, sensitive terminal nerve fibres and cytoplasmic cell extensions which can assume secretory activities, is able to perform a certain number of complex metabolic activities.

Summary

Mature human coronal dentine was studied under the electron microscope in young normal erupted permanent teeth, extracted for orthodontic purposes. The odontoblast appears as an elongated cell with a large nucleus and a cytoplasm containing a pair of centrioles, a well-developed Golgi apparatus, an endoplasmic reticulum in close relationship with mitochondria, ribosomes, clusters of glycogen and numerous fine intracytoplasmic filaments. Laterally the odontoblasts are connected by desmosome and terminal bar-like structures. Collagen bundles are located in the intercellular spaces. At the predentinal level, the odontoblastic process is limited by a cell membrane and contains a cytoplasm rich in fine filaments with occasional endoplasmic reticulum vesicles as well as some secretion vacuoles which have a limiting membrane and contain granular looking material. Interwoven non-calcified collagen fibrils can be observed in the intertubular substance. In the calcified dentine, adjacent to the predentine, large vacuoles can be seen approaching the cell membrane and discharging their content into the periodontoblastic organic space between the calcified wall of the dentinal tubule and the cell membrane through a membrane-fusion phenomenon without any discontinuity in the latter. Non-calcified collagen fibrils can be seen in these spaces. At a more peripheral level in transverse sections, the odontoblastic process assumes an annular outline, related to a peripheral condensation of cytoplasm through a centrally located large and elongated vacuole (over 1 micron in transverse diameter) and filled with a fine granular looking material. The peripherally condensed cytoplasm has a hyaline appearance. Densely calcified peritubular zones separated by intertubular substance surround the odontoblastic processes and in the peripheral layers progressive obliteration of some tubular lumens has been observed thus indicating the possibility of dentine sclerosis in young calcified dentine. *Last but not least,* typical amyelinated sensory nerve fibers could be located for the first time under the electron microscope in the predentine as well as in the calcified dentine, where they are located in the dentinal tubules in close relationship with the odontoblastic processes.

References

Anderson, D. J.: Sensory Mechanisms in Dentine. Oxford: Pergamon Press 1963.

Arwill, T.: Innervation of the teeth. Trans. roy. Schools Dent. Stockholm and Umea **2**, 1 (1958).

Awazawa, Y.: Electron microscope investigation of the dentin with particular regard to the nature of the area surrounding the odontoblast process. J. Nihon Univ. School Dent. **5**, 31 (1962).

BAUD, C. A., et A. J. HELD: Innervation de l'organe dentaire. In Rapports 13ème Congrès ARPA int. GEORG (ed.). Genève 1953, p. 180.

— — Silberfärbung, Röntgenmikrographie und Mineralgehalt der Zahnhartgewebe. Dtsch. zahnärztl. Z. **11,** 309 (1956).

BERNICK, S.: Difference in nerve distribution between erupted and unerupted teeth. J. dent. Res. **43,** 406 (1964).

—, R. F. BAKER, R. L. RUTHERFORD, and O. WARREN: Electron microscopy of enamel and dentin. J. Amer. dent. Ass. **45,** 689 (1952).

BLAKE, G. C.: The peritubular translucent zones in human dentine. Brit. dent. J. **104,** 57 (1958).

BRADFORD, E.: The interpretation of calcified sections of human dentine. Brit. dent. J. **98,** 153 (1955).

— The dentine, a barrier to caries. Brit. dent. J. **109,** 387 (1960).

— An histochemical and biochemical study of the peritubular dentine. Ann. Histochim. **8,** 21 (1963).

DREYFUSS, F., R. M. FRANK et B. GUTMANN: La sclérose dentinaire. Bull. Grp. int Rech. sci. Stomat. **7,** 207 (1964).

DUDLEY, H. R., and D. SPIRO: The fine structure of bone cells. J. biophys. biochem. Cytol. **11,** 627 (1961).

FEARNHEAD, R. W.: Histological evidence for the innervation of human dentine. J. Anat. **91,** 267 (1957).

— The histological demonstration of nerve fibres in human dentine. In Sensory Mechanisms of Dentine. ANDERSON, D. J. (ed.). Oxford: Pergamon Press 1963, p. 15.

FRANK, R. M.: Contributions à l'étude au microscope électronique des tissues calcifiés normaux et pathologiques. Woerth. SUTTER (ed.). 1957.

— Electron microscopy of undecalcified sections of human adult dentine. Arch. oral. Biol. **1,** 29 (1959).

— Microscopie électronique de la genèse du collagène dans la papille dentaire. J. Micr. **4,** 43 (1965).

—, and J. NALBANDIAN: Comparative aspects of development of dental hard structures. J. dent. Res. **42,** 422 (1963 a).

— — Microscopie électronique du mode de sécrétion des corps améloblastiques au cours de l'amélogenèse. C. R. Soc. Biol. **157,** 2297 (1963 b).

HATTYASY, D.: Continuous regeneration of the dentinal nerve-endings. Nature (Lond.) **189,** 72 (1961).

HELMCKE, J. G.: Elektronenmikroskopische Strukturuntersuchungen an gesunden und kranken Zähnen. Dtsch. zahnärztl. Z. **15,** 1461 (1955).

HOHLING, H. J.: Zur Frage der organischen Matrix in bezug auf Dentin, Zement und Knochen. Arch. oral. Biol. Suppl. **8, 265** (1963).

JOHANSEN, E.: Microstructure of enamel and dentin. J. dent. Res. Suppl. **43,** 1007 (1964).

—, and H. F. PARKS: Electron microscopic observations on sound human dentine. Arch. oral. Biol. **7,** 185 (1962).

KEREBEL, B.: Innervation de la prédentine humaine. Actualités odonto-stomat. **18,** 181 (1964).

LENZ, H.: Elektronenmikroskopische Untersuchungen der Dentinentwicklung. Dtsch. Zahn-, Mund-, Kieferheilk. **30,** 367 (1959).

LUFT, J. H.: Improvements in epoxy resin embedding methods. J. biophys. biochem. Cytol. **9,** 409 (1961).

MATHEWS, J. L., H. L. DORMAN, and J. G. BISHOP: Fine structure of the dental pulp. J. dent. Res. **38,** 940 (1959).

MILLER, J.: Microradiographic appearance of dentine. Brit. dent. J. **97,** 7 (1954).

MILLONIG, G.: Advantages of a phosphate buffer for OsO_4 solutions in fixation. J. appl. Phys. **32,** 1637 (1961).

NALBANDIAN, J., et R. M. FRANK: Microscopie électronique de l'odontoblaste humain et de son prolongement au cours de la dentinogenèse. C. R. Soc. Biol. **156,** 1498 (1962).

NOBLE, H. W., A. F. CARMICHAEL, and D. M. RANKINE: Electron microscopy of human developing dentine. Arch. oral Biol. **7,** 395 (1962).

Nylen, M. U., and D. B. Scott: An electron microscopic study of the early stages of dentinogenesis. Washington: Public Health Rep. n° 613, 1958.
— — Electron microscope studies of odontogenesis. J. Indiana dent. Ass. **39**, 406 (1960).
Öhman, A., and H. Engström: Studies on the innervation of human teeth. J. dent. Res. **39**, 799 (1960).
Plackova, A., und J. Stepanek: Zur Kenntnis der peritubulären Zone des Dentins. Z. Zellforsch. **52**, 730 (1960).
Reynolds, E. S.: The use of lead citrate at high pH as an electron-opaque stain in electron microscopy. J. Cell. Biol. **17**, 208 (1963).
Rouiller, C. L.: La gaine de Neumann. Thèse Médecine n° 2064. Genève: Médecine et Hygiène 1951.
Sabatini, D. D., K. Bensch, and R. J. Barnett: The preservation of cellular ultrastructure and enzymatic activity by aldehyde fixation. J. Cell Biol. **17**, 19 (1963).
Scott, D. B.: The electron microscopy of enamel and dentin. Ann. N. Y. Acad. Sci. **60**, 575 (1955).
Stella, A., y A. Fuentes: Inervacion dentinaria intracanalicular. Su demostracion por el método de la hematoxilinaférrica de Heidenhain. An. Fac. Odont. (Montevideo) **9**, 157 (1963).
Symons, N. B. B.: A histochemical study of the intertubular and peritubular matrices in normal human dentine. Arch. oral Biol. **5**, 241 (1961).
Takuma, S.: Electron microscopy of the structure around the dentinal tubule. J. dent. Res. **39**, 973 (1960).
Uchinozo, K., and K. Homma: Electron microscopy of nerves of the human tooth pulp. J. dent. Res. **38**, 1133 (1959).
Watson, M. L., and J. K. Avery: The development of the hamster lower incisor as observed by electron microscopy. Amer. J. Anat. **95**, 109 (1954).
Weill, R.: Etude histochimique de la dentine. La zone translucide de Bradford. La gaine de Neumann. Ann. Histochim. **4**, 59 (1959).
Wislocki, G. B., M. Singer, and C. M. Waldo: Some histochemical reactions of mucopolysaccharides, glycogen, lipids and other substances in teeth. Anat. Rec. **101**, 487 (1948).
Wislocki, G. B., and R. F. Sognnaes: Histochemical reactions of normal teeth. Amer. J. Anat. **87**, 239 (1950).
Wyckoff, R. W. G., and O. Croissant: Microradiography of dentine using characteristic X-rays. Biochem. biophys. Acta **66**, 137 (1963).
Zerosi, C.: Recherches sur l'innervation de la dentine. Bull. Grp. int. Rech. sci. Stomat. **2**, 9 (1959).

Preliminary Studies of the Ultracentrifugal and Free Zone Electrophoresis Characteristics of Neutral Soluble Proteins of Bovine Embryo Enamel

E. P. Katz, G. Mechanic, M. J. Glimcher

Department of Orthopedic Surgery, the Harvard Medical School, and the Massachusetts General Hospital, Boston, Mass., U. S. A.

Introduction

The organic matrix of tooth enamel is the most densely calcified tissue in the body. In order to understand calcification and its many facets, one of the prerequisites is to first learn as much as we can about the chemistry and molecular structure of the fibrous proteins that are involved. Much knowledge has been gained in the past about the physical and chemical properties of collagen but relatively little is known of the fibrous protein that constitutes the organic matrix of dental enamel.

We do know that its X-ray diffraction pattern reveals that embryo-enamel matrix is in a cross-β-configuration (GLIMCHER *et al.*, 1961 a). Recently it has been shown that soluble enamel protein reconstituted from solution also has a well defined cross-β-configuration (BONAR *et al.*, in press). The amino acid composition of enamel matrix is characterized by large amounts of proline, glutamic acid and histidine (GLIMCHER *et al.*, 1961 b). More recently it was shown that decalcified bovine embryo enamel matrix may be solubilized by cold neutral buffer and that essentially the same amino acid composition prevails (GLIMCHER *et al.*, 1964).

This paper presents some of the solution characteristics of bovine premolar-embryo enamel protein.

Experimental and results

In sedimentation velocity experiments the number of schleiren peaks, their apparent sedimentation coefficients, and the distribution of the protein between the

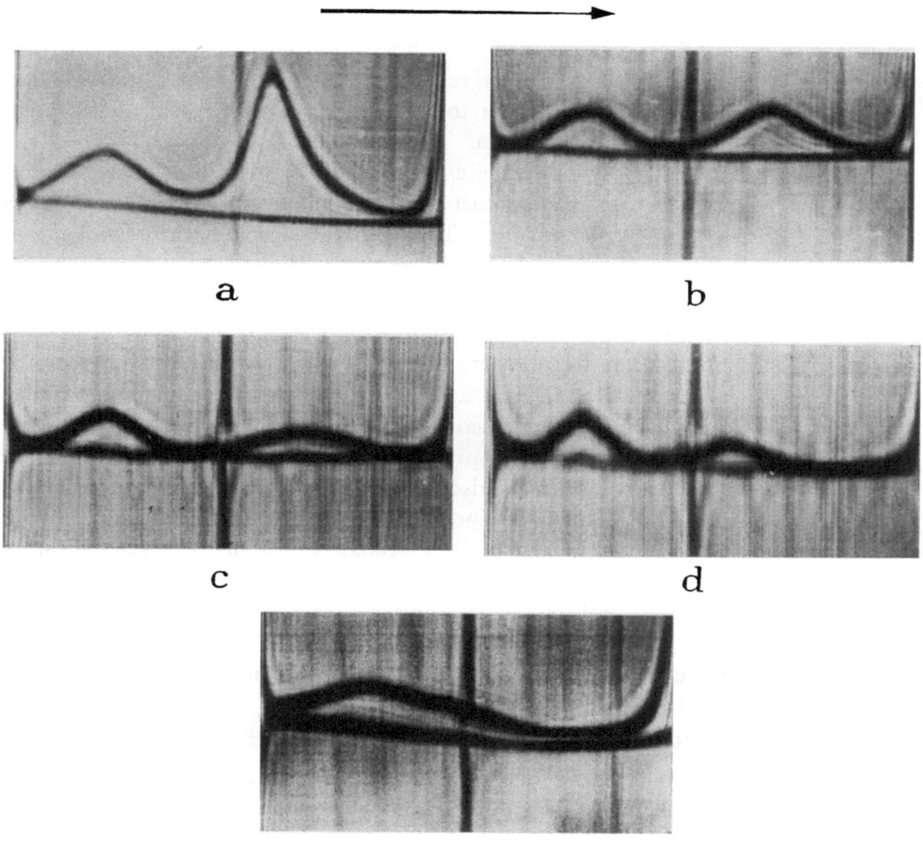

Fig. 1. Synthetic boundary sedimentation velocity experiments at 4°, 0.1 M salt, pH 7.7. The boundary was formed about three-fourths from the bottom of the cell which is on the right. Sedimentation is in the direction of the arrow. a) 1.4% protein solution, 120 min., 42, 040 RPM, phase angle 60°, b) 0.7% protein solution, 50 min., 59, 780 RPM, phase angle 60°, c) 0.35% protein solution, 50 min, 59, 780 RPM, phase angle 50°, d) 0.175% protein solution, 33 min., 59, 780 RPM, phase angle 40°, e) 1.4% protein solution, 150 min., 59, 780 RPM, then 130 min. at 42, 040 RPM, phase angle 50°

peaks are strongly dependent on protein concentration, solvent, pH and the ionic strength of the solution. In so short a paper all these variables on the various parameters characterizing the system are impossible to present or discuss so only representative data will be presented here. Typical sedimentation velocity experiments at various protein concentrations at pH 7.7, 0.1 M NH_4HCO_3 is shown in Fig. 1. Three peaks are evident in Fig. 1 a (1.4% protein) and the apparent distribution of the components is such that 80% is represented by the fast moving peak and about 10% by each of the slower moving peaks. The $S_{20,W}$ value of the major peak is about 9 S, while the two minor peaks have $S_{20,W}$ values of approximately 2 S and 1 S respectively (Fig. 1 e).

As the total protein concentration is decreased there is a redistribution of the material so that progressively less of the protein is represented by the faster sedimenting peak. This is demonstrated in Fig. 1 b, c and d where we see sedimentation patterns of 0.7%, 0.35% and 0.175% protein solutions at pH 7.7 in 0.1 M NH_4HCO_3. Over the concentrations presented here, not only does the apparent ratio of fast to slow moving species change by a factor of 2.4, but also the calculated area of the composite 1—2 S peaks changes with total protein concentration. In other experiments it was found that the relative proportions of the two slower moving peaks appear to be relatively insensitive to total protein concentration.

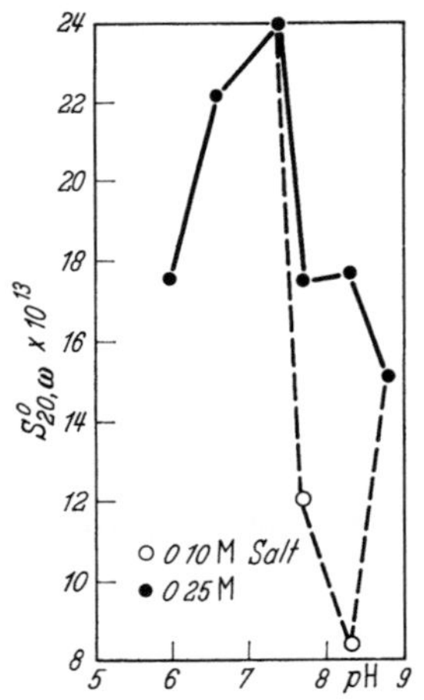

Fig. 2. Plot of $S^0_{20,w}$ at various pH's at 0.1 M and 0.25 M salt

The schleiren patterns in Fig. 1 also demonstrate that the fast sedimenting peak is not resolved from the slower moving ones. This indiates that the three peaks seen apparently constitute one continuous boundary.

At pH's 8.82, 8.3 and 6.04 the sedimentation velocity patterns are similar to those seen in Fig. 1. At pH's 6.04, however, there is a progressive redistribution as more of the material appears in the slower sedimenting peaks. The $S^0_{20,w}$ values of the fast moving peaks changes radically with pH and ionic strength as seen in Fig. 2.

It may also be noted here that high concentrations of urea deaggregate the protein and only slow moving boundary of approximately 1 S may be seen in sedimentation velocity patterns. Upon dialysis against neutral buffer the patterns revert back to their original form shown in Fig. 1 a.

The electrophoretic patterns of a 1.4% protein solution at various pH's are shown in Figs. 3 and 4.

Lowering the protein concentration does not change the distribution of the proteins in either the ascending or descending pattern. At pH 6.04 (Fig. 3 c) the major boundary remains with the δ and ε boundaries indicating the most of the protein is in an isoelectric condition.

At pH 3.61 (Fig. 4 f) there is a marked difference in the patterns obtained from the two arms of the electrophoretic cell. The pattern in which protein is migrating into solution shows a number of hypersharp peaks (ascending pattern) whereas the material migrating through protein solution gives diffuse boundaries (descending pattern).

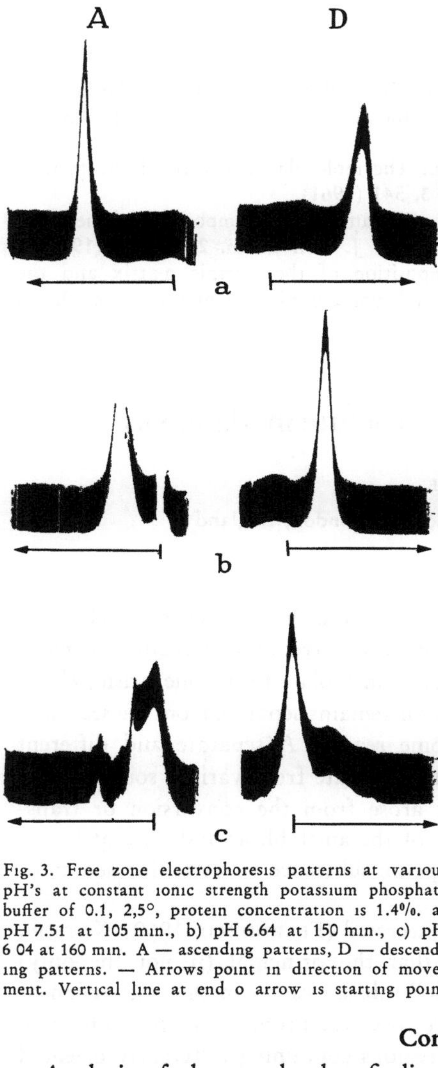

Fig. 3. Free zone electrophoresis patterns at various pH's at constant ionic strength potassium phosphate buffer of 0.1, 2,5°, protein concentration is 1.4%. a) pH 7.51 at 105 min., b) pH 6.64 at 150 min., c) pH 6 04 at 160 min. A — ascending patterns, D — descending patterns. — Arrows point in direction of movement. Vertical line at end o arrow is starting point

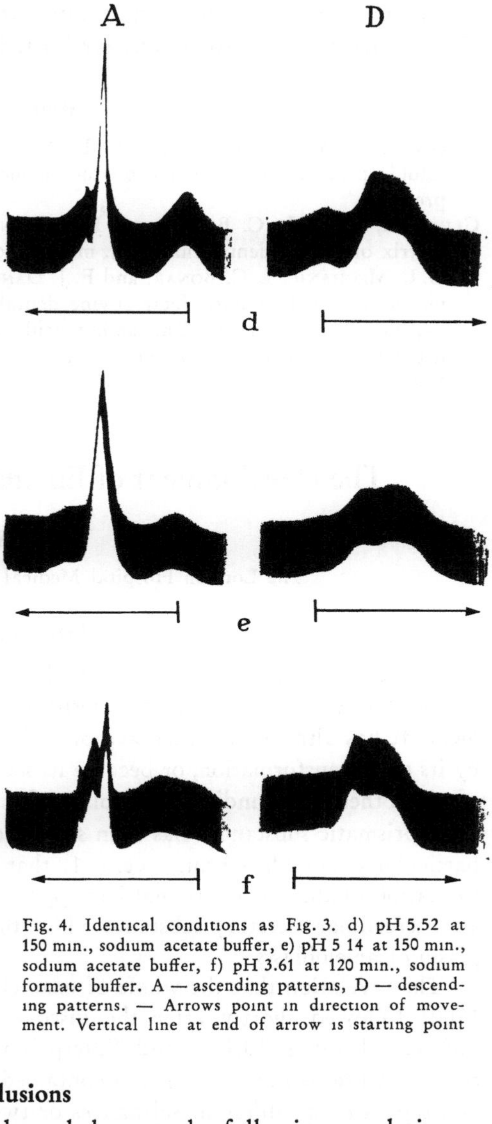

Fig. 4. Identical conditions as Fig. 3. d) pH 5.52 at 150 min., sodium acetate buffer, e) pH 5 14 at 150 min., sodium acetate buffer, f) pH 3.61 at 120 min., sodium formate buffer. A — ascending patterns, D — descending patterns. — Arrows point in direction of movement. Vertical line at end of arrow is starting point

Conclusions

Analysis of these and other findings have led us to the following conclusions. 1. The major portion of the neutral soluble proteins of premolar bovine-embryo enamel matrix exists in aqueous solution as a mixture of labile, reversibly equilibrating species, but that in addition there are minor non-interacting components present. 2. The interacting proteins constitute either a polymerizing multi-component system with rapid re-equilibrating kinetics with respect to transport processes, or a polymerizing single component system whose reaction kinetics are of an intermediate type and are dependent on solution conditions.

Acknowledgements

This work was supported by research grants from the U. S. Public Health Service, National Institutes of Health (AM-06375), and the John A. Hartford Foundation, Inc.

We wish to thank Dr. Karl Schmid for the electrophoretic analyses, and Miss Cathy Rutstein and Mr. Paul Day for technical assistance.

References

Bonar, L. C., M. J. Glimcher, and G. L. Mechanic: The molecular structure of the neutral-soluble proteins of embryonic bovine enamel in the solid state. J. Ultrastruct. Res. (in press).

Glimcher, M. J., L. C. Bonar, and E. J. Daniel: The molecular structure of the protein matrix of bovine dental enamel. J. molec. Biol. **3**, 541 (1961).

—, G. L. Mechanic, L. C. Bonar, and E. J. Daniel: The amino acid composition of the organic matrix of decalcified fetal bovine dental enamel. J. biol. Chem. **236**, 3210 (1961 b).

— —, and U. A. Friberg: The amino acid composition of the organic matrix and the neutral-soluble and acid-soluble components of embryonic bovine enamel. Biochem. J. **93**, 198 (1964).

The Development of Enamel Structure in Mammals

A. Boyde

The London Hospital Medical College, London, England

Introduction

A one to one ratio between the numbers of prisms and the numbers of ameloblasts has been accepted by the great majority of those who have studied enamel development. It has also usually been accepted that one ameloblast forms one prism, either by its own transformation, or because its secretion remains separate from the secretion of the other, surrounding ameloblasts for some reason. A separate and different "interprismatic substance" has been supposed to originate from various sources. Two particularly notable schemes were, 1. that it arose from the conversion or transformation of the inner terminal bar apparatus of the ameloblasts and, 2. that it was an intercellular secretory substance whilst the prism substance was transformed cytoplasm of ameloblasts.

The revelation that the whole of enamel is secreted (Fearnhead, 1960; Watson, 1960) followed shortly after the discovery that the principal (if not the only) difference between "prism" and "interprismatic" substances lay in the orientation of the crystallites which these regions contained. It posed the problem of explaining how two separate and different substances or two regions containing differently oriented crystallites and the "prism sheaths" which separate them could be produced by the same cells. The problem is simplified by the realisation that the prism sheaths in developing enamel only exist as planes at which the crystallite orientation changes quite suddenly between domains (prism or interprism) in which it only changes gradually; the higher organic content of the prism sheaths is only acquired during the increase in mineral content of the bulk of the enamel. The problem then remaining is purely one of crystallite orientation, that is of finding where the orientation is determined, what the orientation is, and hence deducing what sort of controlling factors might be involved.

An early and constant finding of this study was that the crystallites grow very close to the ameloblasts in what Fearnhead (1960) called the mineralising front. The methods which have been used are, therefore, those which would give information about the shape of the mineralising front and the orientation of the crystallites with respect to it.

Materials and methods

Material was obtained from the tooth germs of 20 mammalian species belonging to 9 orders (list in Boyde, 1964). Developing enamel and ameloblasts were fixed in Palade or Dalton fixatives and embedded in 2 : 1 butyl : methyl methacrylate prior to ultra-thin sectioning for electron microscopy.

Crystallite orientation was determined in electronmicrographs by estimating the degree of foreshortening of sectioned crystallite fragments (it having been determined that all the crystallites in enamel are extremely long), and later by examining stereo-pair electron-micrographs of the same material when the orientation of the crystallite fragments with respect to the plane of section could be seen directly.

Half-micron thick sections of the same blocks, stained with crystal violet and basic fuchsin to distinguish enamel from ameloblasts, were used for the preparation of wax reconstructions of the mineralising front. It was thus possible to relate crystallite orientation to the shape of the mineralising front directly.

The surface of the developing enamel was also studied directly by scanning electron microscopy (Boyde and Stewart, 1963).

More recently some success has been obtained with carbon replication of the surface of developing enamel. Tooth germs were fixed in N.F.S. to allow a more perfect stripping of the ameloblasts from this surface, which is then covered with a layer of evaporated carbon. This layer is to constitute the replica: it is peculiarly liable to fracture and therefore very difficult to recover because of the very angular profiles which it contains. The basis of the method of recovery is to destroy the tooth by removing the hydroxyapatite by acid decalcification and the organic matrix with ethylene-diamine. It has been found most satisfactory to remove the organic component first (by refluxing ethylene-diamine in a Soxhlet condensor) leaving the mineral to provide some support for the carbon. The latter is further protected by being competely surrounded by calcium phosphate powder during the extraction process. After washing by distilling water instead, the contents of the Soxhlet condensor are washed into N/2 HCl when the hydroxyapatite of the tooth and the calcium phosphate powder both dissolve. The replica fragments are collected direct on grids, washed in water and dried. Photogrammetric measurements have been made on stereo-pair electron-micrographs of these replicas.

Results and discussion

The surface of developing mammalian enamels contains depressions occupied by the Tomes' processes of the ameloblasts: these depressions are approximately hexagonal in outline at their most superficial level. They do not "fill in" symmetrically. One side (usually the cervical side) of each depression grows most rapidly and is more or less flat. The remaining sides constitute together a continuous curved plane making a sharp angle at the base of the depression where they meet the cervical side — the prism boundary forms here.

The majority of the crystallites develop roughly perpendicular to the surface of the flat cervical sides of the depressions. In the remaining cuspal and lateral sides they diverge to a greater or lesser degree from this perpendicularity rule. However, they always make a large angle with the former group. Thus changes in orientation of the crystallites (the "prism sheaths") are determined by changes in orientation of the mineralising front.

The fact that the crystallites in developing enamel tend to be oriented perpendicular to its mineralising front may be caused by the peculiar growth habit of the crystallites themselves: they grow as very long, thin, flattened hexagons. Mutual interaction between adjacent crystallites might line them up parallel to each other and perpendicular to the mineralising front, or it may just be that only those crystallites which begin to grow in the right direction can continue to grow, since any growing at a significant angle to the perpendicular to the surface of the environment in which they are growing must butt up against another crystal.

Where there are no changes in orientation of the mineralising front all the crystallites are parallel and perpendicular to it and there are no prisms. This situation prevails at the commencement of amelogenesis at the enamel-dentine junction before the ameloblasts acquire their Tomes' processes and at the end of amelogenesis when they lose them again during the formation of the true surface-zone enamel.

A close analysis of the shape of the surface of developing enamel reveals that the *cervical* and *lateral and cuspal reg*ions of the depressions are not equivalent. The cell membrane of Tomes' process must slide past the surface in the latter regions. It seems probable that this is connected with the deficient growth of these surfaces and that it may even cause the deviation of the crystallites which grow in these surfaces from the generalisation that they should be perpendicular to the surface. The crystallites which grow in these *cuspal and lateral* surfaces belong to the "interprismatic regions" of Pattern 1 and 2 enamels (see Fig. 1) or to the cervical extension or "winged Process" of Pattern 3 prisms.

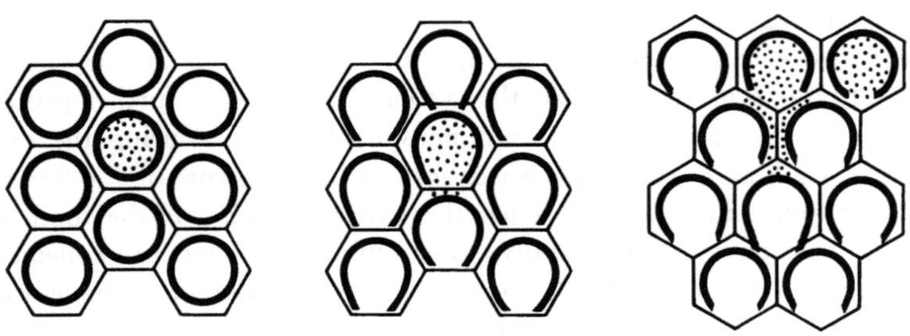

Fig. 1. a) Pattern 1 enamel, Cuspal enamel, Cheiroptera, Insectivora, Sirenia, Odontoceti (Cetacea), Lemuroidea (Primates). b) Pattern 2 enamel, Lateral enamel, Ungulata, Marsupialia, Lagomorpha, Cercopithecoidea (Primates) (also in man!). c) Pattern 3 enamel, Carnivora, Proboscidea, Homo sapiens. — *Prism cross-sectional outlines:* The curved heavier lines represent (sectioned) prism boundary planes of abrupt change in crystallite orientation. There is only a gradual change in crystallite orientation between any two points which can be connected by a line which does not pass through such a boundary plane ("prism sheath"). — *Secretory territories of ameloblasts:* The lighter hexagonal outlines delineate the amounts of enamel produced by separate, single ameloblasts. The dotted areas represent what are conventionally referred to as "prisms"; via this definition it will be seen that "interprismatic regions" can be distinguished in Patterns 1 and 2, and depending on the extent of the prism sheath, perhaps in Pattern 3

The recent studies of stereo electron-micrographs of replicas of the surface of developing enamel have provided additional data which may help to elucidate two unexplained observations made by Boyde (1964). There it was noted that the crystallites in *ungulate* (Pattern 2) enamel prisms diverge less from the mean axis of the prism than do those in Pattern 3 prisms. The cervical (prism body) side of the depressions is concave in pig enamel (Pattern 2) but convex in elephant enamel (Pattern 3). The concave shape of the *cervical* side would encourage parallel orientation — the convex would encourage deviation from the mean prism axis.

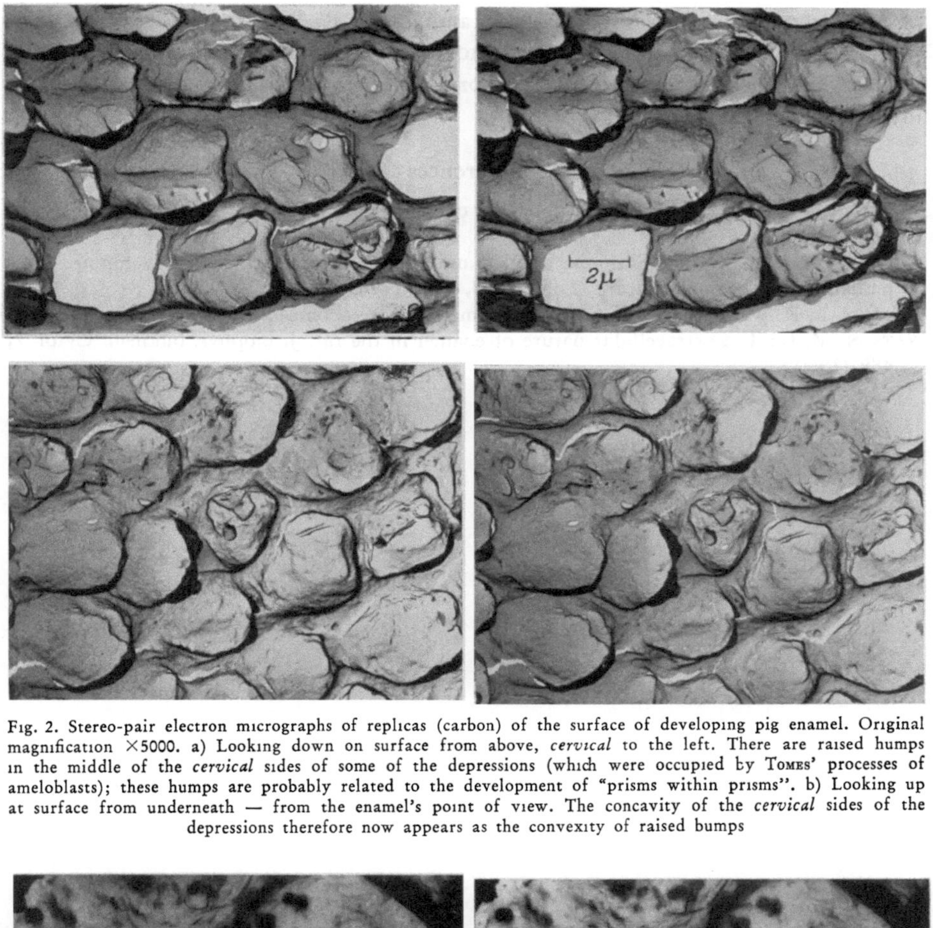

Fig. 2. Stereo-pair electron micrographs of replicas (carbon) of the surface of developing pig enamel. Original magnification ×5000. a) Looking down on surface from above, *cervical* to the left. There are raised humps in the middle of the *cervical* sides of some of the depressions (which were occupied by Tomes' processes of ameloblasts); these humps are probably related to the development of "prisms within prisms". b) Looking up at surface from underneath — from the enamel's point of view. The concavity of the *cervical* sides of the depressions therefore now appears as the convexity of raised bumps

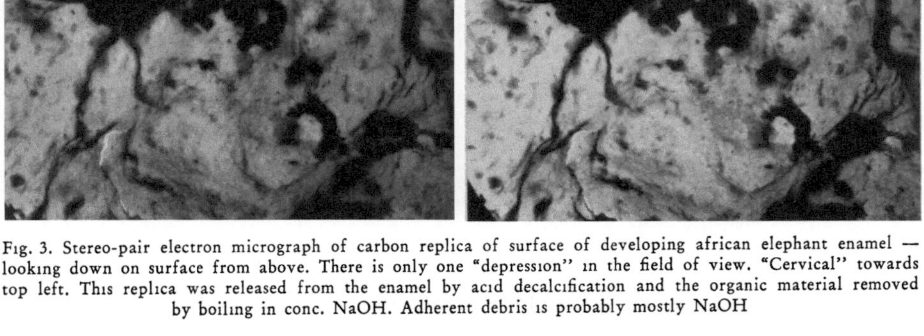

Fig. 3. Stereo-pair electron micrograph of carbon replica of surface of developing african elephant enamel — looking down on surface from above. There is only one "depression" in the field of view. "Cervical" towards top left. This replica was released from the enamel by acid decalcification and the organic material removed by boiling in conc. NaOH. Adherent debris is probably mostly NaOH

Prisms within prisms in pig enamel seem to be related to the development of a sharp, raised hump in the middle of the *cervical* side of the depressions, giving rise to another circumscribed plane of abrupt change of crystallite orientation within the prism.

Acknowledgements

I am very grateful to Mr. R. V. ELY and the M. R. Research Trust for the loan of the Hilger and Watts Stereo-comparator with which the photogrammetric measurements have been made, and to Professor Dr. phil. habil. J. G. HELMCKE for useful advice and discussions.

References

BOYDE, A.: The structure and development of mammalian enamel. Thesis. University of London 1964.

—, and A. D. G. STEWART: Scanning electron microscopy of the surface of developing mammalian dental enamel. Nature (Lond.) **198,** 1102 (1963).

FEARNHEAD, R. W.: Mineralization of rat enamel. Nature (Lond.) **188,** 509 (1960).

WATSON, M. L.: The extracellular nature of enamel in the rat. J. biophys. biochem. Cytol. **7,** 489 (1960).

Gesamtherstellung: Konrad Triltsch, Graphischer Großbetrieb, Würzburg

MIX
Papier aus verantwortungsvollen Quellen
Paper from responsible sources
FSC® C105338

If you have any concerns about our products,
you can contact us on
ProductSafety@springernature.com

In case Publisher is established outside the EU,
the EU authorized representative is:
Springer Nature Customer Service Center GmbH
Europaplatz 3, 69115 Heidelberg, Germany

Printed by Libri Plureos GmbH
in Hamburg, Germany